Success Mantra for
Successful Homoeopathic Prescribing

Tips and Tricks for Successful Practice

By
Dr. V. Krishnaamurthy

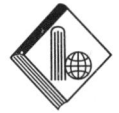

B. Jain Publishers (P) Ltd.
USA — Europe — India

Success Mantra for Successful Homoeopathic Prescribing
First Edition: 2015
4th Impression: 2019

All rights reserved. No part of this book may be reproduced, stored in a retrieval system or transmitted, in any form or by any means, mechanical, photocopying, recording or otherwise, without any prior written permission of the publisher.

© with the Author

Published by Kuldeep Jain for
B. JAIN PUBLISHERS (P) LTD.
B. Jain House, D-157, Sector-63, NOIDA-201307, U.P. (INDIA)
Tel.: +91-120-4933333 • *Email:* info@bjain.com
Website: www.bjain.com

Printed in India

ISBN: 978-81-319-3516-3

A teacher is he who makes difficult things easy.

— *Ralph Waldo Emerson*

Preface

I started my career as a freelance medical journalist. Forty-two years ago, while in New Delhi, when I entered the scene of homoeopathy I noticed one striking thing—while one homoeopath cured most of his patients with one single dose (even obstinate chronic cases), another was giving more than one remedy that too repeatedly, with partial or nil relief. Thus, my journey was towards filling this gap of knowledge among homoeopaths.

I started studying and practicing homoeopathy out of sheer academic interest and after forty-two years of continuous and rigorous study and search got the inspiration to write this book. If the reader keeps this in mind, he would evince much interest in what I am going to write in the following pages.

All the abbreviations used in the book are according to the Textbook of Homoeopathic Therapeutics by Dr. Samuel Lilienthal.

Prof. V. Krishnaamurthy
April 5, 2015
32/56, Kuppaiah Street
West Mambalam, Chennai - 600 033, India
E-mail: jaykrish1966@gmail.com
Phone: 9789069362, 9884612450, 044-24890370

Publisher's Note

Homeopathy is an exact and accurate science. Precision and versatility is its culture. The experiences of various physicians during their course of practice have been penned down through the years of its development.

This work of Dr Krishnaamurthy is another such compilation which provides the readers a practical approach towards homoeopathy. It enlightens the effects of homeopathy in various clinical conditions such as Diabetes, Gout, and Sterility etc. The efficacy of this work is enhanced by the elucidation of the actual treated cases. It may sound unbelievable but the positive result of single homoeopathic dose in various pathological conditions is overwhelming.

We are extremely happy to present this work of Dr Krishnaamurthy to the homeopathic fraternity as it will certainly help the readers to improve their knowledge of homeopathic practice. It will also build a bridge between the theoretical knowledge obtained at the college level and the practical world.

Kuldeep Jain
CEO, B. Jain Publishers

Contents

Preface .... *v*
Publisher's Note .... *vii*

Section 1: An Overview

1. Homoeopathy: Science and Art 3
2. How to find the *similimum*? 5
3. The selection of potency of remedies 7
4. When to repeat? 9
5. Use of repertories. How to translate the words/actions of patients into the rubrics of the repertory? 10
6. How to cure epidemics/endemics/pandemics with a single dose? 13
7. Why does homoeopathy fail? 31
8. Scope and limitations of homoeopathy 33

Section 2: Practical Tools

9. 'Mind' symptoms 37
10. Congestion, Rush of blood, Hyperaemia 38

11.	Lack of reaction—Low vitality—When the indicated remedy fails to act	155
12.	Causations	183
13.	Cross, Crossing	195
14.	Plethora, Plethoric individuals, Precocity	203
15.	Precocious children	214
16.	Old age, Senility, Presenility	216
17.	Diabetes mellitus—Glycosuria	239
18.	Malignant diseases	255
19.	Cancer, Cancerous diathesis, Cancerous constitution, Cancerous cachexia	282
20.	Sterility, Infertility	290
21.	Gout—Retrocedent, Metastatic, Constitutional	296
22.	Treatment of chronic diseases—Miasms—Psora, Sycosis, Syphilis—Constitutional treatment—Generals—General symptoms	349
23.	Habitual—Diseases that have become habitual	386
24.	Nutritional disorders	404
25.	Checked discharges—Suppression of secretions	427
26.	Some useful rubrics of mind	454

Section 3: Actual Cases Treated

27.	Actual Cases Treated	489

Section 4: Materia Medica

28.	Materia medica of valuable and uncommon mind symptoms	535

Bibliography 613

SECTION 1
AN OVERVIEW

- ❖ Homoeopathy: Science and Art
- ❖ How to find Similimum
- ❖ Potency Selection
- ❖ When to Repeat
- ❖ Use of Repertories
- ❖ Epidemics
- ❖ Why does Homoeopathy Fail
- ❖ Scope and Limitations of Homoeopathy

Homoeopathy: Science and Art

We are living in the most semantic period of human history, where people are pragmatic and open minded who readily accept homoeopathy as a medical science. When we go back to Hahnemannian period, we find the intellects were groping in darkness. Speculations and superstitions were ruling the mind of people. Anybody who differed or defied the authority had to pay for it in the form of social boycott or exile. Dr. Hahnemann dared to differ from orthodox medical system in such a scenario when Galileo was punished because he said the earth is round. Despite all such circumstances Hahnemann established homoeopathy as a holistic science which was based on simple but profoundly insightful and infallible Eternal Laws and eternal laws never fail, and never change. These are like sign posts that guide homeopaths through a maze without which they would be lost and forever changing direction. Unfortunately there are many practising homeopaths without having mastered the principal laws and that invariably leads to failure.

Art and science are inseparably bound together. Every art has its foundation in science, and every science finds its expression in art. Man is characterized mainly by his emotions, intellect, sensations, will and understanding. Thus, it is logical that both physical and mental aspects have to be considered. Moreover getting symptoms from an individual is an art and tact of a competent physician. When a physician follows laws correctly and perceives the patients being unprejudiced, success is inexorable for each and every case.

Theory is good so far as it goes. But he, who can infuse theory into practice, lives in, with and for the student.

How to find the *similimum*?

This is the most vital part. So also, case taking. Certain general guidelines must be constantly kept in mind.

1. While treating a mentally deranged patient, concentrate on the physical symptoms of that case to select the remedy for him.
2. While treating a patient with physical symptoms, concentrate more on mind symptoms.
3. The more you keep away from pathology, the closer you are to the similimum. If you think of remedy for 'diabetes' remedy for 'cancer' etc. you cannot get the similimum.
4. The attitude of the patient towards the treatment or towards the doctor may also be of much help in finding the remedy.
5. Look and watch the patient. Is he reflecting every time you ask a question. Does he wander from the topic?
6. Keep in mind the age of the patient. When there is no uncommon symptoms among the symptoms told by the patient, if a female patient is in the age group 11-15 or if the complaints started around puberty, you must write down on the case sheet the word '**chlorosis**'.
7. So also, note the word '**menopause**' if the patient is around 40-46 years of age.
8. The patient may be impatient while sitting in the queue.

9. If he is bargaining in your fees, note down the word **'avarice'**.
10. Do not get annoyed or irritated if he crosses you. This, in itself, becomes a valuable symptom (See Chapter 13—Cross).

The selection of potency of remedies

There is no hard or fast rule for potency selection (see Lilienthal, Boericke and Yingling). Some may say 'Look, Boericke always advises low potencies'. But actually they should thoroughly read the preface and introduction in Boericke's Materia Medica. There we find Boericke telling, "The dosage needs some apology... It is to be *wholly disregarded.*"

SELECTION OF POTENCY: Do not use potencies below 10M in respect of snake poisons, metals, violent poisons and chemicals.

In acute diseases give the 200th. Here too Ars-alb., Lachesis, etc. should not be used below 1M or 10M. If you read Kent's LESSER WRITINGS there you will find that provings of some snake poisons were done by taking one single dose of the 6th potency. If you give snake poisons or metals or chemicals, even one single dose in the 6th or 30th potency, the patient would be proving that for years.

Dr. W. A. Yingling beautifully describes in *The Accoucheur's Emergency Manual* that "Lower potencies do act. But with higher potencies there won't be any need for repetition".

I do not buy, nor keep, potencies below 30th. In the case of poisons, metals and snake points in particular, we do not keep it below the 10M. Of course, you can cure uncomplicated cases of blood cancer, infective hepatitis, septicaemia, hepatitis b-virus, haemophilia with one single dose of Crotalus horridus-200. But after six to ten years there would be a relapse. But if you use 10M or 50M there won't be such a relapse.

The only exception to the above, is the use of the remedy **Calendula** in mother tincture. It is a master remedy being **par excellence** in cases of cut and open injuries. I use it in the following way:

Soak a piece of cotton in hot water and gently squeeze out extra water. Pour a few drops of Calendula Q on the wet cotton and put it on the cut; then apply a bandage tape over it. Now, without removing the bandage, apply Calendula Q (diluted with six parts of hot water) every four hourly. After 3-4 applications the wound heals without leaving a scar. (See Kent's Lectures on Homoeopathic Materia Medica. **Calendula**)

When to repeat?

I give one single dose and wait for a month. After a month, when the patient comes, and

1. reports 'complete cure' we advise the patient to come again after a few months.
2. if there is relapse of same symptoms we give the next high potency of the same remedy and so on and so forth.
3. reports partial relief and/or development of new symptoms, then at this point the section 'Relationship of Remedies' under the remedy last prescribed is helpful. Use Boericke's materia medica and Wilkinson's materia medica for this purpose. Read the remedies given under 'Relationship of Remedies' against the heading 'Remedies Follow Well', 'Compare', 'Complements', 'Similar'. All these mean one and the same thing *viz.,* remedies follow well. Here we ignore 'Antidotes' 'Inimical" ctc.

For example, I have prescribed Sepia-10M, one single dose for a patient and he returned after a month complaining of partial relief. In that case, you can give the next higher potency (one dose only). If there is relief and 'change of symptoms' in such a case I consider the remedies given at the end of Sepia under 'Relationship of Remedies'. We first take the remedies (under these heads) and if there are remedies common to Boericke and Wilkinson **we consider them first and try to select the one remedy suiting the patient's present symptoms (during his second visit).**

Use of repertories.
How to translate the words/actions of patients into the rubrics of the repertory?

Selection of a proper rubric is always a difficult task for both new and experienced practitioners. While selecting a rubric one has to convert patient's language into repertory language, which demands great expertise. Some illustrations have been given here to select a proper rubric from the patient's report. My recommendation to every physician is to go through all the rubrics of mind and generalities in Kent's and Knerr's Reportories.

1. "Doctor, I have come to you as a last resort after finding no cure in the hands of so many doctors. I now entirely rely upon you for the cure of my joint pains..." "Doctor, please cure me somehow. It is my humble request to you. I beg you to cure me". If a patient uses any one of these or similar statements, go to the rubric "Praying, begging" in Kent's Repertory — MIND.

2. We do occasionally come across a child who would do just the opposite of what the parents tell them to do. Go to the rubric "Perverse, refractory..." on page 234 of Lilienthal. (This symptom we see in actual practice but all other existing repertories do not list this).

3. Whenever the patient points out more than one spot with his finger tip or points to an area of suffering by placing his palm on or above along that area, go to the rubric "Gestures" under the chapter MIND in Kent's Repertory. (This you will, of course, take only if you do not have other more valuable mind or general symptom in a given case). A lady of forty-three years complaints of pain in her joints for three years. She uses both her palms and holds it above the ankle, knee etc. to show the affected joints. Then telling that the pain is quite drawing, with both of her hands, she brings it from ankle to her knee as if pulling something from below upwards to show me the type of pain. This is not so much a valuable symptom but in the absence of more valuable symptoms we may use this rubric—'Gesture'.

4. A lady of thirty-two years of age is brought by her friend and it was the friend who was describing her complaint. The patient looked indifferent to the treatment. The friend continued, "Doctor, when I asked her to come to you (the doctor) she just did not come. Even if I forcibly brought her to you, I know she is not going to take the medicines regularly". — 'Indifference' is the rubric for the case.

5. Let us now listen to a patient: "Doctor, I have so much tiredness. My husband is a heart patient and I used to take care of him by regularly giving the tablets etc. Yesterday, he complained of chest pain but it did not remind me to give him the tablet required during the chest pain".

6. In another case, the wife of a patient said, "Doctor, my husband is such an indifferent person. Last week my daughter fell down with profuse bleeding on her leg. He was simply watching it and showed no reaction".

In case (5) and (6) above, it is not 'indifference' because in emergencies no one would be indifferent. This is 'inactivity' of mind. We read all these remedies in the MATERIA MEDICA OF MIND SYMPTOMS (given at the end of this book) and under the remedy *Opium* the following words agree with the above two cases.

...Imbecility of will, as if annihilated...

This cannot be included in the repertory. Better we have to memorize it. The nearest rubric would be 'Torpor'.

The practitioner should know the difference between TORPOR, ABSENTMINDEDNESS, DULLNESS and IMBECILITY mentioned under MIND in Kent's repertory.

7. During case taking, one patient remarked about the corrupt government officials, "Doctor, we must shoot down these corrupt and bribe taking officials".—For this you must take the rubric 'Indignation'.

8. Learn the difference between the rubric "MEN, dread of" and "FEAR of men"

How to cure epidemics/endemics/ pandemics with a single dose?

HOMOEOPATHIC THERAPEUTICS by Dr. Samuel Lilienthal and to a lesser extent Boericke's Materia Medica and Hering's Guiding Symptoms are more than sufficient to treat all epidemics with a single dose. For example, in the case of patients die with lung complications. The killing disease of the lungs is 'pneumonia' and under the chapter 'pneumonia' in HOMOEOPATHIC THERAPEUTICS by Dr. Samuel Lilienthal we find the words 'epidemic pneumonia' under which only two remedies viz., Ferrum metalicum and Mercurius solubilis are mentioned. I have cured several cases of swine flu with one single dose of Mercurius solubilis 10M.

SINGLE DOSE CURE for the present EBOLA, MADRAS EYE etc.

Since 2008, epidemic and pandemic diseases have started spreading one after the other. Having started with Chikungunya, followed by Swine flu and Dengue, now it is the turn of Ebola haunting the world. Yes! In the next seven years, about twenty more epidemic diseases would emerge! Anyone who has been keenly studying the history of medicine till date can predict this.

In homoeopathy cure of a disease is easier than its prevention.

1. Patients affected not only by Dengue, but also those affected by any other types of fever prevalent today have been cured in an hour, with a single dose of the homoeopathic remedy Bryonia alba-200. Many patients who were admitted to the hospitals for fever (whatever be the name of the fever) were cured within an hour of taking Bryonia alba-200 and so they, got voluntary discharge. During the summer season, many people develop 'dryness of lips, thirst for large quantities of water, desire for rest etc.—all being classical symptoms of the remedy 'Bryonia alba'.

2. Likewise, a Swine flu patient admitted to the hospital for weeks, was relieved with single dose of the homoeopathic remedy Mercurius solubilis-1000 and was discharged within an hour.

3. Lachesis-1M has shown excellent results in the treatment of Ebola-infected patients. Three patients suffering from the disease abroad, were discharged from the hospital soon after administration of a single dose of the remedy.

4. For the current epidemic Madras Eye (Conjunctivitis), one single pill of the homoeopathic remedy Cinnabaris-10M completely cures the patient.

Epidemic cholera: Remedies to remember: the general aspect of cholera was like the general aspect of *Cuprum metallicum, Camphor* and *Veratrum album,* and these three remedies are the typical cholera remedies.

- They all have the general feature of cholera, its nature and general aspect.

- They all have the exhaustive vomiting and diarrhoea, the coldness, the tendency to collapse, the sinking from the emptying out of the fluids of the body.

- From what I have said you will see that the Cuprum case is, above all others, the spasmodic case. It has the most intense spasms, and the spasms being the leading feature, they overshadow all the other symptoms of the case. He is full of cramps and is compelled to cry out with the pain from the contractions of the muscles.

- Camphor has the blueness, the exhaustive discharge, though less than Cuprum metalicum and Veratrum album; Cuprum metalicum and Veratrum album patients like to be covered up whereas Camphor patient wants to be uncovered and wants to have the windows open. Let me mention another feature in Camphor - It also has some convulsions which are painful, and during pain he wants to be covered up and wants the windows shut. - If there are cramps in the bowels with the pain, he wants to be covered up.

- So in Camphor, during all of its complaints in febrile conditions (and fever is very rare in Camphor), and during the pains he wants to be covered up and warm, but during the coldness he wants to be uncovered and have the air.

- In cholera, the extreme coldness and blueness indicates Camphor.

- Again, with Camphor there are often scanty as well as copious discharges, so that the cholera patient is often taken so suddenly that he has the coldness, blueness and exhaustion and almost no vomiting or diarrhoea, a condition called dry cholera.

- It simply means an uncommonly small amount of vomiting and diarrhoea.

This is Camphor.

- Another prominent feature is the great coldness of the body without the usual sweat that belongs to the disease.

- Cuprum metallicum and Veratrum album have the cold clammy sweat, and Camphor also has sweat, but more commonly the patient requiring Camphor is very cold, blue and dry and wants to be uncovered. That is the striking feature.

- Veratrum album, is so perfectly adapted to cholera and yet so different. Veratrum is peculiar because of its copious exhaustive discharges, copious sweat, copious discharges from the bowels, copious vomiting, and great coldness of the sweat. There is some cramping and he wants warmth; he is ameliorated by hot drinks, and by the application of hot bottles which relieves pain and suffering.

These three remedies have their own role in collapse and death.

In a nutshell Cuprum metalicum for the cases of a convulsive character, Camphor in cases characterized by extreme coldness and more or less dryness, and Veratrum album when the copious sweat, vomiting and purging are the features.

These features will guide a practitioner to treat an **epidemic** of cholera with confidence.

Epidemic Asiatic Cholera - Sulphur as a preventive, sprinkled into each stocking, boot or shoe, twice a week. 1, Acon., Ars., Camph., Carb-v., Ipec., Cupr., Sec., Veratr.; 2, Bell., Canth., Cham., Cic., Hydr-ac., Jatr., Laur., Merc., Nicotin, Nux-v., Phos., Phos-ac., Ric-aegidi recommends as a preventive for a week, one dose every evening of Chin-mur. 30 and ozonized water. All food must be cooked; raw fruits strictly forbidden.

Epidemic bronchitis or influenza - 1, Acon., Ars., Bell., Caust., Merc., Nux-v., Rhus-tox.; 2, Arn., Bry., Camph., Chin., Ipec., Phos., Puls., Sabad., Seneg., Sil., Spig., Squil., Stict., Veratr.; 3, Agar., Cham., Con., Hyosc., Kalm., Op., Sulph.

Epidemic brain-fever (Meningitis, cerebro-spinalis) Spotted fever - China and Arg. nit. are recommended as prophylactics during an **epidemic**; Gels. at the beginning of the disease; Cic., Cimicif., Crotal., Cupr., Glon., Lyc., Natr., Sulph., Op., Stram., Tab., Veratr. **During the disease; Zinc.**, where depression prevails; Ars. and Bapt. for tendency to decomposition.

Epidemic dysentery - Merc., Ipec., and Acon. are frequently indicated in **epidemic** dysentery that comes in hot weather, and Ipec., Dulc. and Merc. are frequently indicated in the dysentery of cold weather.

Remedies for specific epidemic

Agaricus - Scratching sensation in throat, renewed with every attempt to sing. A professional singer after an **epidemic** influenza.

Ailanthus - Dr. Wells used this remedy in a number of cases, as it was at that time an **epidemic** remedy for scarlet fever, in Brooklyn, and many patients were saved by it. You will often see such a scarlet fever running to a number of other remedies, but this remedy corresponds to one of the most malignant types, and its commonest use will be in an **epidemic** in which the cases largely run to the malignant type.

Allium cepa - Autumnal **epidemics** of spasmodic cough.

Allium cepa - Autumnal **epidemics** of whooping-cough – the symptoms are: hoarse, harsh, dry, ringing, spasmodic cough, causing a raw splitting pain in larynx, so severe that he tries to suppress the cough, worse in a warm room and when lying down; better in the open air, but getting worse again on entering a warm room; copious, fluent, acrid coryza and profuse bland lachrymation; constant sneezing when coming into a warm room; catarrhal ophthalmia; chills run up the back, weakness in hips and loins; lassitude.

Allium cepa - **Epidemics** of autumnal influenza.

Alumen - **Epidemic** membranous croup.

Angustura - **Epidemic** spleen disease of cattle or horses.

Anthracin - this nosode has proven a great remedy in **epidemic** spleen diseases of domestic animals.

Antimonium sulph-aur. - **Epidemic** typhus.

Antimonium tart. - is for **epidemic** intermittent fever (malaria) of winter or early spring, quotidian, tertian and quartan type; tertians anteponing. The symptoms are: intermittents from exposure in damp cellars or basements; nausea, vomiting and anorexia; great sleepiness or irresistible inclination to sleep; < in damp cold weather, motion, lying down at night; chill and heat alternating during the day without thirst; cold skin, trembling and chilliness always from within outward; short chill and long-lasting heat, with somnolence and profuse sweat on forehead; intense thirst and delirium during heat in tertian. Profuse sweat all over, complaints < while sweating, but > after wards. Weariness, lassitude, exhaustion, with great depression of spirits, neither appetite nor thirst during apyrexia.

Apis-mel. - Boy, aged 12, face livid; **epidemic** typhus.

Apis-mel. - In 1858, Dr. C. W. Wolf published a book on bee-poison, declaring it a polychrest, but he also used the tincture from the whole bee. It happened at the time to correspond to the genius **epidemicus** in Berlin, but Wolf recommended it in all intermittent fevers.

Ars-alb. - Paralysis as a sequel of **epidemic** cases of diphtheria; albuminuria. The symptoms are: membrane dry-looking and wrinkled, covering entire fauces; ulcers extending from throat to roof of mouth; tongue white; cervical glands swollen, thin excoriating discharge from nose; sensation as if a hair had lodged in throat; great foetor from the diphtheritic deposits and oozing of blood from under the elevated portions of the thick membrane; sleep broken with a start, crying out, jerking of limbs; great weakness and prostration; great restlessness and anxiety, patient wants to change position often notwithstanding the debility; child wants to be carried from one room to another; cannot bear to be alone; constipation or exhausting watery and offensive diarrhoea; urine frequent or scanty, burning; pulse rapid and weak; thirst, but takes only sips; < after midnight; > from warmth and warm drinks.

Arsenic alb. - In every **epidemic** of malarial fever that I have gone through I have found Arsenicum symptoms more common than those of China.

Arum dracontium - Croupy cough, with hoarseness and rawness of throat, during an **epidemic** influenza.

Baptisia - **Epidemic** influenza.

Belladonna - **Epidemic** chorea; motions of body are generally backward or to and fro; constantly changing emprosthotonos to opisthotonos; boring head into pillow; numbness of fingers; grinding of teeth; moaning; soreness and tenderness of last lumbar vertebrae; flushed face and sore throat. after fright or mental excitement, especially when the flexors are affected and the paroxysms are preceded by numb feeling in muscles, or by a sensation as if a mouse ran over the extremities; dull, heavy, drowsy, stupid; tongue paretic; difficult articulation; violent congestion, throbbing of carotids, dilated pupils, wild look, injected eyes. Reflex chorea from dentition or pregnancy;

Bromium - If there is a diphtheria **epidemic** and the mother bundles up her baby until she overheats him, and keeps in a hot room, and it happens to be a child that is sensitive to being wrapped up, and one whose complaints are worse from being wrapped up, look out.

Cadmium sulph. - Zeitung, and in 1856 in Hirschel's Archiv, vol. ii. These were not followed by any other reports until 1878, when Dr. Hardenstein, of Vicksburg, used the remedy successfully in one of the most murderous **epidemics** of yellow fever, the application of the remedy proving him to be a master in prescribing.

Camphor - Aggravation; during **epidemic** cholera; from hot sun.

Camphor - Miscarriage or abortion during **epidemic** influenza, disposition to catarrhs; pale, loose, cold skin.

Carduus marianus - Contents of stomach and intestines sour. **Epidemic** affection.

Carduus marianus - Cough with stitches in sides of chest, and bloody sputa. **Epidemic** affection.

Carduus marianus - Gastric, catarrhal, or rheumatic fever, with pain in stomach and region of liver, increased by pressing on it; symptoms frequent in **epidemic** influenza.

Carduus marianus - **Epidemic** affection, lasting seven weeks, was lessened to a few days; the longest seven days.

Carduus marianus - Pains in chest going to front part, to shoulders, back, loins and abdomen, combined with urging to urinate. **Epidemic** affection.

Cedron - Considered a specific for bites of venomous serpents, hydrophobia and stings of poisonous insects, in Panama, and used for **epidemic** intermittents.

Chelidonium - Autumn typhus, (**epidemic**) with affection of liver **epidemic** of malarious or other miasm - typhous complications in **epidemic** bronchitis - Whooping cough (**epidemic**) - Widow; **epidemic** influenza - Cutting pain in calves and upper arms, alternating with headache and preventing sleep. **Epidemic** typhus.

Chelidonium - **Epidemics** of malarious or other miasm.

Chelidonium - Widow, aged 75; **epidemic** influenza.

Chininum sulph. - Paralysis of lower extremities, involuntary stools and urination, occurring every other day during fever **epidemic**.

Cina - For intermittent fever (malaria) Cina may be the **epidemic** remedy for children, when adults need other drugs. – The symptoms are: periodicity well marked, at same hour every day, evening; tertian, quartan. Ravenous hunger before and during paroxysm. Chill without thirst, with hot cheeks; shivering creeping over trunk, not relieved by external warmth; cold, pale face, cold sweat on forehead, nose and hands; vomiting during chill. Heat with thirst; face puffed, pale around mouth and nose, with redness of cheeks and thirst for cold drinks, and very short breath. Sweat without thirst, light, followed by vomiting of food and canine hunger, tongue always clean. Apyrexia: worm symptoms; irritable, peevish and obstinate; breath foul.

Cistus can. - An **epidemic** of coryza was prevalent, and this was the strongest symptom - the pain caused by inhaling air, great burning from inhaled air.

Coffea tosta - **Epidemic** cholera infantum.

Colchicum - Gastric, rheumatic genus **epidemicus**.

Colchicum - **Epidemic** or autumnal intermittents (malaria) on a rheumatic or gouty basis. The symptoms are: chills running down the back, even in a warm room, extremities cold, < on motion. Heat with great thirst the whole night, especially on face and extremities. Sweat sour-smelling or absent.

Apyrexia; gastric symptoms, cannot bear the smell of cooked food, nausea.

Colocynthis - Chronic diarrhoea; **epidemic** dysentery.

Corallium rub. - Endemic whooping cough.

Crotalus hor. - Used successfully by Hardenstein in an **epidemic** pyaemia.

Cuprum met. - **Epidemic** pneumonia; after a few-days dry coughing or a diarrhoea, either stitches, mostly in left side of chest, or a pressure behind sternum, or neither, but bronchitic symptoms by auscultation, with headache, fever or great prostration; cannot take a deep breath, the shooting pain prevents it; in some cases dyspnoea, sudden feeling of suffocation, has to sit up, with a pale, collapsed face.

Digitalis - Jaundice and cramps during cholera **epidemic**.

Drosera - Fever occurring when whooping cough is **epidemic**.

Eugenia jambos - **Epidemic** cough among children, with coryza, inflammation of eyes and pain in ears.

Eupatorium perf. - Has been a very useful remedy in intermittent fever, when **epidemic** in the valleys.

Eupatorium perf. - **Epidemic** influenza.

Euphorbium - **Epidemic** influenza.

Ferr-met. - Pneumonia **epidemica** : dyspnoea gradually increased; no pressure under sternum; pale face; stupid; roof of mouth white; skin neither burning nor cold and damp; pulse never hard and full.

Ferr-met. - **Epidemic** pneumonia. The symptoms are: pneumonia senilis; laxity of fibre; pulse soft and quick, or slow and easily compressible; dyspnoea slowly increasing; bloody expectoration; **epidemic** pneumonia, dyspnoea gradually increasing, no pressure under sternum; pale, stupid face;

roof of mouth white; skin neither burning nor cold and damp; pulse never hard and full.

Gelsemium - Dysentery (**epidemic**), malarial or catarrhal.

Grindelia - **Epidemic** rash like Roseola, suffusing face, neck and often whole body, with severe burning and itching.

Gymnocladus - **Epidemic** fevers, typhoid in character.

Ipecacuanha - Has been proved as a useful remedy in **epidemic** dysentery, when the patient is compelled to sit almost constantly upon the stool and passes a little slime, or a little bright red blood; inflammation of the lower portion of the bowel, the rectum and the colon. - It runs through a whole valley and may be **epidemic**; but it commonly relates to endemics.

Ipecacuanha - Night : discharge from eyes agg; sleepless; dry cough agg; pain in molars agg; dry, spasmodic cough; croupy cough; attacks of shooting in chest agg; very profuse sour sweat; disagreeable heat; **epidemic** dysentery agg; cramp in thighs; irritable, irascible; fever agg.

Kali-carb. - The face becomes puffed, the eyes seem to protrude and then there is seen that which is commonly present in Kali-carb., a peculiar sort of a swelling between the eyelids and eyebrows that fills up when coughing. Your attention is called to that peculiar feature, for although there may be bloating nowhere else upon the face that little bagging will appear above the lid and below the eyebrow. It fills up sometimes to the extent of a little water bag. Such a swelling has been produced by Kali-carb., and sometimes that symptom alone guides us to the examination of the remedy for the purpose of ascertaining if Kali-carb. does not fit the rest of the case. Boenninghausen speaks of an **epidemic** of whooping cough in which the majority of cases called for Kali-carb., and this striking feature was present.

Kali-iod. - Furuncular eruption, **epidemic**, of various sizes, from a small pustule to a large boil; often this latter becomes carbuncular and is generally surrounded by little pustules.

Kali-iod. - Furuncular eruption, **epidemic**, of various sizes, from a small pustule to a large boil; often this latter becomes carbuncular and is generally surrounded by little pustules.

Lachesis - Furuncular formation, generally upon lower lip, attended with severe pain and frequently surrounded by erysipelatous areola; rapid and excessive loss of strength, reduced from vigor to absolute prostration within twenty-four hours. **Epidemic** malignant pustule.

Lycopodium - Paroxysms commence between 4 and 8 P.M.; sometimes with chill, again without; thirsty or not; sleepy; fever lasts till midnight or 2 A.M., generally followed by sweat. **Epidemic** intermittent.

Mancinella - Angina following scarlet fever, or during **epidemic** of latter.

Merc., Ipec. and Acon. - are frequently indicated in **epidemic** dysentery that comes in hot weather, and Ipec., Dulc. and Merc. are frequently indicated in the dysentery of cold weather.

Merc-iod-rub. - Glandular swellings; exudation limited, transparent and easily detached; cases attending **epidemic** scarlet fever. Diphtheria.

Merc-sol. - For **epidemic** coryza the remedy is Merc-sol. The symptoms are: frequent sneezing, copious discharge of watery saliva; swelling, redness and rough, scraping soreness of the nose, with itching and pain in the nasal bones on pressing upon them; foetid smell of the nasal mucus; painful heaviness of the forehead; night-sweats, chills and feverish heat; great thirst; pains in the limbs, aggravated by warmth or cold, by dampness.

Merc-sol. - **Epidemic** broncho-pneumonia. The symptoms are: bilious pneumonia (chel.), with blood-streaked expectoration and sharp pains shooting through the lower portion of right lung to back, cannot lie on right side; icteroid symptoms; slimy stools, attended with great tenesmus before, during and after stool (chel., free discharges). Asthenic pneumonia with feeling of weight in lungs, < walking or ascending, short cough and expectoration of bloody saliva; **epidemic** broncho-pneumonia, with deep irritation of the nervous system; nose, larynx and trachea become suddenly dry, dyspnoea sets in with spasmodic cough, < at night, and yellow-green, blood-streaked expectoration; skin burning hot, at times covered with copious sweat; tongue yellow, soon becomes dry; senses dull, violent headache, soporous condition, with light delirium; complains of little or no pain (influenza); infantile lobular pneumonia.

Mer-sol. - Angina: great dryness in mouth and throat; expectoration of masses of mucus from pharynx and choanae; ptyalism; face pale red; left side swollen; dry heat, with confusion of head; burning skin; constant thirst; frequent, strong pulse; severe chill, with drawing in limbs and lassitude; nauseating belching; beating in left praecordia; severe drawing pain in nape and down back; pain in parotid glands and muscles of neck, not agg by motion; fever agg in evening; thick, white coat on tongue; stitching pain in throat when moving jaw; pain extending to ears; vertigo when rising; stitches in occiput, with slight cough; severe headache, particularly in left temple; severe dull pain in occiput; skin of head and face seems tense; fauces of a coppery red color; soft palate and tonsils greatly swollen, dark red and pressed forward; stinging pains from empty swallowing at night and in cold air; agg spring and fall and in wet, cold weather; **epidemic**, young people especially affected; chronic or habitual.

Millefolium - Scarlet fever **epidemic**, with excessive angina and violent fever.

Natrum sulph. - **Epidemic** dysentery.

Nitri spiritus dulcis - **Epidemic** dysentery with lethargy.

Nux moschata - Fall: **epidemic** diarrhoea.

Opium - Woman, aged 30, during **epidemic** of influenza; cough.

Phosphoric-acid. - Cholerine during cholera **epidemic**, especially when patient is debilitated and relaxed by heat of Summer; no pain; lassitude; prostration; general ill-feeling; abdomen bloated, rumbling therein; small painless discharges.

Phosphorus - **Epidemic** influenza : rawness and scraping in pharynx, agg. towards evening; hawking of mucus in morning; fluent coryza with great dullness of head and sleepiness; more during day and after meals; blowing of blood from nose; profuse hemorrhages from nose and mouth; much sneezing; frequent alternation of dry and fluent coryza; sensitiveness in region of liver, with stitches there; hoarseness, rawness in larynx and trachea; cough excited by tickling in chest, generally dry evening and night, with mucous expectoration in morning and during day, agg talking, laughing, crying (children), lying on back or left side; much fever and thirst; lassitude and prostration out of proportion to duration of disease; much heat and great pain in larynx or chest, with dry cough and tendency to diarrhoea.

Phytolacca - Diphtheria : sick and dizzy when trying to sit up; frontal headache; pains shooting from throat into ears, especially on trying to swallow; face flushed; tongue much coated, protruded; thickly coated at back, fiery red at tip; breath fetid, putrid; vomiting; difficulty of swallowing; tonsils swollen, covered with membrane, first upon left, three or four patches; tonsils, uvula and back part of throat covered with ash-colored exudation; tonsils covered with dirty, white, pseudo membrane; small white or yellow spots on tonsils coalesce and form patches of membrane; membrane has appearance of dirty washleather; exudation pearly or greyish white; great thirst; agg from hot drinks; dyspnoea; ropy, offensive mucus lining mouth and throat; glands of neck very tender; pain in neck and back, body sore as if bruised, groans with pain, especially when trying to move or turn in bed; aching limbs; great prostration; violent chill, soon followed by high fever; fever without chill; pulse 120, 140, weak; rash on skin; remarkably nervous phenomena; consecutive paralysis; leaves vision impaired, hearing dull; in cold weather generally **epidemic**; usually of catarrhal or rheumatic origin, brought on by exposure to damp and cold atmosphere or sleeping in damp, ill-ventilated rooms.

Podophyllum - Diarrhoea of children during **epidemic** of cholera; catarrhal affections of respiratory organs sometimes precede attack; all desire for food gone; great thirst; upper part of intestinal tract affected and vomiting more frequent than diarrhoea; copious, foul-smelling, exhausting stools.

Podophyllum - Endemic dysentery.

Polyporus off. (Febris intermittens) - sporadic or endemic fevers at any season except fall. Almost continued fever, though it never runs very high; great languor and aching in all joints. Creeping chills along spine, between shoulder-blades, up the back to nape, intermingled with hot flushes; unusual chilliness in open air, with icy coldness of nose. heat with thirst, face hot and flushed, with prickly sensation; hands, palms, feet hot and dry. Sweat profuse after midnight in old chronic cases, otherwise light. Apyrexia: hepatic pains with jaundice, great lassitude, *constipation and headache;* food passes undigested. Gloom.

Sabadilla - **Epidemic** influenza: great sleepiness during day; chilliness, shivering and horripilations, particularly toward evening; chilliness running upward, from feet to head; lachrymation and redness of eyelids; pressure in eyes, particularly when moving them and when looking upward; pressing headache, particularly in forehead; sore pain in tongue, which is covered with a thick yellow coating; pain in tongue extends into throat; difficult deglutition; frequent sensation as if a skin were hanging loosely in throat; bitter taste in mouth; complete loss of appetite; nausea; dryness of mouth; thirstlessness; constipation with rumbling of flatus or diarrhoea of brown fermented stool, which floats upon the water; urine yellow and turbid; cough with vomiting, headache, sharp stitches in vertex, pain in region of stomach; hoarse cough, often with haemoptysis; painful paralytic weakness of limbs, particularly of knees; all the symptoms agg from cold; aggravation towards afternoon, reaching its height in evening; heat of face with chilliness and coldness of limbs or chilliness running up back, returning every ten minutes; skin dry as parchment; sleep restless; disturbed by anxious dreams; cough immediately on lying down.

Sarcolactic acid - proved by Dr. Wm. B. Griggs, M.D. He found it of great value in the most violent form of **epidemic** influenza, especially with violent and retching and greatest prostration when Arsenic had failed.

Sarracenia - In an **epidemic** occurring in the environs of Wavre it was given to more than two thousand persons living in the very middle of the disease and coming in constant intercourse with it, but all who took it escaped the disease; during the same time more than two hundred cases were treated by the same remedy without the loss of a single patient.

Sarsparilla - An endemic affection occurring in Marienwerder, occasionally with trichoma (plica); patients unwell for a long time; pale-red brownish spots appear on the extremities, rarely on trunk, turn into small, deep ulcers, edges callous, inverted, these heal after a time, but appear on other places; their size is about half an inch, seldom smaller, never larger; they spread in a line like a wreath or garland; the scars elevated, red, winding; later sore throat, pain in nose; inflamed, suppurating spots on soft palate and on septum, soon destroying it; sometimes pains in superficial knots on shin bone and other places; also exostoses.

Secale - After an **epidemic** of the rye disease an unusually large number of cataracts occurred in young people, twenty- three of whom gradually became blind (fifteen men and eight women), associated with headache, vertigo and roaring in ears; of the cataracts two were hard, twelve soft, and nine mixed.

Sinapis nigra - Found of use in Philadelphia with potassium cyanide as a means of prevention in the **epidemic** of smallpox, 1870-71, by Hering, Korndoerfer, Farrington, Knerr, and others.

Stramonium - Rheumatic inflammatory affections of brain with children under seven years, **epidemic** during a Winter season; starting in sleep; moaning with restless motions; when awake they look with staring eyes and despair in their faces, to one point, and either move slowly and shyly backward or run away with a violent, fearful scream; taking hold of things near them; feverish heat, red face; moist skin.

Thuja - Variola; pains in upper arms, fingers and hands, with fulness and soreness of throat; areola around pustules marked and dark-red, pustules milky and flat, painful to touch; especially during suppurative stage where it may prevent pitting; recommended as a preventive as well as a curative by Boenninghausen, who states that it shortened all cases in **epidemic** of 1849, and prevented scars.

Veratrum alb. - Fall and spring: whooping-cough **epidemics**; neuralgia in arms.

Veratrum alb. - **Epidemic** of whooping-cough (spring and fall). The symptoms are: deep, hollow, ringing cough, excited by a tickling in the lowest branches of bronchi, seeming as if it came from abdomen, at night without, in daytime with, expectoration of yellow, tenacious mucus, of a bitter salty, or sour and putrid taste; worse from coming from a cold into a warm air, from getting warm, damp cold weather, eating and drinking cold things; neck too weak to hold head up; cold sweat on forehead; great craving for acids and acid fruits.

Viola odorata - **Epidemic** dysentery, characterized by spasmodic tenesmus, intestinal spasms, tympanitis, etc.

Xanthoxylum - **Epidemic** dysentery, characterized by spasmodic tenesmus, intestinal spasms, tympanitis, etc.

Zincum met. - **Epidemic** membranous croup.

Zincum met. - **Epidemic** meningitis cerebro-spinalis; short breathing, anguish, pressure in chest, and frequently returning dry tussiculation, pulse remarkably slow; pulse small, frequent, very changeable, breathing irregular; short, dry, spasmodic cough; mental disturbance.

From the above list we can easily find out and say that **Polyporus officinale (Boletus laricis) is the specific for chikungunya.**

Why does homoeopathy fail?

From the time of origin of homoeopathy by Dr. Hahnemann till today, it has survived the tests of time. In many countries homoeopathy has been recognised as an authentic system of medicine. Today, more and more people are becoming aware of it and are experiencing its wonderful cures. Its phenomenal success has been witnessed and appreciated not only in India but also all over the world.

The World Health Organization (WHO) has recognized Homoeopathy as an accepted system of medicine and as the second largest system of medicine in the world. However, homoeopathy has been a victim of constant onslaught from various agencies all around the globe against time to time. The fact is that homoeopathy does not fail; it is the homoeopathy practitioner who fails. Research orientation is what we need today; there is a researcher and scientist in every one of us. We must be open minded and an "active contributor" to the development of science. We must use every possible resource to explore new things, and make Homoeopathy an acceptable and accessible science to all. We must avoid the ignorance of Section 153 of the Organon which says that we have to prescribe on 'uncommon-rare-strange' or 'peculiar' symptoms.

Failures are because many have taken homoeopathy as a backdoor entry to medical practice. Homoeopathy is not to do away with the knowledge of *diagnosis and differential diagnosis*. When a physician is aware of 'common' symptoms of disease then only he will be able to understand what are 'uncommon' and work out the cases. Thus, here the Encyclopaedia of Common and Uncommon Symptoms affords excellent help.

SECTION 2
PRACTICAL TOOLS

- Mind Symptoms
- Congestion, Rush of Blood, Hyperaemia
- Cachexia, Cachectic, Dyscrasia
- Lack of Reaction — Low Vitality —When the Indicated Remedy Fails to Act
- Cause of Diseases
- Cross, Crossing
- Plethora, Plethoric Individuals, Precocity
- Precocious Children
- Old Age, Senility, Presenility
- Diabetes Mellitus — Glycosuria
- Malignant diseases
- Cancerous Diathesis, Cancerous Constitution, Cancerous Cachexia
- Sterility, Infertility
- Gout—Retrocedent, Metastatic, Constitutional
- Treatment of Chronic Diseases—Miasms—Psora, Sycosis, Syphilis—Constitutional Treatment—Generals—General Symptoms
- Diseases That Have Become Habitual
- Nutritional Disorders
- Checked Discharges - Suppression Of Secretions
- Some Useful Rubrics of Mind

Scope and limitations of homoeopathy

Unless there is a doctor-patient relationship you cannot treat/cure a patient. This is because we do not treat the disease (by giving insulin for diabetes etc.) but we treat the patient. Again, 'uncommon-rare-strange-peculiar' symptoms *are told by the patient in the clinic only and nowhere else.* Thus and therefore, difficulties would be seen in prescribing for your relatives who demand medicine over phone without coming as a patient to the practitioner.

The practitioner should always ask the patient to come physically at least once so that the physician can carefully note what all the patient tells and based on those symptoms he should try to find out the similimum. Many a time the homeopath gets surprised to find a valuable symptom which his relative did not tell him. There is lot of difference between telling symptoms to a doctor and talking to a relative.

A suggestion to treat far off patients: ask them to write down on paper in their own handwriting, scan it and send it to you. (No direct typing in the computer). A homeopath should note that during provings the provers were asked TO WRITE DOWN symptoms felt by them.

'Mind' symptoms

The most commonly misunderstood topics in homoeopathy are 'mind symptoms' (section 213 of the Organon) and 'uncommon-rare-strange-peculiar-symptoms' (Section 153). When Section 213 is read with section 153 we can conclude that we should take only those mind symptoms which we have never heard before normally/commonly/usually in any patient.

'Mind Symptoms' and 'uncommon symptoms' (for selecting the remedy) are not what you have learnt but they are, in reality, something different which you have to learn by rote.

Again, most of the valuable 'mind' or 'uncommon' symptoms cannot be classified under any head in the repertories and an honest and conscious homoeopath has to learn them by rote. ('rote' means mechanical or habitual repetition). Dr. Hahnemann advises that without prescribing on mind symptoms a cure is not possible (Section 213 of the *Organon*). Refer to cases 5 to 16 on page no. 493-501).

Congestion, Rush of blood, Hyperaemia

Many terms are unique to homoeopathic practice. Homoeopaths should restrain from being a symptom-coverer. Bernard Shaw wrote that if a homoeopath looks at a Chinese he would prescribe him for jaundice (because the colour of the skin of Chinese people is yellow). No one need get offended by this statement. I am only trying to carefully lift all mysterious clouds enveloping our science.

Let us now learn some terminologies most useful in selecting the remedy.

Congestion: When two or more symptoms are in one and the same part of the body, instead of considering each symptom separately you should take the rubric **'congestion'**. For example, a patient came in complaining of headache, dandruff and hairfall; he had been having this for several years. A naïve physician would take 'dandruff' 'hairfall' and 'headache' for finding the remedy. But when these three symptoms are found together at one place *viz.*, head, we should not take the three symptoms separately but as one whole unit and the term is 'congestion'. For this do not take the list of remedies under CONGESTION in the Chapter 'Head' in **Kent's Repertory** but you must go to the Chapter GENERALITIES at the end of **Kent's Repertory** and there also you find a rubric CONGESTION. You must take this for chronic diseases.

A patient is having varicose veins in legs, pain in knee, corns on sole, cramps in feet. All these complaints are on the lower limb. Here too we must use the rubric 'congestion'.

'Congestion' — other examples

When pain or some other symptom is felt in a part while exerting another part, e.g., headache while coughing, involuntary urination or urging to urinate when excited etc.

'Worry causes headache'. 'Mental tension causes or aggravates skin complaints'. (For this we have the term neurotic eczema. See the remedy *Anacardium orientale* in Boericke's Materia Medica. In that remedy under the paragraph Skin we find the following: Intense itching, eczema, with mental irritability... neurotic eczema).

Instead of the term congestion some materia medicas use the term 'rush of blood' or 'hyperaemia'.

Following are from Lilienthal:

Rush of blood of plethoric individuals requires: 1, Acon., Aur., Bell., Calc., Lyc., Phos., Sep., Sulph. 2. Arn., Bry., Chin., Ferr., Nat-mur., Nux-vom., Rhus-tox, Thuj.

Rush of blood complained of by plethoric, debilitated, hypochondriac, or nervous individuals. The principal remedies are: 1, Acon., Aur., Calc., Hep., Kalm., Kreos., Lyc., Phos., Sep., Sulph.; 2, Amb., Amm., Arn., Bell., Bry., Carb-v., Caust., Croc., Chin., Fer., Iod., Natr-m., Nux-v., Op., Petr., Phos-ac., Rhus, Samb., Sarsap., Senn., Sil., Stann., Thuj.

Rush of blood of nervous, very irritable individuals: 1. Acon, Arn., Bell., Chin., Nux-v.; 2. Amb., Aur., Calc., Fer., Lyc., Petr., Samb.

(Memory weak, inability to think) - if by congestion of blood to the head: Chin., Melilot., Merc., Rhus, Sulph.

Remedies having the symptom 'congestion' 'rush of blood' or 'hyperaemia'

Agaricus (Hepatic derangements) - congested, enlarged liver.

Absithinium (Delirium) - sleeplessness in typhoid with congestion at the base of brain.

Actea spicata - active sanguineous congestions.

Adrenalin - therapeutically, adrenalin has been suggested in acute congestion of lungs, asthma, grave's and addison's diseases, arterio-sclerosis, chronic aortitis, angina pectoris, haemophilia chlorosis, hay fever, serum rashes, acute urticaria, etc.

Aesculus hip - venous congestion, especially portal and hemorrhoidal. - follicular pharyngitis connected with hepatic congestion. - torpor and congestion of the liver and portal system, with constipation. - very painful, dark purple, external haemorrhoids, with constipation and vertigo and portal congestion.

Aesculus hip (Haemorrhoids) - depressed and irritable. angina granulosa, a dark-red congestion of fauces, with dryness and soreness, from abdominal plethora.

Aesculus hip (Hepatic derangements) - congestion of liver and portal system.

Aesculus hip (Vertigo, dizziness) - derangement of the portal system, producing nervous congestion in the brain.

Agaricus (Paralysis) - paraplegia from congestion of lumbar cord

Ailanthus - passive congestion: headaches.

Ailanthus (Hay fever, Catarrhus aestivus) - eyes suffused and congested.

Ailanthus (Headache) - passive congestive headache and dizziness, face red and hot, > by nosebleed (Arn.).

Aletris (Haemorrhage from uterus) - menorrhagia in consequence of congested condition of uterus and ovaries.

Aloe (Haemorrhoids) - constipation of old people of sedentary habits and given to high living. Uterine congestion and prolapsus with heaviness in abdomen and back.

Aloe (Uterus complaints) - uterine congestion and prolapsus, with fulness and heaviness and labor-like pains in loins and groins, < standing.

Aloe - congestion to head and chest, but especially to portal system. there is no remedy richer in symptoms of portal congestion and none that has given better clinical results, both for the primary pathological condition and secondary phenomenon.

Alumen (Vertigo, dizziness) - rush of blood to head.

Alumina - rush of blood to face after eating.

Alumina silicata - congestion of brain.

Aluminium (Headache) - headache, attended with nausea, oppression in forehead, rush of blood to eyes and nose, epistaxis, pale face and languor.

Ambra - rush of blood to head, when listening to music.

Amm-brom (Epilepsy) - tinnitus aurium from congestion of the labyrinth.

Amm-brom (Headache) - tinnitus aurium from congestion of labyrinth.

Amm-brom (Sore throat) - fauces dark-red, congestion.

Amm-carb (Sore throat) - enlarged tonsils, congested, covered with membrane.

Ammoniac. - anxiety, with congestion of lungs. Ammonium brom. - cerebral congestion. Ammonium carb. - tip of nose congested. Ammonium mur. - chronic congestion of liver.

Amygdalus. - congestion or turgescence of vessels of brain; general effusion on both hemispheres; dura mater gorged.

Amyl nit. - superficial arterial hyperaemia.

Amyl nit. (Headache) - congestive headache.

Amyl nit. (Sunstroke) - congestive stage of sunstroke.

Antimonium-sul-aur - congestion of upper lobe of left lung.

Antipyrinum - acts especially on the vaso-motor centers, causing dilation of capillaries of skin and consequent circumscribed patches of hyperaemia and swelling.

Ant-tart (Asthma) - suffocative cough or congestion of blood to chest and palpitation of heart.

Apis-mel. (Amenorrhoea) - suppressed menses, with congested or inflamed ovaries.

Apis-mel. (Haemorrhage from uterus) - red spots on body, stinging like bee-stings, often the result of active congestion of ovaries.

Apis-mel. (Meningitis, cerebro-spinalis) - stupor from effusion (Op. from congestion).

Apis-mel. (Meningitis, encephalitis) - meningitis from suppression or spread of erysipelas or other exanthemata. Congestion to the head and face, with fullness, burning and throbbing in brain.

Apis-mel. (Uterus complaints) - menses suppressed or diminished, with congestion to head.

Apis. - delirium: with congestion; eruptions; heat; during sleep.

Apocynum cannabinum - takes cold easily, nostrils become congested and blocked up easily.

Arg-met - in society indisposed to talk; he complains of rush of blood to head and cheeks, singing in ears; itching in reddened eyes.

Arg-nit. - great melancholy and weakness of mind with congestion to head.

Arg-nit. (Asthma) - any bodily exertion brings on a fit with palpitation and congestion of face.

Arg-nit. (Blennorrhoea of the lachrymal sac) - conjunctiva congested.

Arg-nit. (Fever, relapsing) - excessive congestion of blood to head, with throbbing of carotid arteries.

Arg-nit. (Kidney/bladder stone) - nephralgia from congestion of kidney or from passage of little stones.

Arg-nit. (Nephralgia, renal colic) - nephralgia from congestion of kidneys or from passage of calculi.

Arg-nit. (Ophthalmia) - great hyperaemia of conjunctiva.

Arg-nit. (Vision complaints) - marked hyperaemia of conjunctiva with mucous discharge and redness of inner canthi.

Arg-nit. (Dacryo-cystitis) - caruncula swollen, looking like a lump of raw flesh, conjunctiva congested.

Aristolochia serpentaria virginia (symptoms of intestinal tract; colliquative diarrhoea, meteorism. Flatulent dyspepsia. brain congestion. Distention and cutting pains in abdomen. Symptoms like those of poison-oak).

Arnica - noises in ear caused by rush of blood to the head. - coma, insensibility. - congestive chills, meningitis, etc. - in cases of sanguine plethoric people with lively expression, very red face, disposed to cerebral congestion. - prolapsus uteri.

Arnica (Haemorrhages) - pain causes a rush of blood to the head, which feels very hot to the patient

Arnica (Hearing, defective) - noises in ears, as if caused by rush of blood to the head.

Arnica (Otitis and otorrhoea) - noises in ears from rush of blood to head

Arnica (Sore throat) - whole throat congested

Ars-alb. (Bronchitis chronica) - dyspnoea, from more or less extensive emphysema and consecutive pulmonary congestions. Difficulty of breathing continues during the intervals upon coughing, and returns periodically, especially at night

Ars-alb. (Haemorrhage from uterus) - chronic endometritis and passive hyperaemia, based on atony.

Artemisia - congestion of brain and spine. - congestion of brain.

Artemisia (Vertigo, dizziness) - great heaviness of head and congestion of all cerebro-spinal vessels.

Asafoetida (Heart diseases) - beating of heart, with faintness, rush of blood to head, flushing of face, anxiety and slow breathing

Asafoetida (Vertigo, dizziness) - congestion of the portal system and pulsation of the veins

Asafoetida - venous pulsations; congestion of portal vein; congestive fulness about heart and chest, with asthma; heat of face and ears, after eating; pressure on chest, etc.; copious discharges; all signs of fulness of venous system.

Asarum europ (Vision complaints) - asthenopia accompanied by congestive headaches.

Asclepias cornuti (Dropsy) - post-scarlatinal dropsy, or from suppressed perspiration, from renal or cardiac affections.

Congestive headaches with dullness and stupidity, scanty urine during headache, profuse after.

Asclepias cornuti (Headache) - congestive headache from suppression of sweat or urine and fever.

Asterias (Apoplexy) - cerebral congestion with obstinate constipation.

Aur-mur.-nat. (Ophthalmia) - retinal congestion.

Aurum met. - erethism or vascular fulness characterizes nearly all complaints; thus ruddy with scrofula, vascular leukoma, congestive asthma, ebullitions, erections, congested kidneys and liver-all from hypertrophied heart. - congestion to head.

Aurum met. (Asthma) - asthma from congestion to chest.

Aurum met. (Headache) - congestion to and heat in the head, with sparks before eyes, with nausea and bilious vomiting, < from any mental exertion or motion, ideas become confused, roaring in head.

Aurum met. (Headache) - congestive headaches.

Aurum met. (Heart diseases) - pure cardiac hypertrophy without dilatation, with increased force of heart-stroke and hyperaemia of lungs, < from any exertion, as walking up hill, and feeling of a crushing weight under sternum and as if blood would burst through chest, if he does not cease walking.

Aurum met. (Hepatic derangements) - hepatic congestion consecutive to cardiac disease, with burning and cutting in right hypochondrium, ending in cirrhosis and fatty degeneration with dropsy. Chronic hepatitis with suicidal melancholy, averse to motion.

Aurum met. (Insanity) - often asks questions, jumping from one thing to another, without waiting for a reply. Rush of blood to head, palpitations, pollutions, otherwise patient in fair physical health, and > in fresh air and out-door exercise.

Aurum met. (Labor) - congestion to head and chest, palpitation of heart.

Aurum met. (Love pangs) - congestion of blood to the chest and anxious beating of the heart. - congestion of blood to the head.

Aurum met. (Mind Symptoms) - rush of blood to head, roaring in ears.

Aurum mur. - hyperemia from overaction of heart; consequent congestion of liver, kidneys, genitals.

Baptisia (Heart diseases) - palpitations with congestion to head.

Baryta mur. (Tonsillitis) - elongation of uvula with hyperaemia and blennorrhoea.

Baryta mur. (Uvula, affections of) - elongated uvula, with hyperaemia and blennorrhoea.

Belladonna (Coxalgia, hip-disease) - congestion to head.

Belladonna (Croup) - hoarseness with flushed face and congested eyes.

Belladonna (Delirium) - congestion to brain with great drowsiness, but inability to sleep.

Belladonna (Diaphragm, diseases of) - in puerperal affections with painful headache from active hyperaemia (Atrop.).

Belladonna - Belladonna acts upon every part of the nervous system, producing active congestion, furious excitement, perverted special senses, twitching, convulsions and pain. - dry, as if glazed; angry-looking congestion (ginseng); red, worse on right side. Eustachian tube and tympanic congestion.

- fundus congested. stupefaction, with congestion to head, pupils enlarged; delirium.

Belladonna (Amenorrhoea) - suppression of menses followed by hyperaemia, rush of blood to the head, wakefulness and throbbing of carotids and temples.

Belladonna (Apoplexy) - the first stage of the disease, with grinding and gnashing of teeth before attack, where severe congestive symptoms are still present, or at a later period, when the extravasation causes severe inflammatory reaction.

Belladonna (Bronchitis acute) - stitches in chest, congestion to head, hot skin, inclined to be moist.

Belladonna (Chlorosis) - painful menstruation, with rush of blood to head.

Belladonna (Chorea) - violent congestion, throbbing of carotids, dilated pupils, wild look, injected eyes. Reflex chorea from dentition or pregnancy.

Belladonna (Cinchona, ill effects of) - congestion of blood to the head, with heat in the face.

Belladonna (Colic) - congestion of blood to the head.

Belladonna (Dentition, morbid) - numerous turgid blood vessels in congested gums.

Belladonna (Enteritis) - anguish, with congestion to the head and dimness of vision.

Belladonna (Gastritis) - difficult breathing, anguish, with congestion of blood to the head, dimness. of sight, faintishness, restless and sleepless.

Belladonna (Haematemesis, gastrorrhagia) - congestive delirium and convulsions. - warmth and even congestive burning in stomach with desire for acid drinks.

Belladonna (Haemorrhage from the lungs, haemoptysis) - bloody expectoration mixed with mucus. Active congestion. - congestion of blood to head and chest.

Belladonna (Haemorrhages) - congestion to head, eyes, eyeballs, which are red.

Belladonna (Headache) - congestion of blood to head, with danger of apoplexy

Belladonna (Heart diseases) - congestion of blood to various parts, violent palpitations, reverberating to the head.

Belladonna (Hepatic derangements) - congestion of the head.

Belladonna (Infantile remittent fever) - great heat and cerebral congestion.

Belladonna (Iris, affections of) - congested face. - congestion of conjunctiva, ciliary neuralgia, photophobia.

Belladonna (Jaundice) - congestion to head.

Belladonna (Measles) - congestion to head.

Belladonna (Menses complaints) - too early and too profuse, of hot, bright-red blood, containing dark, offensive clots, or the blood thick, decomposed and of a dark-red color, the discharge feeling hot as it passes before: dysmenorrhoea depending on a congested or inflamed ovary, more often the right one, with dragging and pressing downward pains and cutting from behind forward or vice versa, passing through the horizontal diameter of pelvis and not around circumference (as sep. and plat. do).

Belladonna (Migraine) - violent hyperaemia, with throbbing carotids, red face, intolerance of least jar, noise or light.

Belladonna (Miscarriage, abortion) - cerebral congestion and moaning, which gives her temporary relief.

Belladonna (Neuralgia) - congestion of head, with bright-red face and delirium.

Belladonna (Ophthalmia) - blindness, following severe congestive headaches. - hyperaesthesia and hyperaemia of the optic nerve and retina, apoplexy of retina, with suppressed menses.

Belladonna (Pericarditis) - acute stage with cerebral congestion and delirium.

Belladonna (Rheumatism) - stitching, burning and throbbing pains, with high fever, hot, dry skin, thirst, congestion to head, with throbbing headache and pulsations of carotids.

Belladonna (Scarlatina) - tympanum markedly congested, and congestion extending to external auditory canal.

Belladonna (Sleeplessness) - sleeplessness, especially of plethoric children, from nervous excitement, from local congestion, from irritation in various parts.

Belladonna (Synovitis) - congestion to head, flushed cheeks, etc.

Belladonna (Tonsillitis) - intense congestion, throbbing of carotids.

Belladonna (Uterus complaints) - cervical mucous membrane very much congested and reddened

Belladonna (Vertigo, dizziness) - epileptiform vertigo, often reflex from congestion of sexual organs or spinal cord.

Bellis per. - venous congestion, due to mechanical causes.

Benzinum nit. - venous hyperaemia of the brain and general venous engorgement.

Bromium (Tuberculosis of lungs) - congestion to head and chest, > by nosebleed.

Bryonia (Dropsy) - congestion of the head.

Bryonia (Dyspepsia, weakness of stomach) - congestive headaches.

Bryonia (Headache) - > by tying up the head, pressure and closing eyes. gastric, rheumatic and congestive headaches.

Bryonia (Headache) - congestive headaches, as if forehead would split open, with nosebleed, commencing in morning, not on waking, but after opening eyes and lasting till evening.

Bryonia (Menses complaints) - too early, too profuse, dark-red, smelling badly. Before: congestion to head and chest, pinching in abdomen.

Bryonia (Nails, diseases of) - tight, compressed feeling with pressing-out sensation, as if the finger needed more room, dark, congested part.

Bufo sahytiensis (Headache) - congestive headaches, < after breakfast, > by nosebleed.

Cactus - congestions; irregular distribution of blood. - congestive headaches, periodical, threatening apoplexy.

Cactus (Apoplexy) - vertigo from sanguineous congestions to the head.

Cactus (Asthma) - sanguineous congestion in chest, preventing free speech, < when lying down in bed.

Cactus (Haemorrhoids) - constipation as from haemorrhoidal congestion.

Cactus (Headache) - from sanguineous congestion or rheumatism, < by eating, any sudden motion or deep inspiration.

Cactus (Hearing, defective) - hardness of hearing from congestion

Cactus (Heart diseases) - sanguinous congestion to chest. endocarditis and pericarditis.

Cactus (Sunstroke) - vertigo, from sanguineous congestion to the head.

Cactus (Vertigo, dizziness) - vertigo from sanguineous congestion to the head, frequently caused by derangement of the heart. great nervous excitability, < from physical exertion, turning in bed, stooping, rising from recumbent position or deep breathing.

Cactus (Vision complaints) - hyperaemia of fundus, sight blurred, cannot see at a distance.

Cactus - sanguineous congestions in persons of plethoric habit.

Cactus (Diaphragm, diseases of) - rush of blood to chest.

Calcarea ars. - epilepsy with rush of blood to the before attack; aura felt in region of heart; flying sensation. - violent rush of blood to with vertigo.

Calc-ars. (Epilepsy) - epilepsy proceeding from cardiac affections, commencing with a pain in heart or constriction, rush of blood to the head, loss of speech and unconsciousness.

Calc-carb. - congestions: head; eyes; ears; nose; face; chest; abdomen, limbs; plethora.

Calc-carb. (Headache) - congestion of head, hammering through forehead and base of brain.

Camphor - internal congestions.

Camphor (Sunstroke) - severe headache, congestion of brain, fainting, delirium, convulsions.

Canchalagua - congested.

Carbo animalis - causes local congestions without heat. - rush of blood with confusion.

Carbo-veg. (Headache) - congestion of head from overheated rooms, > followed by nosebleed.

Carbo-veg. (Headache) - congestion of head from overheated rooms, heat on top of head during climaxis.

Carbon-sulph. - paralysis with intense congestion of nerve centres.

Carboneum oxygen. - cerebral congestion; hallucination of vision, hearing and touch.

Carduus - dropsical conditions depending on liver disease, and when due to pelvic congestion and hepatic disease.

Carduus (Hepatic derangements) - portal hyperaemia.

Carduus (Ulcers) - oedema of feet, portal hyperaemia, haemorrhoids, constipation.

Caulophyllum (Leucorrhoea) - menses suppressed from nervous causes in young girls or in nervous, debilitated women with relaxed, flabby uterus or displaced and passively congested uterus, especially after miscarriage.

Caulophyllum (Menses complaints) - neuralgic and congestive dysmenorrhoea with spasmodic, irregular and very severe pains, especially the first two days of menses.

Caulophyllum (Paralysis) - paraplegia from retroversion and congestion of womb after childbirth, with partial loss of sensation in affected limbs.

Causticum (Vertigo, dizziness) - congestion of the blood to the head, with heat and dimness of sight.

Causticum - disposition to hyperemia and congestion depending on diminished action of motor nerves on muscular coat of blood vessels. —aphonia.

Cedron (Prosopalgia) - patient nervous, excitable, with cold hands, feet and nose, congestion to head.

Chamomilla (Ophthalmia) - the tissue so much congested that blood oozes out from between the swollen lids, especially upon any attempt to open them.

Chelidonium (Chorea) - congestion to cerebellum.

Chelidonium (Dyspepsia, weakness of stomach) - great longing for wine, which does not cause congestion or heat in head as formerly.

Chelidonium (Hepatic derangements) - abdominal plethora from simple congestion to positive inflammation.

Chelidonium - congestion of liver and kidneys; mucous membranes. (spasm of smooth muscle everywhere, intestinal colic, uterine colic, bronchial spasm, tachycardia, etc.) boldo boldoa fragrans (bladder atony; cholecystitis and biliary calculus. bitter taste, no appetite; constipation, hypochondriasis languor, congestion of liver; burning weight in liver and stomach. painful hepatic diseases. disturbed liver following malaria.) elemuy gauteria (stones in kidneys and bladder; grain doses of powdered bark in water or 5 drops of tincture. pellagra). - Calc. brom. removes inflammatory products from uterus; children of lax fiber, nervous and irritable, with gastric and cerebral irritation. Tendency to brain disease. insomnia and cerebral congestion.

China-carbonaceous caries, commencing with a black spot, scrofulous or tuberculous subjects; the pain is throbbing, of a congestive nature, or caused by abuse of mercury. - has a special affinity for liver and spleen, producing hyperemia and congestion.

China (Amenorrhoea) - rush of blood to the head, with pulsation of the carotids.

China (Anaemia) - palpitations with rush of blood to head, and redness of face with cold hands.

China (Asthma) - pressure in chest as if from rush of blood, with violent palpitation of the heart, easy perspiration.

China (Heart diseases) - palpitation, with rush of blood to face, with cold hands.

China (Menses complaints) - menses too early, too profuse, with discharge of dark, coagulated blood, or watery, pale blood, with coagula. Before: congestion to uterus, with sensation of fulness and painful pressure towards genitals, especially when walking. during: abdominal cramps, congestion to uterus and chest. after: great weakness, trembling debility, convulsions, fainting fits.

China-ars. (Angina pectoris) - angina pectoris, with dropsical symptoms, venous hyperaemia and cyanosis.

China-sul. (Otitis and otorrhoea) - tinnitus aurium and impairment of hearing from paralysis of the vessels, with congestion and exudation, especially of labyrinth and tympanum.

China-sulph. - periodical recurrence of nervous and congestive paroxysms, trismus, paraplegia, ophthalmia, pulmonary hemorrhage, etc. - pruritus and congested conditions of the rectum.

Chloralum - passive cerebral hyperaemia (use 30th) - comatose for days, ending in cerebral congestion. - delirium tremens, when brain is congested.

Chloralum (Pemphigus) - vesicles surrounded by marked capillary hyperaemia.

Cicuta (Cholera) - congestion of blood to the head or chest.

Cicuta (Epilepsy) - concussion of brain, congestion at the base of the brain and in the medulla oblongata, at first the patient is rigid, opisthotonos or emprosthotonos, with fixed, staring eyes, bluish face and frothing at the mouth, followed by shocks passing from head through body.

Cicuta (Headache) - semilateral headache, like pressure as from congestion of blood to the head, with sunken features.

Cicuta - congestions to brain and spinal cord, also to lungs and abdominal viscera.

Cimicifuga (Angina pectoris) - cerebral congestion.

Cimicifuga (Glaucoma) - congestive headaches.

Cimicifuga (Headache) - rush of blood to head, brain feels too large for cranium.

Cimicifuga (Heart diseases) - unconsciousness, cerebral congestion.

Cimicifuga (Ophthalmia) - hyperaemia of conjunctiva, iris, choroid and retina, due to prolonged exertion of myopic or hypermetropic eyes.

Cimicifuga (Tuberculosis of lungs) - intercurrent congestive state from exposure, with dry, harassing cough, diarrhoea, night-sweats.

Cinnabaris - congestion to head; face purple red.

Coccinella - rush of blood to face.

Coccinella (Headache) - redness and heat of cheeks, congestion in face as from hot flashes.

Cocculus (Asthma) - hysteric asthma with rush of blood to chest and difficult breathing as if the throat were constricted.

Cocculus (Ophthalmia) - rheumatic glaucoma, with venous hyperaemia, dilated pupils, insensibility to light, haziness of lens and vitreous humor, severe pain in and around the eyes.

Coccus cacti (Albuminuria) - general lassitude, pulmonary congestions during acute desquamative nephritis, with profuse mucous secretion and suffocative spasmodic cough.

Collinsonia - pelvic and portal congestion, resulting haemorrhoids and constipation, especially in females.

Collinsonia (Constipation) - congestive inertia of the bowels, weight and pressure in rectum, with intense irritation and itching in ano. pelvic congestion.

Collinsonia (Haemorrhage from the lungs, haemoptysis) - bleeding caused by cardiac affections or portal congestion.

Collinsonia (Haemorrhage from uterus) - congested condition of uterus.

Collinsonia (Haemorrhoids) - congestion of pelvic organs and catarrh of bladder, with piles.

Colocynth - neuralgia of the small branches of the infraorbital nerves, in plethoric, choleric, irritable men, from 40 to 50 years of age, and disposed to hemorrhoidal and gouty affections and to congestions towards head; most frequent cause was vexation, but sometimes too close application to business; but once produced, this neuralgia was apt to recur many days successively at same hour, in forenoon.

Conium - such a condition is often found in old age, a time of weakness, languor, local congestions, and sluggishness.

Conium (Chronic catarrh of the head) - heat of face, congestion to head, with catarrhal sensation.

Conium (Ophthalmia) - great dread of light with very little visible inflammation, conjunctiva unnaturally bloodless, and the globe of the eye has a pearly aspect, palpebral conjunctiva alone congested, striated, or studded with granulations.

Conium (Photophobia) - pale redness of the eyeball, with congested vessels of the conjunctiva, suitable to scrofulous subjects.

Conium (Prosopalgia) - heat in face, with congestion to head, lacerating in right half of face, which feels as if excoriated.

Convallaria - pulmonary congestion.

Convallaria (Uterus complaints) - diabetes, with intense itching at introitus and hyperaemia, > by cold water.

Corallium - congestion of face after dinner.

Crocus sat. (Chorea) - congestion to the head with epistaxis of dark and stringy blood.

Crocus sat. (Haemorrhage from uterus) - haemorrhage from overloading of uterine vessels with blood, a passive congestion.

Crocus sat. - boy, aged 10, whose father died suddenly in insane asylum; a febrile condition with congestion to head, followed by cerebral disturbances, after awaking from a sleep. - child sits or stands up in bed making various quick movements without being conscious of what he is doing; this is followed by a short interval of quietness, in which he may regain consciousness, but without any knowledge of what has passed; this remission followed by another attack, and so on; febrile condition with congestion to head; eyes fixed and bright; redness and heat of face; urine pale and scanty; desires neither food nor drink.

Crotalus hor. (Albuminuria) - passive renal congestion, when from embarrassed circulation, as from obstructive heart disease, asthma, chronic bronchitis, etc., especially during its course, or as sequelae of zymotic diseases.

Crotalus hor. (Headache) - congestive headaches, especially on right side (lach., left), with abdominal ailments, bilious vomiting, constipation, < by lying down again after rising.

Crotalus hor. (Hepatic derangements) - pressive hepatic congestion, especially when from heart disease or from imperfect performance of uterine functions, or if a sequel of malarial fever. acute yellow atrophy.

Crotalus hor. - cortical substance of brain, and membranes of brain in a state of engorgement, with dark, fluid, degraded blood; the cortex highly congested and stained a deep brown color; the arachnoid thickened, tough, opaque and adherent to the pia mater, and the meshes of the latter distended with serum; extravasation and ecchymosis.

Cuprum acet. (Meningitis, cerebro-spinalis) - congestion of brain, with convulsive motions of extremities.

Cuprum met. (Amenorrhoea) - rush of blood to the head, with a strange tingling pain in the crown of the head, or pale face with blue margins around the eyes, or burning redness of the face with red eyes.

Cuprum met. (Paralysis) - congestion in chest, palpitation of heart, pulse slow, weak and small.

Curare (Headache) - congestion of blood to the head, with pulsative vibrating pains and loss of consciousness.

Cyclamen (Chlorosis) - periodical congestion to head, with pallor of countenance.

Digitalis - chronic bronchitis; passive congestion of the lungs, giving bloody sputum due to failing myocardium. - Mrs. f., aged 69; heart disease, with extensive congestion to lung. - with drunkards congestion of blood to head and heart.

Digitalis (Aneurism) - passive congestion of lungs, depending on a weakened, dilated heart.

Digitalis (Heart diseases) - suffocative spells with painful constriction of chest as if internal parts of chest were grown together, passive congestion of lungs with cyanosis, must sometimes sit up in order to get breath. pericarditis, pericardial effusion with consequent dropsy.

Digitalis (Meningitis, encephalitis) - amaurotic congestion of retina.

Drosera (Laryngitis and laryngeal phthisis) - local congestion of these parts.

Duboisia - hyperaemia of retina with weakness of accommodation, fundus red, blood-vessels full and tortuous; pupils dilated, with dim vision.

Duboisin (Ophthalmia) - chronic hyperaemia of palpebral conjunctiva.

Dulcamara - congestive headache, with neuralgia and dry nose.

Dulcamara (Paralysis) - paresis and hyperaemia of spinal cord from lying on damp cold ground.

Epiphegus - subinvolution, with painful menstruation and congestion.

Erigeron. - produces active congestion of various organs, with a tendency to hemorrhage therefrom.

Eryngium - renal colic. (Pareira; Calc.) congestion of kidneys with dull pain in back, running down the ureters and limbs.

Eucalyptus - dull congestive headache.

Euonymus - passive congestion and torpor of liver; chronic catarrhal affections of stomach and intestines.

Fagopyrum - cerebral hyperaemia.

Ferr-met. (Headache) - frequent congestive headaches, with pulsating pain in head, usually < after midnight, face fiery red during attack, feet cold. - headache of anaemic, debilitated persons, especially with congestion to head and chest

Ferr-met. (Heart diseases) - anaemia masked behind plethora and congestions, pale color of mucous membranes, with nun's murmur.

Ferr-met. (Mind Symptoms) - anaemia and debility with congestion to head and chest.

Ferr-phos. (Heart diseases) - hyperaemia from relaxation of muscular fibres of blood vessels. - palpitation from congestion with full, quick pulse.

Ferr-phos. (Infantile remittent fever) - hyperaemia of the brain.

Ferr-phos. (Insanity) - transitory mania depending upon hyperaemia of the brain.

Ferr-phos. (Menses complaints) - excessive congestion at monthlies, blood bright-red.

Ferr-phos. (Neuralgia) - congestive neuralgia from chill or cold, with pain as if a nail were being driven in, accompanied by flushed face, burning or diffused heat, feeling of weight and pressure.

Ferr-phos. (Otitis and otorrhoea) - first stage of inflammation or even only hyperaemia of membrana tympani and redness of meatus.

Ferr-phos. (Vertigo, dizziness) - congestion to parts of brain.

Ferrum met. - pseudo-plethora; congestions, etc., yet anemic; face is earthy, flushing easily. - hammering, pulsating, congestive headache; pain extends to teeth, with cold extremities.

Ferrum phos. - hyperaemia of optic disc and retina, with blurred vision.

Ferrum phos. - In pale, anaemic subjects, with violent local congestions. congestions of lungs.

Ferrum pyrophosph. - congestion of brain and headache following great loss of blood; tarsal cysts.

Ferrum sulph. (watery and painless stools; menorrhagia pressing, throbbing between periods with rush of blood to head. basedow's disease. erethism. pain in gall-bladder; toothache; acidity; eructation of food in mouthfuls).

Fluoric acid. (Hepatic derangements) - ascites from hepatic induration and portal congestion.

Franciscea (Pericarditis) - (e. m. hale). - intense headache, like a band around the head, with symptoms of cerebral congestion.

Gambogia. - congestion to head, lungs and female sexual organs.

Gelsemium (Apoplexy) - intense passive congestion to the head with nervous exhaustion.

Gelsemium (Back pain–spinal irritation) - spinal congestion.

Gelsemium (Glaucoma) - choroidal and venous congestions, either with or without serous effusion. amaurotic symptoms, with dilatation of pupils, disturbed accommodation, pain in eyes, with or without lachrymation.

Gelsemium (Headache) - passive congestion in the brain. - sensation as if a band were tied around forehead (passive arterial congestion).

Gelsemium (Hepatic derangements) - passive congestion of liver, bilious diarrhoea and relaxed gall-ducts.

Gelsemium (Jaundice) - passive congestion of liver, bilious diarrhoeas and relaxed gall-ducts.

Gelsemium (Measles) - abdominal and thoracic congestion.

Gelsemium (Meningitis, cerebro-spinalis) - at the very onset of the disease, severe chill followed by congestion of the brain and spinal cord, livid cheeks, dilated pupils, little or no thirst. perfect loss of strength and great exhaustion, staggering gait, dullness of speech, icy coldness of hands and feet, pulse very weak or hardly perceptible.

Gelsemium (Meningitis, encephalitis) - intense and overwhelming congestion of the brain in children, during dentition.

Gelsemium (Menses complaints) - delayed and painful, suppressed. before: congestion to head and face. - vomiting, with bearing-down pains in abdomen. during: neuralgic and congestive dysmenorrhoea, with sharp, labor-like pains in uterus alternating with other neuralgic pains.

Gelsemium (Neurasthenia) - congestion of spine, muscles feel bruised and will not obey the will.

Gelsemium (Uterus complaints) - neuralgic and congestive dysmenorrhoea, with frontal headache and dim vision.

Gelsemium (Vision complaints) - after apoplexy, congestion of the head.

Gelsemium. - active or passive congestion of brain, spinal cord, lungs, liver and other organs. - congestions, arterial or venous, with sluggish circulation. - in scarlet fever it determines the eruption to the surface, controls the pulse, calms the nervous erethism, and lessens the cerebral congestion. - Miss?—, aged 19, had two years ago severe attack of congestive intermittent fever, quotidian type; facial neuralgia.

Glonoine - any exertion brings on rush of blood to heart and fainting spells. - rush of blood in pregnant women.

Glonoine (Albuminuria) - brain feels too large, congested.

Glonoine (Amenorrhoea) - amenorrhoea with great congestion in head, < by shaking head.

Glonoine (Epilepsy) - alternate congestion of heart and head.

Glonoine (Epilepsy) - convulsions from cerebral congestion.

Glonoine (Headache) - bad sequelae of cutting hair. Intense congestion of the brain in plethoric constitutions, with persistent sensation of pulsation, from sudden suppression of menses, after anxiety and worry with sleeplessness. - congestive headache, sensation of fluttering in head, of constriction in vessels of head, expansive pressure, flushed face, drowsiness, venous congestion to abdomen.

Glonoine (Heart diseases) - alternate congestion to heart and head.

Glonoine (Insanity) - congestion alternately to head and heart.

Glonoine (Labor) - congestive form.

Glonoine (Meningitis, cerebro-spinalis) - congestion of chest, with labored action of heart.

Glonoine (Meningitis, cerebro-spinalis) - violent congestion of head, with sense of expansion.

Glonoine (Ophthalmia) - venous hyperaemia or congestion of retina and optic nerve.

Glonoine (Prosopalgia) - cold sweat on face during congestion to head.

Graphites - rush of blood to with flushed face also with nose bleed and distension and flatulence.

Graphites (Chlorosis) - tendency to rush of blood to head with flushing of face, following a sudden shock about heart.

Graphites (Distension of abdomen and flatulence) - abdomen distended with flatus and rush of blood to head.

Graphites (Headache) - pain as if head were numb and pithy, as if constricted, especially in occiput, extending to nape of neck, with pains on looking up as if neck were broken. during amenorrhoea frequent congestion to head and chest, dark-red cheeks, oppression and anguish when lying down.

Graphites (Leucorrhoea) - induration and congestion of cervix.

Graphites (Neurasthenia) - rush of blood to chest and head, but not from true plethora.

Gratiola - rush of blood with vanishing of sight.

Gratiola (Nymphomania) - irritable condition of sexual organs with congestions.

Grindelia - there is practically no difference in their action, although the g. squarrosa is credited with more splenic symptoms, dull pains and fullness in left hypochondrium; chronic malaria; gastric pains associated with splenic congestion.

Hamamelis - middle-aged man, with congested liver; bleeding piles. passive congestion, or venous stagnation of skin and mucous membranes. - purpura hemorrhagica with epistaxis and congestion of conjunctiva. - venous congestion, hemorrhoids, conjunctival vascularity, ciliary neuralgia, photophobia, lachrymation. - venous congestions; hemorrhages. - ovarian congestion and neuralgia; feel very sore. - venous congestion, haemorrhages, varicose veins, and haemorrhoids, with bruised soreness of affected parts, seem to be the special sphere of this remedy.

Hamamelis (Cornea, diseases of) - keratitis dependent upon a blow or burn, especially when complicated with haemmorrhage into anterior chamber (hyperaemia).

Hamamelis (Glaucoma) - venous congestion, haemorrhoids, conjunctival vascularity, ciliary neuralgia, photophobia, lachrymation.

Hamamelis (Haematuria, haemorrhage from urinary organs) haemorrhoids of bladder, passive congestions.

Hamamelis (Haemorrhage from uterus) - haemorrhage from portal congestion.

Hamamelis (Ovaries, diseases of) - congestion, inflammation and neuralgia of ovaries, with cutting, tearing pains in swollen and tender ovary, < at menses, with retention of urine.

Hedeoma - leucorrhoea, with itching and burning ovaries congested and painful; bearing-down spasmodic contractions.

Helianthus - vomiting, black stools, congestion and dryness of mouth and pharynx, redness and heat of skin.

Helleborus (Albuminuria) - congestion of kidneys with extensive effusion of serum in abdominal cavity and tissue of lower extremities.

Helleborus (Nephritis) - congestion of kidneys with extensive effusion of serum in abdominal cavity and tissues of lower extremities.

Helonias - it seems as if the monthly congestion, instead of venting itself as it should through the uterine vessels, had extended to the kidneys. - the menses are often suppressed and the kidneys congested.

Helonias (Amenorrhoea) - suppression of menses when the kidneys are congested, urine scanty and turbid.

Helonias (Leucorrhoea) - old chronic cases without congestion.

Hepar sulph. (Haemorrhoids) - great want of vital power of expulsion from the congested condition of the veins in rectum.

Hepar sulph. (Menses complaints) - uterus enlarged and anteverted, with congestion of ovaries.

Hepar sulph. (Pharyngitis) - chronic venous congestion of pharyngolaryngeal mucous membrane.

Hydrastis (Haemorrhage from uterus) - metrorrhagia and menorrhagia from deficient contraction of bloodvessels, uterus enlarged, relaxed and congested.

Hydrastis (Ophthalmia) - mucous membrane of eyelids much congested.

Hydrastis (Prolapsus of rectum) - simple prolapsus in children, with congestion and swelling of the mucous membrane and marked constipation.

Hydrastis (Scrofulosis) - constipation from weakened and congestive state of the lower bowel.

Hydrocyanic acid. - acts upon cerebral veins, producing congestion; secondarily upon heart, nerves, etc. - marked cyanosis; venously congested lung.

Hyoscyamus (Haemorrhages) - constant flow of bright-red blood, with bluish face, congested eyes, twitching of muscles.

Hyoscyamus (Headache) - unconsciousness from congestion of blood to the head, with delirium, answers all questions properly.

Hyoscyamus (Insanity) - epileptoid spasms, rush of blood to head with sparkling eyes and fixed look.

Hyoscyamus (Mania) - very little rush of blood to head Hyoscyamus (Mind Symptoms) - nervous irritability without hyperaemia.

Hyoscyamus (Scarlatina) - great nervous excitability, without much cerebral hyperaemia.

Hypericum - congestion to head, lungs or heart. - local congestions; nervous erethism, with or without hemorrhage; great nervous depression following wounds.

Ignatia - after catamenia, which came at night time, symptoms of insanity; believes herself married and pregnant; is tormented by remorse for imagined crimes; seeks constantly to escape to drown herself; terrible anxiety from rush of blood to head and heart; is only quiet when lying undisturbed and brooding over her troubles, which she rehearses in a doleful tone; if disturbed, screams, strikes and tears things, crying all the while "I am neglecting my duty, breaking my vow;" face pale and distorted; desire for sour things; difficulty to get her to eat; conscientious scruples after eating; menses suppressed. - congestive headaches following anger or grief; worse, smoking or smelling tobacco, inclines forward.

Ignatia (Menses complaints) - dysmenorrhoea from irritation of nervous system, and not from uterine congestion.

Ignatia (Ophthalmia) - the eyes are more painful than congested, with sensation as of sand in eyes.

Indigo. - congestive condition of head and lungs, with palpitation of heart.

Iodum - throbbing; rush of blood, and feeling of a tight band.

Iodum (Apoplexy) - chronic congestion to brain from hypertrophy of right ventricle or from compression of blood-vessels around the neck from a struma.

Iodum (Dyspepsia, weakness of stomach) - large, full pulse and cerebral congestions.

Iodum (Haemorrhage from uterus) - chronic menorrhagia in thin, delicate women subject to corrosive leucorrhoea, with other indications of congested uterus and ovaries.

Iodum (Leucorrhoea) - corrosive discharge in thin, delicate women, between menses, who suffer from chronic congestion or inflammation of uterus and ovaries (right side).

Iodum (Ovaries, diseases of) - chronic congestion, usually with leucorrhoea.

Iodum (Tuberculosis of lungs) - suitable to young persons who grow too rapidly and subject to frequent congestions to the chest, with dry cough excited by tickling all over chest, < in warm room, with expectoration of stringy, transparent mucus, sometimes streaked with blood.

Iodum (Uraemia) - chronic congestive headache in old people.

Ipecac (Sore throat) - congestion of blood to head, with pale face.

Iridum - compare: iridium chloride. (produces salivation and stiffness of jaws followed by and nervous symptoms. Congestion of nares and bronchi. Dragging pain in lower back. Headache worse right side, heavy feeling as of liquid lead).

Jonosia asoka - unilateral headache; reflex uterine, congestive headache, better open air and by free flow.

Juniperus communis - compare : sabina; juniperus virginianus red cedar (violent tenesmus vesical. Persistent dragging in back; hyperaemia of the kidneys; pyelitis and cystitis; dropsy of the aged with suppressed urine. Dysuria, burning, cutting pain in urethra when urinating. Constant urging apoplexy, convulsions, strangury, uterine haemorrhage). - renal hyperaemia. (eucalyptol.)

Kali-bich. - congestion of kidneys; nephritis, with scanty, albuminous urine and casts.

Kali-bich. (Bronchitis chronica) - bronchitis oscillating between acute and torpid inveterate bronchitis, with a certain degree of irritation, vascular congestion and moderate mucopurulent secretion, frequently accompanied by periosteal or rheumatic pains. cough resonant, whistling, with nausea and expectoration of thick mucus.

Kali-bich. (Hoarseness) - subacute and chronic inflammatory processes in larynx or bronchial tubes, with congestion and swelling of the tubes, and increased secretion of a glutinous mucus which veils and alters the voice.

Kali-bich. (Laryngitis and laryngeal phthisis) - iod., scrofulous, with congestion, swelling of the tissues and increased secretion of a glutinous fluid, < mornings, when the tough mucus nearly strangles him.

Kali-bich. (Pharyngitis) - chronic congestion of fauces and pharyngeal mucous membrane, follicles looking like little tubercles on pharyngeal wall.

Kali-bich. (Sore throat) - chronic congestion of fauces and pharyngeal mucous membrane.

Kali-brom. - congestion of uvula and fauces.

Kali-carb. (Headache) - congestion to head with throbbing and humming.

Kali-iod. - irritable; congestion to head, heat and throbbing.

Kali-mur. (Albuminuria) - alternate states of sadness and cheerfulness with congestion, > by nosebleed.

Kali-mur. (Albuminuria) - congestion to heart, slow pulse, twitching of face.

Kali-mur. (Albuminuria) - congestive vertigo, < after violent exercise. portal congestion and enlarged liver.

Kali-mur. (Dyspepsia, weakness of stomach) - portal congestion.

Kali-mur. (Insanity) - intoxication from the smallest quantity of wine or beer, causing congestion, > from nosebleed.

Kali-mur. (Uterus complaints) - chronic congestion of uterus.

Kali-nit. - acute exacerbations in phthisis; congestion of lungs.

Kali-sil. - congested, blood surges from body to head.

Kali-iod (Ovaries, diseases of) - severe burning, tearing and twitching pains in the ovarian region, especially right side. Sensation of congestion and swelling of the ovaries, with pain as from a corrosive tumor there. Affections connected with syphilis.

Kali-mur. - alternate states of sadness and cheerfulness, associated with congestion, > from nosebleed. - congestions; in second stage, interstitial exudation; causes swelling or enlargement of parts, white coated tongue or white sputa. - disturbed action of vasomotor nerves, congestions, with tension, or coldness.

Kalmia (Headache) - neuralgic paroxysmal pains, especially right side (glon., congestive, steady pain), > by profuse micturition.

Koch's lymph (acute and chronic parenchymatous nephritis; produces pneumonia, broncho-pneumonia, and congestion of the lungs in tuberculous patients, and is a remarkably efficacious remedy in lobular pneumonia-broncho-pneumonia); avian-tuberculin from birds-(acts on the apices of the lungs; has proved an excellent remedy in influenzal bronchitis; symptoms similar to tuberculosis; relieves the debility, diminishes the cough, improves the appetite, and braces up the whole organism; acute broncho-pulmonary diseases of children; itching of palms and ears; cough, acute, inflammatory, irritating, incessant, and tickling; loss of strength and appetite); hydrast. (to fatten patients after tuberc.).

Lac-can. (Menses complaints) - congestion of ovaries. During: great distress in pelvic region, with sensation as if abdomen would burst, slightly > from leaning back.

Lac-can. (Ovaries, diseases of) - heat in the ovarian and uterine region (with menses). inflammatory and congestive condition of the ovaries before menses, especially of the right ovary, with extreme soreness and sensitiveness, which makes every motion and position, even breath, painful.

Lac-can. (Uterus complaints) - congested condition of uterus, with extreme soreness and tenderness, making every motion, position, even breathing painful.

Lachesis (Apoplexy) - the paroxysms are preceded by frequent absence of mind, or vertigo with rush of blood to the head.

Lachesis (Leucorrhoea) - uterine congestion with prolapsus uteri.

Lachesis - woman, aged 48, 18 months after climaxis, catamenia had been copious, very dark, had been subject to congestion towards head and chest; swelling of right ovary.

Lactic-acid. (Diarrhoea of infants) - stools undigested, curdy, watery, mixed with bright grass-green mucus, great jerking of muscles, rush of blood to head and face.

Ledum (Haemorrhage from the lungs, haemoptysis) - congestion to chest and head.

Ledum (Heels, pains in) - soles painful when walking, as if congested with blood.

Leptandra - chronic congestion and other chronic disorders of liver.

Lilium tig. (Heart diseases) - frequent sensation as if the heart stopped, followed by rush of blood to heart, violent palpitations and sharp pain going from left nipple through chest to back, > by lying on left side and in open air.

Lilium tig. (Urinary difficulties) - if desire is not attended to, feeling of congestion to chest.

Lilium tig. - heart feels full to bursting, from congestion; much fluttering; reflex heart symptoms. - ceases when resting.

(Sep.; Lac. c.; Bell.) congestion of uterus, prolapse, and anteversion.

Lilium tigrinum (Cystitis, inflammation of bladder) - continuous pressure on bladder and, if not complied with, congested sensation in chest.

Limulus - difficult to remember names, confused with heat of face, rush of blood to face, worse when meditating.

Lithium carb. - lithium bromatum (cerebral congestion, threatened apoplexy, insomnia and epilepsy).

Lonicera - congestion of and chest; coma.

Lycopersicum - always shows signs of acute congestion.

Lycopodium (Bronchitis chronica) - congestion of liver, flatulency, constipation, cachectic complexion, red gravel, acid dyspepsia.

Lycopodium (Coffee and its therapeutics) - coffee makes him sick and brings on aversion to it, a symptom often found in portal congestion and hepatic disorders.

Lycopodium (Rheumatism) - chronic forms, especially of old people, with painful rigidity of muscles and joints, and feeling of numbness in affected parts, forgetfulness, vertigo, congestion to head, sour belching, early nausea, flatulence, oppression of chest, palpitation, etc.

Lycopodium. - distrustful, suspicious and fault finding. — dyspepsia. –chronic hepatic congestion. —excess of lithic gravel.

Lycopus - lessens tonicity of bloodvessels, with consequent congestions; heart muscle weakened.

Mag-carb. (Headache) - congestion of blood to head, especially when smoking.

Mag-mur. (Bronchitis acuta) - congestion of blood to the chest from bathing in the sea, causing spasmodic cough and bloody expectoration, < at night, with tension and constriction of chest.

Mag-mur. (Headache) - congestive and hysterical headaches, with sensation as if boiling water in cranium, pains in temples, > by firm pressure with the hands and from wrapping the head up warmly.

Mag-mur. (Hysteria) - congestive headaches with sensation as if boiling water in cranium, especially about temples, > by pressure and by wrapping up the head warmly (Sil.).

Mag-mur. (Menses complaints) - congestion of blood to head, with painful undulation and whizzing as of boiling water on side on which she rests.

Magnesia-mur. - woman, aged 58, had been subject to repeated attacks of biliousness and disturbance of functions of liver for several years, attended with dyspepsia and constipation; enlargement and congestion of liver. - women after suffering months or years from attacks of indigestion or biliousness; enlargement and congestion of liver.

Manganum acet. - feels large and heavy, with rush of blood; pain from above downward.

Melilotus - compare : melilotus alba-(white clover) practically the same action. (haemorrhages, congestive headaches, engorged blood vessels, spasms.) - congestions and haemorrhages seem to be the special manifestations of this drug. - violent congestive and nervous headaches. - congestion relieved by hemorrhage. Congestive or nervous headaches; engorgements of blood vessels in any part or organ; spasms, infantile, eclampsia and epilepsy; insanity, to relieve brain from pressure and irritation. - man, aged 20, lymphatic temperament; congestive headaches.

Melilotus (Dentition, morbid) - highly congested.

Melilotus (Headache) - congestive headaches with violent palpitations and prolapsus uteri. violent congestive headache with sensation as if brain would burst through forehead (Glon.), driving the patient almost frantic.

Melilotus (Headache) - face highly congested, almost livid.

Melilotus (Neuralgia) - violent congestion of head, profuse and frequent epistaxis.

Mentha pip. - asthmatic breathing, with congestive headache.

Mephitis - awakes at night with rush of blood to lower legs.

Merc-sol. (Amenorrhoea) - rush of blood to the head.

Merc-sol. (Hepatic derangements) - rush of blood to head.

Merc-sol. (Jaundice) - jaundice with violent rush of blood to head, bad taste, tongue moist and furred, yellow.

Merc-sol. (Menses complaints) - dry heat and rush of blood to head. During: anxiety, red tongue with dark spots, salty taste, scorbutic gums, teeth feel sharp.

Mercurius cor. - frontal pain, congestion of with burning in cheeks.

Mercurius sol. - mercur. acet. (congestion with stiffness, dryness and heat of parts affected. Inflamed, burn and itch. lack of moisture. Dry, talking difficult. Pressure in lower sternum; chancre in urethra; tenia capitis favosa margin of ulcers painful).

Mezereum - compare : dirca palustris-leather wood (a gastrointestinal irritant inducing salivation, emesis and purgation; cerebral hyperaemia; neuralgic pains, with depression, palpitation, and dyspnoea).

Millefolium - coffee causes congestion to head. - congestions.

Mitchella - bladder symptoms accompany complaints, especially uterine congestion.

Moschus (Hysteria) - rush of blood to head, with staring eyes.

Moschus (Vertigo, dizziness) - congestion of blood to the head. Vertigo, with violent rush of blood to the head, relieved in the open air.

Murex - woman, aged 30, sanguine lymphatic temperament, mother of two children, was subject in infancy to violent attacks of cough, caused by congestion to lungs, the result of a psoric taint (retrocession of itch), these attacks ceased to appear about the time of her first pregnancy, since when he has been suffering; uterine affection.

Muriatic-acid. (Scarlatina) - rush of blood to head, with bright-red face and great drowsiness.

Natrum ars. (Coryza) - burning of eyes and congestion of conjunctiva.

Natrum carb. (Chronic catarrh of the head) - violent sneezing with rush of blood to the head.

Natrum carb. (Sexual complaints) - passive congestion.

Natrum hypochlor. - in congested and atonic states of the uterus and its ligaments, with hepatic disorders.

Natrum mur. (Tuberculosis of lungs) - congestion to head, with hectic flush and general malaise after least exertion.

Natrum mur. - chronic headache, semi-lateral, congestive, from sunrise to sunset, with pale face, nausea, vomiting; periodical; from eye-strain; menstrual. - coldness of legs with congestion to head, chest, and stomach.

Natrum sulph. (Hepatic derangements) - congestion of liver with soreness and sharp, sticking pains.

Natrum sulph. [Migraine (headache)] - congestion of blood to head, with fulness.

Nux vomica (Asthma) - rush of blood to the chest, with orgasm of the blood, heat, warmth and palpitation.

Nux vomica (Fainting) - and generally when nausea, pale face, scintillations before the eyes or obscuration of sight, pains in the stomach, anguish, trembling, and congestion of blood to the head or chest are present.

Nux vomica (Gastralgia) - neurotic and congestive gastralgia.

Nux vomica (Haematemesis, gastrorrhagia) - portal congestion, dyspepsia.

Nux vomica (Headache) - congestive and abdominal headaches, with nausea and vomiting, worse by coughing and stooping.

Nux vomica (Leucaemia) - congestion to head, and red, bloated face.

Nux vomica (Menses complaints) - congestive headache with vertigo.

Nux vomica (Vertigo, dizziness) - congestion of blood, with heat and redness of the face, also with violent pains in the forehead, with vertigo and fainting.

Nux mos. - Mrs. c., aged 35, subject to hemorrhage from rectum, cured a year ago by sulph.; pregnant, four months; pelvic congestion.

Nux vom. - Nux patients are easily chilled, avoid open air, etc. congestive headache, associated with haemorrhoids. - boy, aged 11, sanguine temperament; congestion of liver. - congestion of blood to head, chest or abdomen. - is sullen and obstinate; would not eat nor speak; eyes large, congested; urine high colored, with mealy sediment. —mania. - man, aged 48, secretary to countess st. — choleric temperament, often troubled with congestion to head and disorders of digestive organs, younger brother died in asylum; insanity. - miss?— aged 48, nervous temperament, suffering six years, after disappearance of congestive headaches; morning diarrhoea. - woman, small stature, frequently suffering from congestions, flushes of heat and epistaxis, for last fourteen days has had a pressure in scrobiculum; hematemesis.

Oleum jec. - gadus morrhua cod - (frequent breathing, with flapping of alae nasi; rush of blood to chest; pain in lungs and cough; dry heat in palms.).

Onosmodium - vision blurred; optic disc hyperaemic, and retinal vessels enlarged.

Opium - serous apoplexy-venous, passive congestion. - venous congestion, with dark red surface.

Opium (Amenorrhoea) - suppression, with congestion of blood to the head, which feels heavy.

Opium (Asthma) - congestion of blood to the chest, or pulmonary spasms, with deep, stertorous, rattling breathing.

Opium (Constipation) - beating and sensation of heaviness in abdomen, rush of blood to head, sleepiness, bed feels hot, hot sweat. Constipation in connection with ovaritis or ovaralgia.

Opium (Delirium) - venous congestion with dark-red face.

Opium (Diabetes) - face bloated, congested or sunken and pale.

Opium (Emotions, ill effects of-fear, dread, fright) - immediate effect of fright, stupefied, with internal heat, rush of blood to head, dim sight with twitches and starting.

Opium (Haemorrhage from the lungs, haemoptysis) - rush of blood to chest.

Opium (Headache) - somnolence after meals from passive cerebral congestion.

Opium (Meningitis basilaris) - congested face.

Opium (Meningitis, cerebro-spinalis) - stupefaction, with or without pain, delirium, mania, heaviness, with great congestion to head, occiput feels as heavy as lead, the head falling back constantly.

Opium (Otitis and otorrhoea) - haemotorrhoea, congestion of ears

Oxalic-acid. - woman, aged 50; congestion of left lung; later pneumonia.

Oxytropis - congestion of spine and paralysis.

Paeonia - rush of blood to and face.

Pareira - compare : parietaria (renal calculi; nightmare, patient dreaming of being buried alive); chimaphila (chronic catarrhal congestion following cystitis; acute prostatitis; feeling of a ball in perineum when sitting); fabiana, see pichi (dysuria; post-gonorrhoeal complications; gravel; vesical catarrh); uva.; hydrang.; berber.; ocim.; hedeom.

Petroleum - congestions; hemorrhages, blood light red, from internal organs.

Phellandrium (Headache) - crushing feeling on top of head, with aching and burning in temples and above the eyes, which are congested.

Phosphoric acid. (homesickness, nostalgia) - chronic congestions to the head.

Phosphoric acid, (Tuberculosis of lungs) - tickling cough, seemingly from pit of stomach, with burning in chest and passive congestion, followed by great weakness in chest and dyspnoea, < from least exposure.

Phosphorus (Albuminuria) - congestion of the right heart, and hence venous congestion of kidneys.

Phosphorus (Dyspepsia, weakness of stomach) - congestion to head.

Phosphorus (Headache) - in washer-women fear of washing, as it causes rush of blood to head, red face and eyes, heat in head.

Phosphorus (Heart diseases) - nervous palpitations, especially of old maids, from emotions, as from the sudden entrance into the room of an unexpected visitor, welcome or unwelcome, from motion, from rush of blood to the chest. Vertigo, with tendency to fall to the left side.

Phosphorus (Hepatic derangements) - hyperaemia, at first enlargement, fatty degeneration and finally atrophy of the liver with jaundice and dropsy.

Phosphorus (Meningitis, cerebro-spinalis) - congestion to head.

Phosphorus (Prosopalgia) - pains from forehead into eyes (right) and from vertex and temples down upon zygoma, with bloatedness of face, congestion to head, vertigo and ringing of ears, < from talking, stooping or external pressure, > while eating, lying down, after sleeping, from heat. Neuralgia accompanied by much nervous waste, especially in nervous and nervo-sanguineous temperaments.

Phosphorus (Vision complaints) - retinal hyperaemia.

Phosphorus - ebullitions and congestions. - man, aged 24, tall, strong, florid complexion, subject to congestions of head and chest, had pneumonia and an inflammatory affection of heart, since then suffering; heart disease. - man, very stout, plethoric, worker in a brewery, suffering three months; hepatic congestion. - Mrs. M., aged 30, has a permanent hard protuberance on left side of head, also one on metacarpal bone of left hand and one on right foot; congestion of blood to head.

Physostigma - congestion of eyes. - uncommon mental activity. During climacteric change, after severe mental suffering (lost three children), palpitation of heart; beats irregular; some three months ago, at time for return of menstruation, was suddenly taken with a feeling of partial faintness, loss of memory, face very red, eyes congested, violent pain all over and through head, constant disposition to talk, which made her cough, feeling as if stomach were full, even up to pit of throat, belching of wind; sensation of heart beating hard and furiously, yet its motion could hardly be discovered, and in a few moments a violent tonic spasm, lasting nearly an hour; every muscle in body rigid, no loss of consciousness; when passing off roaring in ears, great dyspnoea and excessive soreness of muscles of whole body.

Physostigma (Calabar) (Myelitis acuta, inflammation of the spinal cord) -congestion of spinal cord, with tetanic spasms - congestive state of paralysis of the spinal cord.

Picric-acid. (Diabetes) - cortex of brain congested.

Picric-acid. (Paralysis) - during first stage intense occipital headache after severe mental effort, congestion of spine with tonic and clonic spasms, keeps his legs wide apart when standing, looks steadily at objects as if unable to make them out, followed by paresis. Brain-fag, limbs become too weak to support the body. Will-power as if suspended.

Piper-meth. (Back pain–spinal irritation) - congestion of posterior part of brain and spinal cord, with feeling as though he must move or head and neck would be compressed.

Piper-meth. (Sleeplessness) - occipital congestion, sore inside and tender outside.

Podophyl. (Hepatic derangements) - fullness in right hypochondrium, hyperaemia of the liver, with flatulence, pain and soreness.

Podophyl. (Jaundice) - jaundice from torpor of liver, from gall-stones, from hyperaemia of liver with fullness, soreness and pain in hepatic region, > by rubbing and stroking hypochondrium with hands.

Podophyl. (Leucorrhoea) - congestion of portal system.

Podophyllum - hepatic and intestinal congestion.

Polyporus pinicola - great lassitude, congestion of head, with vertigo, face hot and flushed, prickling sensation all over; restless at night from pain in wrists and knee; rheumatic pains; profuse perspiration.

Primula veris. - cerebral congestion, with neuralgia; migraine; rheumatic and gouty pains.

Psorinum (Apoplexy) - congestion of blood to the head with heat

Psorinum (Headache) - congestion of blood to the head, with red, hot cheeks and nose, with great anxiety every afternoon after dinner (during pregnancy).

Psorinum (Vertigo, dizziness) - congestions of blood to the head, with red, hot cheeks and nose, redness of the eruption on the face, with great anxiety, every afternoon after dinner.

Ptelea - mucous membranes are congested and irritated, with sense of roughness, smarting or prickling; causes congestion of liver, stomach and bowels and secondarily of lungs; is indicated briefly when there are irritability, and dull, confused frontal headache; bitter taste, eructations like rotten eggs or bitter; swollen liver, relief from lying on right side, bilious stools; languor; muscular soreness.

Ptelea (Hepatic derangements) - jaundice, with hyperaemia of the liver.

Pulsatilla - congestion to single parts. - sleepless nights on account of great fear and anxious restlessness; despairs of her salvation and seeks aid in constant prayer; irregular catamenia; heat and congestion to head and face; headache, precordial weight and backache.

Ricinus - vertigo, occipital pain, congestive symptoms, buzzing in ears.

Sabadilla - intermit (Kreos.; Puls.) (due to transient and localized congestion of womb alternating with chronic anaemic state).

Sabina - compare : sanguisorba (venous congestion and passive haemorrhages; varices of lower extremities; dysentery. Long lasting profuse menses with congestion to and limbs in sensitive, irritable patients. Climacteric haemorrhages).

sanguisuga. - rush of blood to head and face.

Salicylic acid. (Vertigo, dizziness) - rush of blood to head, excited mood.

Salix nigra - ovarian congestion and neuralgia.

Sanguinaria can. (Apoplexy) - sanguineous apoplexy from venous congestion. Pain like a flash of lightning on the back of the head.

Sanguinaria can. (Headache) - rush of blood with dizziness in head, she feels as if she would fall when she attempts to rise from a sitting position, with nausea and vomiting.

Sanguinaria can. (Ophthalmia) - retinal congestion, with flushed face and congestive headache.

Sanguinaria can. - chronic rhinitis; membrane dry and congested.

Sanguisorba officinals - a member of the rosaceae family, (profuse, long-lasting menses, especially in nervous patients with congestive symptoms to limbs. Passive hemorrhages at climacteric. Chronic metritis. hemorrhage from lungs. Varices and ulcers).

Saponaria - congestions to head; tired feeling in nape.

Sarracenia - congestion to head, with irregular heart action.

Secale - passive, congestive pain (rises from back of head), with pale face.

Secale (Leucorrhoea) - leucorrhoea, brownish, offensive, like cream, from weakness and venous congestion.

Senecio - backaches of congested kidneys.

Senega - old asthmatics with congestive attacks.

Sepia - acts especially on the portal system, with venous congestion. Venous congestion of the fundus.

Sepia (Amenorrhoea) - in some, tendency to cough, to congestion and pain in the apex of one or both lungs.

Sepia (Amenorrhoea) - pain in loins from uterine and other abdominal congestion.

Sepia (Anaemia) - pelvic congestion.

Sepia (Cancer) - indurations, ulcerations and congestion of the os and cervix uteri.

Sepia (Constipation) - constipation of females, with pain and pressure in iliac regions, from uterine or abdominal congestion.

Sepia (Cough) - coughs from passive congestions and obstructions in the portal systems.

Sepia (Gastritis) - congestion and heat of the head.

Sepia (Haemorrhage from uterus) - chronic congestion of uterus with sense of weight as if all would come out of the vulva.

Sepia (Heart diseases) - congestion of blood to chest with violent palpitation, an occasional hard thump of the heart, sensation of a ball in inner parts.

Sepia (Ovaries, diseases of) - congestion, stinging pains in ovarian region running around from the back over each hip, bearing-down pains from uterus.

Sepia (Prosopalgia) - intermittent faceache, with congestion of the eyes and head.

Sepia (Uterus complaints) - venous passive congestion, chronic metritis, displacements, especially retroversion.

Sepia (Uterus, subinvolution after childbirth) - venous congestion of uterus, stitching pains felt mostly in neck of uterus or extending to abdominal cavity.

Silicea - children or young people suffering during growth with fever, violent pains in joints, swelling of limbs and congestions.

Silicea (Migraine) - rush of blood to head, great sensitiveness of hair, falling out of hair, perspiration on head, pains running from neck up into head, paroxysms end with profuse urination.

Solanum nig. - congestive headache.

Solidago - backache of congested kidneys. (Senec-aur.)

Spiranthes - is an anti-phlogistic remedy akin to Acon. Its symptoms showing congestion and inflammation.

Spongia (Headache) - congestive headaches from dry cold weather, after intoxication.

Spongia (Heart diseases) - rapid, hard breathing. Rheumatic pericarditis, after effusion took place (Acon. during stage of hyperaemia).

Spongia (Meningitis basilaris) - congestion of blood to head with pressing, knocking and pulsating pains in forehead.

Spongia (Tuberculosis of lungs) - tuberculosis pulmonum, first stage, with hard, ringing cough, rush of blood to chest, palpitations and sudden weakness while walking.

Spongia tosta - rush of blood; bursting headache; worse, forehead.

Staphisagria. - for sixteen years attacks of mental disturbance, every four years, beginning on the 4th of January, always lasting two months; great restlessness, would go about house in search of something, not knowing what, but if attracted by any object, would put it in his pocket if possible, and, if not, would hide it in his coat; excessive loquaciousness;

inability to read, on account of letters running together; firmly believed he would lose his fortune, constantly told his wife to be careful that they did not starve; thinks his wife will run away from him; sleep greatly disturbed, lies down a few moments, and suddenly jumps from bed to middle of room, stands there about a minute, scratches his head, and looks about as if a new idea had struck him; constant chilliness, sits by fire for hours without getting warm, amuses himself by throwing into the fire any article near at hand, regardless of value; at times more violent, strikes at any one coming near him, although he is conscious something is the matter with him, and tells his wife he will try not to kill any one; great thirst; canine hunger, eats anything set before him, complete loss of taste; general appearance is marked by extreme nervous excitement; face wears an anxious expression; shuffling gait; hands tremble, cannot retain anything in their grasp, not even long enough to drink water without spilling it; all symptoms < about midnight; in intervals between attacks, feeling of pressure over nape of neck; at times this disappears, and is followed by a throbbing sensation, and a rush of blood to crown of head; vertigo, especially when walking in open air; from slightest gust of wind legs feel as if they were going out from under him, and that he will fall backward.

Stellaria media - induces a condition of stasis, congestion, and sluggishness of all functions.

Stramonium - rush of blood to head; staggers with tendency to fall forward and to the left. Rush of blood to head, with furious loquacious delirium.

Stramonium (Diaphragm, diseases of) - mixture of hyperaemia and spasm, of affection of spinal cord and of diaphragm.

Strontium (Apoplexy) - violent congestion to head, with hot and red face from every exertion, as walking, smothered feeling about heart, allowing no rest.

Strophanthus - lungs congested. Menorrhagia; uterine haemorrhage; uterus heavily congested.

Sulfonalum - congestion of lungs; stertorous breathing.

Sulphur (Back pain–spinal irritation) - spinal congestion from suppression of menses or haemorrhoidal flow.

Sulphur (Chronic catarrh of the head) - portal congestions (Sep.) sense of congestion in nose in open air.

Sulphur (Haematemesis, gastrorrhagia) - portal congestion with engorged liver.

Sulphur (Haemorrhoids) - suppressed haemorrhoids, with colic, palpitation, congestion of lungs.

Sulphur (Hearing, defective) - rush of blood to head.

Sulphur (Myelitis acuta, inflammation of the spinal cord) - congestion of lumbar spine, followed by retention of urine and paraplegia.

Sulphur (Neurasthenia) - paraplegia from spinal congestion.

Sulphur (Ophthalmia) - hypopion, cataract, chorioiditis and chorioretinitis, if accompanied by darting pains and where the disease is based upon abdominal venosity, stagnation in portal circulation, habitual constipation, cerebral congestion, or upon metastasis of chronic or suppressed skin diseases.

Sulphur (Pharyngitis) - venous congestion, piles, constipation.

Sulphur (Tuberculosis of lungs) - congestion towards head and chest, with palpitations of heart.

Sulphur (Vision complaints) - retinitis caused by overuse of eyes, congestion of optic nerve.

Sulphur - adapted to persons of scrofulous diathesis, subject to venous congestions, especially of portal system. - after meals congestion to head, with throbbing and forgetfulness; feels as if crazy; does not know whether she has done what she intended or whether objects seen are really there, or whether she only imagines them to be, until she has touched them; menses scanty and late. Congestion to single parts; eyes, nose, chest, abdomen, arms, legs, etc.

Tabacum - rapid blindness without lesion followed by venous hyperaemia and atrophy of optic nerve. - congestion to and nape of neck, followed by weakness and faintness in stomach.

Tarentula hisp. (Mind Symptoms) - hyperaemia and hyperaesthesia of female sexual organs.

Tarentula hisp. (Uterus complaints) - hyperaemia and hyperaesthesia of sexual organs.

Terebinth. - congestion and inflammation of viscera; kidneys, bladder, lungs, intestines and uterus.

Terebinth. (Albuminuria) - congestion of kidneys with rupture of the fine capillaries and consequent pouring out of blood into the pelvis of kidneys.

Thuja (Menses complaints) - burning pain in vagina, < by walking. After: rush of blood to head, nightmare, sleeplessness, leucorrhoea from one menstrual period to the other.

Thyreoidinum - dry, congested, raw, burning; worse left side.

Trifolium - feeling of fullness with congestion of salivary glands, followed by increased copious flow of saliva. White clover. Prophylactic against mumps, feeling of congestion in salivary glands, pain and hardening, especially submaxillary; worse, lying down. Filled with watery saliva, worse lying down. Taste of blood in mouth and throat. Sensation as if heart would stop, with great fear, better sitting up or moving about; worse, when alone, with cold sweat on face.

Trillium cernuum (Menses complaints) - discharge dark, thick, clotted and exhausting the women. Before: congestion to head, shortness of breath.

Trombidium - congestion of the liver, with urgent, loose, stools on rising.

- gentleman of full habits, subject to attacks of rheumatism and congestion of liver; diarrhoea.

Usnea barbata - is a remedy in some forms of congestive headache; sunstroke.

Ustilago - vascular system of ovaries is most powerfully affected, producing congestion, enlargement, and great irritation, with ovaralgia, dysmenorrhoea, and especially menorrhagia.

Ustilago (Eczema) - whole skin dry, hot, congested.

Ustilago (Sore throat) - tonsils congested, inflamed.

Verat-alb. - puerperal mania and convulsions, with violent cerebral congestion; bluish and bloated face; protruded eyes; wild shrieks, with disposition to bite and tear.

Veratrum alb. (Febris flava, yellow fever) - raising the head causes convulsions, vomiting, collapse with intense congestion.

Veratrum alb. (Hepatic derangements) - hyperaemia of liver, with gastric catarrh, putrid taste, disgust for warm food, great pressure in hepatic region, alternating with vomiting or diarrhoea.

Veratrum alb. (Labor) - violent cerebral congestion, bluish-bloated face, shrieks, tearing the clothes, puerperal mania.

Veratrum alb. (Meningitis, cerebro-spinalis) - choleraic collapse simultaneously with intense congestion.

Veratrum vir. (Apoplexy) - congestive apoplexy. Intensely congestive headaches. Convulsions from intense congestion of the capillary vessels of the brain.

Veratrum vir. (Headache) - excessive congestion to head, flushed face, diplopia, ringing ears.

Veratrum vir. (Hearing, defective) - congestion, nausea, vomiting.

Veratrum vir. (Heart diseases) - fluttering of heart, feels as if she would die, < from slightest exertion, so that she sits down to catch her breath, face bluish-cold or flushed. Congestion to heart and lungs with violent fever, rapid respiration, heart's action and pulse suddenly increase to strong and loud action, throbbing carotids, congestion to head without delirium, constant burning pain in chest and sensation of a heavy load there, sometimes changing gradually to the reverse, pulse and heartbeat becoming fluttering, soft, slow, weak, intermittent, finally filiform.

Veratrum vir. (Insanity) - insanity from cerebral congestion.

Veratrum vir. (Labor) - profound cerebral congestion, between convulsions she remains unconscious and lies in a deep sleep, face red, eyes injected.

Veratrum vir. (Mind Symptoms) - cerebral hyperaemia with coldness of whole body.

Veratrum vir. (Menses complaints) - suppressed menses with cerebral congestion.

Veratrum vir .(Paralysis) - cerebral hyperaemia, causing paralysis and tingling in limbs.

Veratrum vir. (Rheumatism) - cardiac oppression, with passive congestion.

Veratrum vir. (Scarlatina) - intense arterial excitement during febrile state, with cerebral congestion or irritation of the spinal centres.

Veratrum vir.(Tetanus and trismus) - cerebral congestion.

Veratrum vir. (Vertigo, dizziness) - congestions of the brain from vascular irritation.

Veratrum vir - congestion intense, almost apoplectic.

Veratrum viride (Cough) - spasmodic cough from spinal congestion or cerebral irritation with spasms.

Verbena - passive congestion and intermittent fever.

Viburnum op. - ovarian region feels heavy and congested. Spasmodic and congestive affections, dependent upon ovarian or uterine origin.

Vipera (Heart diseases) - violent congestion to heart, he tears his clothing open, with excessive sensation of sickness in abdomen.

Vipera (Hepatic derangements) - hyperaemia of liver, after failure of lach.

Wyethia - rush of blood to head.

Yohimbinum - causes hyperaemia of the milk glands and stimulates the function of lactation. Congestive conditions of the sexual organs.

Zincum met. - a teacher of leuco-phlegmatic habit, frequent vertigo for several months, an involuntary, periodically appearing fit of laughing, which he cannot suppress; fits appear several times a day and cause severe convulsions of chest and abdomen, rush of blood to head and brain; a tendency to constipation and apoplexy.

Zincum met. (Constipation) - venous congestion in abdominal organs.

Zincum met. (Ophthalmia) - amblyopia, green halo around the evening light, with rush of blood to head.

Diseases associated with 'congestion'

(Abscesses) a. For acute abscesses, to: 1, Bell., Hep., Merc., Sil.; 2, Apis, Ars., Asa., Bry., Cepa, Cham., Hep., Lach., Led., Mez., Phos., Puls., Sulph-b. for chronic abscesses, whether cold or occasioned by **congestions**, to: Asa., Aur., Calc., Carb-v., Con., Hep., Iod., Laur., Lyc., Mang., Merc., Merc-cor., Nitr-ac., Phos., Sep., Sil., Sulph.

(Albuminuria) Coccus cacti. - general lassitude. Pulmonary **congestions** during acute desquamative nephritis, with profuse mucous secretion and suffocative spasmodic cough.

(Albuminuria) Crotalus hor. - passive renal **congestion**, when from embarrassed circulation, as from obstructive heart disease, asthma, chronic bronchitis, etc., especially during its course, or as sequelae of zymotic diseases.

(Albuminuria) Glonoine - brain feels too large, congested.

(Albuminuria) Helleborus - **congestion** of kidneys with extensive effusion of serum in abdominal cavity and tissue of lower extremities.

(Albuminuria) Kali-mur. - alternate states of sadness and cheerfulness with **congestion**, > by nosebleed - **congestion** to heart, slow pulse, twitching of face - congestive vertigo, < after violent exercise - portal **congestion** and enlarged liver.

(Albuminuria) Phosphorus - **congestion** of the right heart, and hence venous **congestion** of kidneys.

(Albuminuria) Terebinth. - **congestion** of kidneys with rupture of the fine capillaries and consequent pouring out of blood into the pelvis of kidneys.

(Amenorrhoea) Apis mel. - suppressed menses, with congested or inflamed ovaries.

(Amenorrhoea) Belladonna - suppression of menses followed by **hyperaemia, rush of blood** to the head, wakefulness and throbbing of carotids and temples.

(Amenorrhoea) China - **rush of blood** to the head, with pulsation of the carotids.

(Amenorrhoea) Cuprum met. - **rush of blood** to the head, with a strange tingling pain in the crown of the head, or pale face with blue margins around the eyes, or burning redness of the face with red eyes.

(Amenorrhoea) Glonoine - amenorrhoea with great **congestion** in head, < by shaking head.

(Amenorrhoea) Helonias - suppression of menses when the kidneys are congested, urine scanty and turbid.

(Amenorrhoea) Merc-sol. - **rush of blood** to the head.

(Amenorrhoea) Opium - suppression, with **congestion** of blood to the head, which feels heavy.

(Amenorrhoea) Sepia - in some, tendency to cough, to **congestion** and pain in the apex of one or both lungs - pain in loins from uterine and other abdominal **congestion.**

(Anaemia) China - palpitations with **rush of blood** to head, and redness of face with cold hands.

(Anaemia) Sepia - pelvic **congestion.**

(Aneurism) Digitalis - passive **congestion** of lungs, depending on a weakened, dilated heart (Angina pectoris) China ars - angina pectoris, with dropsical symptoms, venous **hyperaemia** and cyanosis.

(Angina pectoris) Cimicifuga - cerebral **congestion.**

(Apoplexy) Asterias - cerebral **congestion** with obstinate constipation.

(Apoplexy) Belladonna - the first stage of the disease, with grinding and gnashing of teeth before attack, where severe congestive symptoms are still present, or at a later period, when the extravasation causes severe inflammatory reaction.

(Apoplexy) Cactus - vertigo from sanguineous **congestions** to the head.

(Apoplexy) Gelsemium - intense passive **congestion** to the head with nervous exhaustion.

(Apoplexy) Iodum - chronic **congestion** to brain from hypertrophy of right ventricle or from compression of blood-vessels around the neck from a struma.

(Apoplexy) Lachesis - the paroxysms are preceded by frequent absence of mind, or vertigo with **rush of blood** to the head.

(Apoplexy) Psorinum - **congestion** of blood to the head with heat.

(Apoplexy) Sanguinaria can - sanguineous apoplexy from venous **congestion**. Pain like a flash of lightning on the back of the head.

(Apoplexy) Strontium - violent **congestion** to head, with hot and red face from every exertion, as walking, smothered feeling about heart, allowing no rest.

(Apoplexy) Veratrum vir. - congestive apoplexy. Intensely congestive headaches - convulsions from intense **congestion** of the capillary vessels of the brain.

(Asthma) Ant-tart. - suffocative cough or **congestion** of blood to chest and palpitation of heart.

(Asthma) Arg-nit. - any bodily exertion brings on a fit with palpitation and **congestion** of face.

(Asthma) Aur-met. - asthma from **congestion** to chest.

(Asthma) Cactus - sanguineous **congestion** in chest, preventing free speech, < when lying down in bed.

(Asthma) China - pressure in chest as if from **rush of blood**, with violent palpitation of the heart, easy perspiration.

(Asthma) Cocculus - hysteric asthma with **rush of blood** to chest and difficult breathing as if the throat were constricted.

(Asthma) Kali-mur. - **congestion** of chest with cold feet.

(Asthma) Nux vomica - **rush of blood** to the chest, with orgasm of the blood, heat, warmth and palpitation.

(Asthma) Opium - **congestion** of blood to the chest, or pulmonary spasms, with deep, stertorous, rattling breathing.

(Asthma) - For asthma from **congestion** of blood to the chest: 1, Acon., Aur., Bell., Merc., Nux-v., Phos., Spong., Sulph.

(Back pain–spinal irritation) Gelsemium - spinal **congestion**.

(Back pain–spinal irritation) Piper meth. - **congestion** of posterior parts of brain and spinal cord, with feeling as though he must move or head and neck would be compressed.

(Back pain–spinal irritation) Sulphur - spinal **congestion** from suppression of menses or haemorrhoidal flow.

(Blennorrhoea of the lachrymal sac) Arg-nit. - conjunctiva congested.

(Bronchitis acuta) Belladonna - stitches in chest, **congestion** to head, hot skin, inclined to be moist.

(Bronchitis acuta) Mag-mur. - **congestion** of blood to the chest from bathing in the sea, causing spasmodic cough and bloody expectoration, < at night, with tension and constriction of chest.

(Bronchitis chronica) Ars-alb. - dyspnoea, from more or less extensive emphysema and consecutive pulmonary **congestions**. Difficulty of breathing continues during the intervals upon coughing, and returns periodically, especially at night.

(Bronchitis chronica) Kali-bich. Bronchitis oscillating between acute and torpid inveterate bronchitis, with a certain degree of irritation, vascular **congestion** and moderate mucopurulent secretion, frequently accompanied by periosteal or rheumatic pains. Cough resonant, whistling, with nausea and expectoration of thick mucus.

(Bronchitis chronica) Lycopodium - **congestion** of liver, flatulency, constipation, cachectic complexion, red gravel, acid dyspepsia.

(Cancer) Sepia - indurations, ulcerations and **congestion** of the os and cervix uteri.

(Chlorosis) Belladonna - painful menstruation, with **rush of blood** to head.

(Chlorosis) Cyclamen - periodical **congestion** to head, with pallor of countenance.

(Chlorosis) Graphites - tendency to **rush of blood** to head with flushing of face, following a sudden shock about heart.

(Cholera) Cicuta - **congestion** of blood to the head or chest.

(Chorea) Belladonna - violent **congestion**, throbbing of carotids, dilated pupils, wild look, injected eyes. Reflex chorea from dentition or pregnancy.

(Chorea) Chelidon. - **congestion** to cerebellum.

(Chorea) Crocus sat. - **congestion** to the head with epistaxis of dark and stringy blood.

(Chronic catarrh of the head) Conium - heat of face, **congestion** to head, with catarrhal sensation.

(Chronic catarrh of the head) Natrum carb. - violent sneezing with **rush of blood** to the head.

(Chronic catarrh of the head) Sulphur - portal **congestions** (Sep.). Sense of **congestion** in nose in open air.

(Cinchona, ill effects of) Belladonna - **congestion** of blood to the head, with heat in the face.

(Coffee and its therapeutics) Lycopodium - coffee makes him sick and brings on aversion to it, a symptom often found in portal **congestion** and hepatic disorders.

(Colic) Belladonna - **congestion** of blood to the head.

(Constipation) Collinsonia - congestive inertia of the bowels, weight and pressure in rectum, with intense irritation and itching in ano pelvic **congestion**.

(Constipation) Opium - beating and sensation of heaviness in abdomen, **rush of blood** to head, sleepiness, bed feels hot, hot sweat. Constipation in connection with ovaritis or ovaralgia.

(Constipation) Sepia - constipation of females, with pain and pressure in iliac regions, from uterine or abdominal **congestion**.

(Constipation) Zincum met. - venous **congestion** in abdominal organs.

(Cornea, diseases of) Hamamelis - keratitis dependent upon a blow or burn, especially when complicated with haemmorrhage into anterior chamber (**hyperaemia**).

(Coryza) Natrum ars. - burning of eyes and **congestion** of conjunctiva.

(Cough) Sepia - coughs from passive **congestions** and obstructions in the portal systems.

(Cough) Veratrum viride - spasmodic cough from spinal **congestion** or cerebral irritation with spasms.

(Coxalgia, hip-disease) Bell. - **Congestion** to head.

(Croup) Bell. - hoarseness with flushed face and congested eyes.

(Cystitis, inflammation of bladder) Lilium tigrinum - continuous pressure on bladder and, if not complied with, congested sensation in chest.

(Dacryo-cystitis) Arg-nit. Caruncula swollen, looking like a lump of raw flesh, conjunctiva congested.

(Delirium) Absinthium - sleeplessness in typhoid with **congestion** at the base of brain.

(Delirium) Bell. - **congestion** to brain with great drowsiness, but inability to sleep.

(Delirium) Opium - venous **congestion** with dark-red face.

(Dentition, morbid) Belladonna - numerous turgid blood vessels in congested gums.

(Dentition, morbid) Melilotus - highly congested.

(Diabetes) Opium - face bloated, congested or sunken and pale.

(Diabetes) Pic-acid. - cortex of brain congested.

(Diaphragm, diseases of) Bell. - In puerperal affections with painful headache from active **hyperaemia** (Atrop.).

(Diaphragm, diseases of) Cactus. - **rush of blood** to chest.

(Diaphragm, diseases of) Stramonium - mixture of **hyperaemia** and spasm, of affection of spinal cord and of diaphragm.

(Diarrhoea of infants) Lactic-acid. - stools undigested, curdy, watery, mixed with bright grass-green mucus, great jerking of muscles, **rush of blood** to head and face.

(Distension of abdomen and flatulence) Graphites - abdomen distended with flatus and **rush of blood** to head.

(Dropsy) Asclepias cornuti - post-scarlatinal dropsy, or from suppressed perspiration, from renal or cardiac affections. Congestive headaches with dullness and stupidity, scanty urine during headache, profuse after.

(Dropsy) Bryonia - **congestion** of the head.

(Dyspepsia, weakness of stomach) Arnica - after a meal sensation of impending apoplectic **congestion** of brain, with throbbing headache and drowsiness.

(Dyspepsia, weakness of stomach) Bryonia - congestive headaches.

(Dyspepsia, weakness of stomach) Chelidonium - great longing for wine, which does not cause **congestion** or heat in head as formerly.

(Dyspepsia, weakness of stomach) Iodum - large, full pulse and cerebral **congestions**.

(Dyspepsia, weakness of stomach) Kali-mur. - portal **congestion**.

(Dyspepsia, weakness of stomach) Phosphorus - **congestion** to head.

(Eczema) Anacardium - itching vesicles, rapidly becoming pustular, large, flat, later confluent, discharging a yellowish transparent fluid, hardening to a crust in the open air as the epidermis peels off, surface swollen, hyperaemic and suppurating, spreading from right to left and affecting chiefly fingers, eyelids, face and scrotum, chest and around neck.

(Eczema) Ustilago - whole skin dry, hot, congested.

(Emotions, ill effects of-fear, dread, fright) Opium - immediate effect of fright, stupefied, with internal heat, **rush of blood** to head, dim sight with twitches and starting.

(Enteritis) Belladonna - anguish, with **congestion** to the head and dimness of vision.

(Epilepsy) Amm-brom. - tinnitus aurium from **congestion** of the labyrinth.

(Epilepsy) Calc-ars. - epilepsy proceeding from cardiac affections, commencing with a pain in heart or constriction, **rush of blood** to the head, loss of speech and unconsciousness.

(Epilepsy) Cicuta - concussion of brain, **congestion** at the base of the brain and in the medulla oblongata. At first the patient is rigid, opisthotonos or emprosthotonos, with fixed, staring eyes, bluish face and frothing at the mouth, followed by shocks passing from head through body.

(Epilepsy) Glonoine - alternate **congestion** of heart and head; convulsions from cerebral **congestion**.

(Fainting) Nux vomica - and generally when nausea, pale face, scintillations before the eyes or obscuration of sight, pains in the stomach, anguish, trembling, and **congestion** of blood to the head or chest are present.

(Gastralgia) Nux vomica - neurotic and congestive gastralgia.

(Gastritis) Belladonna - difficult breathing, anguish, with **congestion** of blood to the head, dimness of sight, faintness, restless and sleepless.

(Gastritis) Sepia - **congestion** and heat of the head.

(Glaucoma) Belladonna - eyes injected, pupils dilated, fundus hyperaemic and pain both in and around eye, severe and throbbing, may come and go suddenly, < afternoon and evening.

(Glaucoma) Cimicifuga - congestive headaches.

(Glaucoma) Gelsemium - choroidal and venous **congestions**, either with or without serous effusion. Amaurotic symptoms, with dilatation of pupils, disturbed accommodation, pain in eyes, with or without lachrymation.

(Glaucoma) Hamamelis - venous **congestion**, haemorrhoids, conjunctival vascularity, ciliary neuralgia, photophobia, lachrymation.

(Glaucoma) Phosphorus - fundus hyperaemic and hazy, halo around light, and various lights and colors (especially red) before eyes.

(Glaucoma) Prunus spinosa - fundus hyperaemic.

(Haematemesis, gastrorrhagia) Belladonna - congestive delirium and convulsions. - Warmth and even congestive burning in stomach with desire for acid drinks.

(Haematemesis, gastrorrhagia) Nux vomica - portal **congestion**, dyspepsia.

(Haematemesis, gastrorrhagia) Sulphur - portal **congestion** with engorged liver.

(Haematuria, haemorrhage from urinary organs) Hamamelis haemorrhoids of bladder, passive **congestion**.

(Haemorrhage from the lungs, haemoptysis) Belladonna - bloody expectoration mixed with mucus. Active **congestion**. - **congestion** of blood to head and chest.

(Haemorrhage from the lungs, haemoptysis) Collinsonia - bleeding caused by cardiac affections or portal **congestion**.

(Haemorrhage from the lungs, haemoptysis) Ledum - **congestion** to chest and head.

(Haemorrhage from the lungs haemoptysis) Opium - **rush of blood** to chest (Haemorrhage from uterus) Aletris menorrhagia in consequence of congested condition of uterus and ovaries.

(Haemorrhage from uterus) Apis-mel. - red spots on body, stinging like bee-stings, often the result of active **congestion** of ovaries.

(Haemorrhage from uterus) Ars-alb. chronic endometritis and passive **hyperaemia**, based on atony.

(Haemorrhage from uterus) Collinsonia - congested condition of uterus.

(Haemorrhage from uterus) Crocus sat. - haemorrhage from overloading of uterine vessels with blood, a passive **congestion**.

(Haemorrhage from uterus) Hamamelis - haemorrhage from portal **congestion**.

(Haemorrhage from uterus) Hydrastis - metrorrhagia and menorrhagia from deficient contraction of blood vessels, uterus enlarged, relaxed and congested.

(Haemorrhage from uterus) Iodum - chronic menorrhagia in thin, delicate women subject to corrosive leucorrhoea, with other indications of congested uterus and ovaries.

(Haemorrhage from uterus) Sepia - chronic **congestion** of uterus with sense of weight as if all would come out of the vulva.

(Haemorrhages) Arnica - pain causes a **rush of blood** to the head, which feels very hot to the patient.

(Haemorrhages) Belladonna - **congestion** to head, eyes, eyeballs, which are red.

(Haemorrhages) Hyoscyamus - constant flow of bright-red blood, with bluish face, congested eyes, twitching of muscles.

(Haemorrhoids) Aesculus hip. - depressed and irritable. Angina granulosa, a dark-red **congestion** of fauces, with dryness and soreness, from abdominal plethora.

(Haemorrhoids) Aloe - constipation of old people of sedentary habits and given to high living. Uterine **congestion** and prolapsus with heaviness in abdomen and back.

(Haemorrhoids) Belladonna - **congestion** of blood to head.

(Haemorrhoids) Cactus - constipation as from haemorrhoidal **congestion.**

(Haemorrhoids) Collinsonia - **congestion** of pelvic organs and catarrh of bladder, with piles.

(Haemorrhoids) Hepar-sulph - great want of vital power of expulsion from the congested condition of the veins in rectum.

(Haemorrhoids) Sulphur - suppressed haemorrhoids, with colic, palpitation, **congestion** of lungs.

(Hay fever, catarrhus aestivus) Ailanthus - eyes suffused and congested.

(Headache) Ailanthus - passive congestive headache and dizziness, face red and hot, > by nosebleed (Arn.).

(Headache) Aluminium - headache, attended with nausea, oppression in forehead, **rush of blood** to eyes and nose, epistaxis, pale face and languor.

(Headache) Amm-brom. - tinnitus aurium from **congestion** of labyrinth.

(Headache) Amyl-nit. - congestive headache.

(Headache) Asclepias cornuti - congestive headache from suppression of sweat or urine and fever.

(Headache) Aur-met. - **congestion** to and heat in the head, with sparks before eyes, with nausea and bilious vomiting, < from any mental exertion or motion, ideas become confused, roaring in head - congestive headaches.

(Headache) Belladonna - **congestion** of blood to head, with danger of apoplexy.

(Headache) Bryonia - > by tying up the head, pressure and closing eyes. Gastric, rheumatic and congestive headaches - congestive headaches, as if forehead would split open, with nosebleed, commencing in morning, not on waking, but after opening eyes and lasting till evening.

(Headache) Bufo - congestive headaches, < after breakfast, > by nosebleed.

(Headache) Cactus - from sanguineous **congestion** or rheumatism, < by eating, any sudden motion or deep inspiration.

(Headache) Calc-carb. - **congestion** of head, hammering through forehead and base of brain.

(Headache) Carbo-veg. - **congestion** of head from overheated rooms, > followed by nosebleed - **congestion** of head from overheated rooms, heat on top of head during climaxis.

(Headache) Character - congestive: Acon., Ailanth., Alum., Ammcarb., Amyl-nitr., Arn., Asclep., Aur., Bell., Bry., Bufo, Cact., Calc., Carb-v., Cham., Cimicif., Cocc., Curare, Dig., Fer., Fer-phos., Gels., Glon., Hep., Hyosc., Ign., Lach., Lil., Lyc., Magn-carb., Magn-mur., Melilot., Nux, Op., Phos., Puls., Psor., Rhus, Sang., Spong., Veratr., Veratr-vir.

(Headache) Cicuta - semilateral headache, like pressure as from **congestion** of blood to the head, with sunken features.

(Headache) Cimicifuga - **rush of blood** to head, brain feels too large for cranium.

(Headache) Coccinella - redness and heat of cheeks, **congestion** in face as from hot flashes.

(Headache) Crotalus hor. - congestive headaches, especially on right side (Lach., left), with abdominal ailments, bilious vomiting, constipation, < by lying down again after rising.

(Headache) Curare - **congestion** of blood to the head, with pulsative vibrating pains and loss of consciousness.

(Headache) Ferr-met - frequent congestive headaches, with pulsating pain in head, usually < after midnight, face fiery red during attack, feet cold. - headache of anaemic, debilitated persons, especially with **congestion** to head and chest.

(Headache) Gelsemium - Passive **congestion** in the brain -sensation as if a band were tied around forehead (passive arterial **congestion**).

(Headache) Glonoine - bad sequelae of cutting hair. Intense **congestion** of the brain in plethoric constitutions, with persistent sensation of pulsation, from sudden suppression of menses, after anxiety and worry with sleeplessness. - congestive headache, sensation of fluttering in head, of constriction in vessels of head, expansive pressure, flushed face, drowsiness, venous **congestion** to abdomen.

(Headache) Graphites - pain as if head were numb and pithy, as if constricted, especially in occiput, extending to nape of neck, with pains on looking up as if neck were broken. During amenorrhoea frequent **congestion** to head and chest, dark-red cheeks, oppression and anguish when lying down.

(Headache) Hyoscyamus - unconsciousness from **congestion** of blood to the head, with delirium, answers all questions properly.

(Headache) Kali-carb. - **congestion** to head with throbbing and humming.

(Headache) Kalmia - neuralgic paroxysmal pains, especially right side (glon., congestive, steady pain), > by profuse micturition.

(Headache) Mag-carb. - **congestion** of blood to head, especially when smoking.

(Headache) Mag-mur. - **congestive** and hysterical headaches, with sensation as if boiling water in cranium, pains in temples, > by firm pressure with the hands and from wrapping the head up warmly.

(Headache) Melilotus - congestive headaches with violent palpitations and prolapsus uteri. Violent congestive headache with sensation as if brain would burst through forehead (Glon.), driving the patient almost frantic - face highly **congested,** almost livid.

(Headache) Nux vomica - congestive and abdominal headaches, with nausea and vomiting, worse by coughing and stooping.

(Headache) Opium - somnolence after meals from passive cerebral **congestion**.

(Headache) Phellandrium - crushing feeling on top of head, with aching and burning in temples and above the eyes, which are congested (Headache) Phosphorus - in washer-woman fear of washing, as it causes **rush of blood** to head, red face and eyes, heat in head.

(Headache) Psorinum - **congestion** of blood to the head, with red, hot cheeks and nose, with great anxiety every afternoon after dinner (during pregnancy).

(Headache) Pulsatilla - passive **congestion**, pale face, palpitations.

(Headache) Sanguinaria can. - **rush of blood** with dizziness in head, she feels as if she would fall when she attempts to rise from a sitting position, with nausea and vomiting.

(Headache) Spongia - congestive headaches from dry cold weather, after intoxication.

(Headache) Veratrum vir. - excessive **congestion** to head, flushed face, diplopia, ringing ears.

(Hearing, defective) Arnica - noises in ears, as if caused by **rush of blood** to the head.

(Hearing, defective) Cactus - hardness of hearing from **congestion**

(Hearing, defective) if caused by **congestion** of blood, with buzzing, etc.: 1, Aur., Bell., Caust., Graph., Merc., Phos., Puls., Sil., Sulph.

(Hearing, defective) Sulphur - **rush of blood** to head.

(Hearing, defective) Veratrum vir. - **congestion**, nausea, vomiting.

(Heart diseases) Asafoetida - beating of heart, with faintness, **rush of blood** to head, flushing of face, anxiety and slow breathing.

(Heart diseases) Aur-met. - pure cardiac hypertrophy without dilatation, with increased force of heart-stroke and **hyperaemia** of lungs, < from any exertion, as walking up hill, and feeling of a crushing. Weight under sternum and as if blood would burst through chest, if he does not cease walking.

(Heart diseases) Baptisia - palpitations with **congestion** to head.

(Heart diseases) Belladonna - **congestion** of blood to various parts, violent palpitations, reverberating to the head.

(Heart diseases) Cactus - sanguinous **congestion** to chest. Endocarditis and pericarditis.

(Heart diseases) China - palpitation, with **rush of blood** to face, with cold hands.

(Heart diseases) Cimicifuga - unconsciousness, cerebral **congestion.**

(Heart diseases) Digitalis - suffocative spells with painful constriction of chest as if internal parts of chest were grown together, passive **congestion** of lungs with cyanosis, must sometimes sit up in order to get breath. Pericarditis, pericardial effusion with consequent dropsy.

(Heart diseases) Ferr-met. - anaemia masked behind plethora and **congestion**, pale color of mucous membranes, with nun's murmur.

(Heart diseases) Ferr-phos. - **hyperaemia** from relaxation of muscular fibres of blood vessels - palpitation from **congestion** with full, quick pulse.

(Heart diseases) Glonoine - alternate **congestion** to heart and head.

(Heart diseases) Lilium-tig. - frequent sensation as if the heart stopped, followed by **rush of blood** to heart, violent palpitations and sharp pain going from left nipple through chest to back, > by lying on left side and in open air.

(Heart diseases) Phosphorus - nervous palpitations, especially of old maids, from emotions, as from the sudden entrance into the room of an unexpected visitor, welcome or unwelcome, from motion, from **rush of blood** to the chest. Vertigo, with tendency to fall to the left side.

(Heart diseases) Sepia - **congestion** of blood to chest with violent palpitation, an occasional hard thump of the heart, sensation of a ball in inner parts.

(Heart diseases) Spongia - Rapid, hard breathing. Rheumatic pericarditis, after effusion took place (Acon. during stage of **hyperaemia**).

(Heart diseases) Valvular affections: with **congestion** to head: Bapt., Chin.

(Heart diseases) Veratrum vir. - fluttering of heart, feels as if she would die, < from slightest exertion, so that she sits down to catch her breath, face bluish-cold or flushed. **Congestion** to heart and lungs with violent fever, rapid respiration, heart's action and pulse suddenly increase to strong and loud action, throbbing carotids, **congestion** to head without delirium, constant burning pain in chest and sensation of a heavy load there, sometimes changing gradually to the reverse, pulse and heartbeat becoming fluttering, soft, slow, weak, intermittent, finally filiform.

(Heart diseases) Vipera - violent **congestion** to heart, he tears his clothing open, with excessive sensation of sickness in abdomen.

(Heels, pains in) Ledum - soles painful when walking, as if congested with blood.

(Hepatic derangements) Agaricus - Congested, enlarged liver.

(Hepatic derangements) Aesculus hip. - **congestion** of liver and portal system.

(Hepatic derangements) Aur-met. - hepatic **congestion** consecutive to cardiac disease, with burning and cutting in right hypochondrium, ending in cirrhosis and fatty degeneration with dropsy. Chronic hepatitis with suicidal melancholy, averse to motion.

(Hepatic derangements) Belladonna - **congestion** of the head.

(Hepatic derangements) Carduus mar. - portal **hyperaemia.**

(Hepatic derangements) Chelidon. - abdominal plethora from simple **congestion** to positive inflammation.

(Hepatic derangements) Crotalus hor. - pressive hepatic **congestion**, especially when from heart disease or from imperfect performance of uterine functions, or if a sequel of malarial fever. Acute yellow atrophy.

(Hepatic derangements) Fluoric-acid - ascites from hepatic induration and portal **congestion.**

(Hepatic derangements) Gelsemium - passive **congestion** of liver, bilious diarrhoea and relaxed gall-ducts.

(Hepatic derangements) Merc-sol. - **rush of blood** to head.

(Hepatic derangements) Natrum sulph. - **congestion** of liver with soreness and sharp, sticking pains.

(Hepatic derangements) Phosphorus - **hyperaemia**, at first enlargement, fatty degeneration and finally atrophy of the liver with jaundice and dropsy.

(Hepatic derangements) Podophyl. - fullness in right hypochondrium, **hyperaemia** of the liver, with flatulence, pain and soreness.

(Hepatic derangements) Ptelea - jaundice, with **hyperaemia** of the liver.

(Hepatic derangements) Veratrum alb. - **hyperaemia** of liver, with gastric catarrh, putrid taste, disgust for warm food, great pressure in hepatic region, alternating with vomiting or diarrhoea.

(Hepatic derangements) Vipera - **hyperaemia** of liver, after failure of lach.

(Hoarseness) Kali-bich. - subacute and chronic inflammatory processes in larynx or bronchial tubes, with **congestion** and swelling of the tubes, and increased secretion of a glutinous mucus which veils and alters the voice.

(Homesickness, nostalgia) Phosphoric acid. - chronic **congestions** to the head.

(Hysteria) Mag-mur. - Congestive headaches with sensation as if boiling water in cranium, especially about temples, > by pressure and by wrapping up the head warmly (Sil.).

(Hysteria) Moschus - **rush of blood** to head, with staring eyes.

(Infantile remittent fever) Belladonna - great heat and cerebral **congestion**.

(Infantile remittent fever) Ferr-phos. - **hyperaemia** of the brain.

(Insanity) Aur-met. - often asks questions, jumping from one thing to another, without waiting for a reply. **Rush of blood** to head, palpitations, pollutions, otherwise patient in fair physical health, and > in fresh air and out-door exercise.

(Insanity) Ferr-phos. - transitory mania depending upon **hyperaemia** of the brain.

(Insanity) Glonoine - **congestion** alternately to head and heart.

(Insanity) Hyoscyamus - epileptoid spasms, **rush of blood** to head with sparkling eyes and fixed look (Insanity) Kali-mur - intoxication from the smallest quantity of wine or beer, causing **congestion**, > from nosebleed.

(Insanity) Veratrum vir. - insanity from cerebral **congestion.**

(Iris, affections of) Belladonna - congested face. - **congestion** of conjunctiva, ciliary neuralgia, photophobia.

(Jaundice) Belladonna - **congestion** to head.

(Jaundice) Gelsemium - passive **congestion** of liver, bilious diarrhoeas and relaxed gall-ducts.

(Jaundice) Merc-sol. - jaundice with violent **rush of blood** to head, bad taste, tongue moist and furred, yellow.

(Jaundice) Podophyl. - jaundice from torpor of liver, from gallstones, from **hyperaemia** of liver with fulness, soreness and pain in hepatic region, > by rubbing and stroking hypochondrium with hands.

(Kidney/bladder stone) Arg-nit. - nephralgia from **congestion** of kidney or from passage of little stones.

(Laryngitis and laryngeal phthisis) Drosera - local **congestion** of these parts.

(Laryngitis and laryngeal phthisis, Kali-bich. - Iod., scrofulous), with **congestion**, swelling of the tissues and increased secretion of a glutinous fluid, < mornings, when the tough mucus nearly strangles him.

(Leukemia) Nux vomica - **congestion** to head, and red, bloated face.

(Leucorrhoea) Caulophyl. - menses suppressed from nervous causes in young girls or in nervous, debilitated women with relaxed, flabby uterus or displaced and passively congested uterus, especially after miscarriage

(Leucorrhoea) Graphites - induration and **congestion** of cervix.

(Leucorrhoea) Helonias - old chronic cases without **congestion.**

(Leucorrhoea) Iodum - corrosive discharge in thin, delicate women, between menses, who suffer from chronic **congestion** or inflammation of uterus and ovaries (right side).

(Leucorrhoea) Lachesis - uterine **congestion** with prolapsus uteri.

(Leucorrhoea) Podophyl - **congestion** of portal system.

(Leucorrhoea) Secale - leucorrhoea, brownish, offensive, like cream, from weakness and venous **congestion**.

(Love pangs) Aur-met. - **congestion** of blood to the chest and anxious beating of the heart. - **congestion** of blood to the head.

(Mania) Hyoscyamus - very little **rush of blood** to head (Measles) Belladonna - **congestion** to head.

(Measles) Gelsemium - abdominal and thoracic **congestion**.

(Mind symptoms) Aur-met. - **rush of blood** to head, roaring in ears

(Mind symptoms) Ferr-met. - anaemia and debility with **congestion** to head and chest.

(Mind symptoms) Hyoscyamus - nervous irritability without **hyperaemia**.

(Mind symptoms) Tarentula hisp. - **hyperaemia** and hyperaesthesia of female sexual organs.

(Mind symptoms) Veratrum vir. - cerebral **hyperaemia** with coldness of whole body.

(Memory weak, inability to think) - if by **congestion** of blood to the head: Chin., Melilot., Merc., Rhus, Sulph.

(Meningitis basilaris) Opium - congested face.

(Meningitis basilaris) Spongia - **congestion** of blood to head with pressing, knocking and pulsating pains in forehead.

(Meningitis, cerebro-spinalis) Apis mel. - stupor from effusion (op from **congestion**).

(Meningitis, cerebro-spinalis) Cuprum acet. - **congestion** of brain, with convulsive motions of extremities.

(Meningitis, cerebro-spinalis) Gelsemium - at the very onset of the disease, severe chill followed by **congestion** of the brain and spinal cord, livid cheeks, dilated pupils, little or no thirst. Perfect loss of strength and great exhaustion, staggering gait, dullness of speech, icy coldness of hands and feet, pulse very weak or hardly perceptible.

(Meningitis, cerebro-spinalis) Glonoine - **congestion** of chest, with labored action of heart. - violent **congestion** of head, with sense of expansion.

(Meningitis, cerebro-spinalis) Opium - stupefaction, with or without pain, delirium, mania, heaviness, with great **congestion** to head, occiput feels as heavy as lead, the head falling back constantly.

(Meningitis, cerebro-spinalis) Phosphorus - **congestion** to head.

(Meningitis, cerebro-spinalis) Veratrum alb. - choleraic collapse simultaneously with intense **congestion**.

(Meningitis, encephalitis) Apis-mel. - meningitis from suppression or spread of erysipelas or other exanthemata. **Congestion** to the head and face, with fullness, burning and throbbing in brain.

(Meningitis, encephalitis) Digitalis - amaurotic **congestion** of retina.

(Meningitis, encephalitis) Gelsemium - intense and overwhelming **congestion** of the brain in children, during dentition.

(Menses complaints) Belladonna - too early and too profuse, of hot, bright-red blood, containing dark, offensive clots, or the blood thick, decomposed and of a dark-red color, the discharge feeling hot as it passes before: dysmenorrhoea depending on a congested or inflamed ovary, more often the right one, with dragging and pressing downward pains and cutting from behind forward or vice versa, passing through the horizontal diameter of pelvis and not around circumference (as Sep. and Plat. do).

(Menses complaints) Bryonia - too early, too profuse, dark-red, smelling badly. Before: **congestion** to head and chest, pinching in abdomen.

(Menses complaints) Calc-carb. - congestive headache, < on ascending or when rising from a stooping position, with coldness of limbs.

(Menses complaints) Caulophyl. - neuralgic and congestive dysmenorrhoea with spasmodic, irregular and very severe pains, especially the first two days of menses.

(Menses complaints) China - menses too early, too profuse, with discharge of dark, coagulated blood, or watery, pale blood, with coagula. Before: **congestion** to uterus, with sensation of fullness and painful pressure towards genitals, especially when walking.

During: abdominal cramps, **congestion** to uterus and chest. After: great weakness, trembling debility, convulsions, fainting fits.

(Menses complaints) Ferr-phos. - excessive **congestion** at monthlies, blood bright-red.

(Menses complaints) Gelsemium - delayed and painful, suppressed. Before: **congestion** to head and face - vomiting, with bearing-down pains in abdomen. During: neuralgic and congestive dysmenorrhoea, with sharp, labor-like pains in uterus alternating with other neuralgic pains.

(Menses complaints) Hepar sulph. - uterus enlarged and anteverted, with **congestion** of ovaries.

(Menses complaints) Ignatia - dysmenorrhoea from irritation of nervous system, and not from uterine **congestion**.

(Menses complaints) Lac can. - **congestion** of ovaries. During: great distress in pelvic region, with sensation as if abdomen would burst, slightly > from leaning back.

(Menses complaints) Mag-mur. - **congestion** of blood to head, with painful undulation and whizzing as if boiling water on side on which she rests.

(Menses complaints) Merc-sol. - dry heat and **rush of blood** to head. During: anxiety, red tongue with dark spots, salty taste, scorbutic gums, teeth feel sharp.

(Menses complaints) Nux vomica - congestive headache with vertigo.

(Menses complaints) Thuja - burning pain in vagina, < by walking. After: **rush of blood** to head, nightmare, sleeplessness, leucorrhoea from one menstrual period to the other.

(Menses complaints) when the menses are attended with **congestion** of blood to the head, vertigo: Caust., Gels., Iod., Merc., Phos., Veratr.

(Menses complaints) Trillium - discharge dark, thick, clotted and exhausting the women. Before: **congestion** to head, shortness of breath.

(Menses complaints) Veratrum vir. - suppressed menses with cerebral **congestion.**

(Migraine) Belladonna - violent **hyperaemia**, with throbbing carotids, red face, intolerance of least jar, noise or light.

(Migraine) Natrum sulph. - **congestion** of blood to head, with fullness.

(Migraine) Silicea - **rush of blood** to head, great sensitiveness of hair falling out of hair, perspiration on head, pains running from neck up into head, paroxysms end with profuse urination.

(Miscarriage, abortion) Belladonna - cerebral **congestion** and moaning, which gives her temporary relief.

(Myelitis acuta, inflammation of the spinal cord) Physostigma (Calabar) - **congestion** of spinal cord, with tetanic spasms - congestive state of paralysis of the spinal cord.

(Myelitis acuta, inflammation of the spinal cord) Sulphur **congestion** of lumbar spine, followed by retention of urine and paraplegia.

(Nails, diseases of) Bryonia - tight, compressed feeling with pressing-out sensation, as if the finger needed more room, dark, congested part.

(Nephralgia, renal colic) Arg-nit. - nephralgia from **congestion** of kidneys or from passage of calculi.

(Nephritis) Helleborus - **congestion** of kidneys with extensive effusion of serum in abdominal cavity and tissues of lower extremities.

(Neuralgia) Belladonna - **congestion** of head, with bright-red face and delirium.

(Neuralgia) Ferr-phos. - congestive neuralgia from chill or cold, with pain as if a nail were being driven in, accompanied by flushed face, burning or diffused heat, feeling of weight and pressure.

(Neuralgia) Melilotus - violent **congestion** of head, profuse and frequent epistaxis.

(Neurasthenia) Gelsemium - **congestion** of spine, muscles feel bruised and will not obey the will.

(Neurasthenia) Graphites - **rush of blood** to chest and head, but not from true plethora.

(Neurasthenia) Sulphur - paraplegia from spinal **congestion.**

(Nymphomania) Gratiola - irritable condition of sexual organs with **congestion.**

(Ophthalmia) Arg-nit. - great **hyperaemia** of conjunctiva.

(Ophthalmia) Aur-mur.-nat. - retinal **congestion.**

(Ophthalmia) Belladonna - blindness, following severe congestive headaches - hyperaesthesia and **hyperaemia** of the optic nerve and retina, apoplexy of retina, with suppressed menses.

(Ophthalmia) Chamomilla - the tissue so much congested that blood oozes out from between the swollen lids, especially upon any attempt to open them.

(Ophthalmia) Cimicifuga - **hyperaemia** of conjunctiva, iris, choroid and retina, due to prolonged exertion of myopic or hypermetropic eyes.

(Ophthalmia) Cocculus - rheumatic glaucoma, with venous **hyperaemia**, dilated pupils, insensibility to light, haziness of lens and vitreous humor, severe pain in and around the eyes.

(Ophthalmia) Conium - great dread of light with very little visible inflammation, conjunctiva unnaturally bloodless, and the globe of the eye has a pearly aspect, palpebral conjunctiva alone congested, striated, or studded with granulations.

(Ophthalmia) Duboisin - chronic **hyperaemia** of palpebral conjunctiva.

(Ophthalmia) Glonoine - venous **hyperaemia** or **congestion** of retina and optic nerve.

(Ophthalmia) Hydrastis - mucous membrane of eyelids much congested.

(Ophthalmia) Ignatia - the eyes are more painful than congested, with sensation as if sand in eyes.

(Ophthalmia) Sanguinaria can. - retinal **congestion**, with flushed face and congestive headache.

(Ophthalmia) Sulphur - hypopion, cataract, choroiditis and chorioretinitis, if accompanied by darting pains and where the disease is based upon abdominal venosity, stagnation in portal circulation, habitual constipation, cerebral **congestion**, or upon metastasis of chronic or suppressed skin diseases.

(Ophthalmia) Zincum met. - amblyopia, green halo around the evening light, with **rush of blood** to head.

(Otitis and otorrhoea) Arnica - noises in ears from **rush of blood** to head.

(Otitis and otorrhoea) China sul. - tinnitus aurium and impairment of hearing from paralysis of the vessels, with **congestion** and exudation, especially of labyrinth and tympanum.

(Otitis and otorrhoea) Ferr-phos. - first stage of inflammation or even only **hyperaemia** of membrana tympani and redness of meatus.

(Otitis and otorrhoea) Opium - haemotorrhoea, **congestion** of ears.

(Ovaries, diseases of) Hamamelis - **congestion**, inflammation and neuralgia of ovaries, with cutting, tearing pains in swollen and tender ovary, < at menses, with retention of urine.

(Ovaries, diseases of) Iodum - chronic **congestion**, usually with leucorrhoea.

(Ovaries, diseases of) Kali-iod. - severe burning, tearing and twitching pains in the ovarian region, especially right side. Sensation of **congestion** and swelling of the ovaries, with pain as from a corrosive tumor there. Affections connected with syphilis.

(Ovaries, diseases of) Lac-can. Heat in the ovarian and uterine region (with menses). - Inflammatory and congestive condition of the ovaries before menses, especially of the right ovary, with extreme soreness and sensitiveness, which makes every motion and position, even breath, painful.

(Ovaries, diseases of) Sepia - **congestion**, stinging pains in ovarian region running around from the back over each hip, bearing-down pains from uterus.

(Paralysis) Agaricus - paraplegia from **congestion** of lumbar cord.

(Paralysis) Caulophyllum - paraplegia from retroversion and **congestion** of womb after childbirth, with partial loss of sensation in affected limbs.

(Paralysis) Cuprum met. - **congestion** in chest, palpitation of heart, pulse slow, weak and small.

(Paralysis) Dulcamara - paresis and **hyperaemia** of spinal cord from lying on damp cold ground.

(Paralysis) Picric-acid. - during first stage intense occipital headache after severe mental effort, **congestion** of spine with tonic and clonic spasms, keeps his legs wide apart when standing, looks steadily at objects as if unable to make them out, followed by paresis. Brain-fag, limbs become too weak to support the body. Will-power as if suspended.

(Paralysis) Veratrum vir. - cerebral **hyperaemia**, causing paralysis and tingling in limbs.

(Pemphigus) Chloralum - vesicles surrounded by marked capillary **hyperaemia**.

(Pericarditis) Belladonna - acute stage with cerebral **congestion** and delirium.

(Pericarditis) Franciscea - (e. m. hale). - intense headache, like a band around the head, with symptoms of cerebral **congestion.**

(Pharyngitis) Hepar-sulph. - chronic venous **congestion** of pharyngolaryngeal mucous membrane.

(Pharyngitis) Kali-bich. - Chronic **congestion** of fauces and pharyngeal mucous membrane, follicles looking like little tubercles on pharyngeal wall.

(Pharyngitis) Sulphur - Venous **congestion**, piles, constipation.

(Photophobia) Conium - pale redness of the eyeball, with congested vessels of the conjunctiva, suitable to scrofulous subjects.

(Prolapsus of rectum) Hydrastis - simple prolapsus in children, with **congestion** and swelling of the mucous membrane and marked constipation.

(Prosopalgia) Cedron - patient nervous, excitable, with cold hands, feet and nose, **congestion** to head.

(Prosopalgia) Conium - heat in face, with **congestion** to head, lacerating in right half of face, which feels as if excoriated.

(Prosopalgia) Glonoine - cold sweat on face during **congestion** to head.

(Prosopalgia) Phosphorus - pains from forehead into eyes (right) and from vertex and temples down upon zygoma, with bloatedness of face, **congestion** to head, vertigo and ringing of ears, < from talking, stooping or external pressure, > while eating, lying down, after sleeping, from heat. Neuralgia accompanied by much nervous waste, especially in nervous and nervo-sanguineous temperaments.

(Prosopalgia) Sepia - intermittent faceache, with **congestion** of the eyes and head.

(Rheumatism) Belladonna - stitching, burning and throbbing pains, with high fever, hot, dry skin, thirst, **congestion** to head, with throbbing headache and pulsations of carotids.

(Rheumatism) Lycopodium - chronic forms, especially of old people, with painful rigidity of muscles and joints, and feeling of numbness in affected parts, forgetfulness, vertigo, **congestion** to head, sour belching, early nausea, flatulence, oppression of chest, palpitation, etc.

(Rheumatism) Veratrum vir. - cardiac oppression, with passive **congestion**.

(Scrofulosis) Hydrastis - constipation from weakened and congestive state of the lower bowel.

(Sexual complaints) Natrum carb. - passive **congestion**.

(Sleeplessness) Belladonna - sleeplessness, especially of plethoric children, from nervous excitement, from local **congestion**, from irritation in various parts.

(Sleeplessness) Piper meth. - occipital **congestion**, sore inside and tender outside.

(Smallpox) Belladonna - during first stage, high fever with cerebral **congestion**.

(Sore throat) Amm-brom. - fauces dark-red, **congestion**.

(Sore throat) Amm-carb. - enlarged tonsils, congested, covered with membrane.

(Sore throat) Arnica - whole throat congested.

(Sore throat) Ipecac. - **congestion** of blood to head, with pale face.

(Sore throat) Kali-bich. - chronic **congestion** of fauces and pharyngeal mucous membrane.

(Sore throat) Ustilago - tonsils congested, inflamed.

(Suffocative catarrh) Ant-tart., Ars., Carb-v., Chin., Ipec., Phos., Puls., Samb. - **hyperacmia** and hypostasis pulmonum.

(Sunstroke) Amyl-nit. - congestive stage of sunstroke.

(Sunstroke) Cactus - vertigo, from sanguineous **congestion** to the head.

(Sunstroke) Camphor - severe headache, **congestion** of brain, fainting, delirium, convulsions.

(Synovitis) Belladonna - **congestion** to head, flushed cheeks, etc.

(Tetanus and trismus) Veratrum vir. - cerebral **congestion**.

(Tonsillitis) Baryta mur. - elongation of uvula with **hyperaemia** and blennorrhoea.

(Tonsillitis) Belladonna - intense **congestion**, throbbing of carotids

(Tuberculosis of lungs) Bromium - **congestion** to head and chest, > by nosebleed.

(Tuberculosis of lungs) Cimicifuga - intercurrent congestive state from exposure, with dry, harassing cough, diarrhoea, night-sweats.

(Tuberculosis of lungs) Hamamelis - cannot lie down because of difficulty of breathing from **congestion**.

(Tuberculosis of lungs) Iodum - suitable to young persons who grow too rapidly and subject to frequent **congestions** to the chest, with dry cough excited by tickling all over chest, < in warm room, with expectoration of stringy, transparent mucus, sometimes streaked with blood.

(Tuberculosis of lungs) Natrum mur. - **congestion** to head, with hectic flush and general malaise after least exertion.

(Tuberculosis of lungs) Phosphoric acid. - tickling cough, seemingly from pit of stomach, with burning in chest and passive **congestion**, followed by great weakness in chest and dyspnoea, < from least exposure.

(Tuberculosis of lungs) Phosphorus - **rush of blood** to head and chest.

(Tuberculosis of lungs) Spongia - tuberculosis pulmonum, first stage, with hard, ringing cough, **rush of blood** to chest, palpitations and sudden weakness while walking.

(Tuberculosis of lungs) Sulphur - **congestion** towards head and chest, with palpitations of heart.

(Ulcers) Carduus mar. - oedema of feet, portal **hyperaemia**, haemorrhoids, constipation.

(Uraemia) Ars., Aur., Cann. Ind., Carbol. ac., Cupr., Hydr-ac., Iod., Nicotin, Phos., Tereb., where uraemic blood-poisoning complicates morbus Brightii; but we must not neglect to use the catheter twice or three times a day. In acute uraemia, during accouchement or complicating zymotic affections, especially scarlatina, with prevailing cerebral **hyperaemia**: Amm.-carb., Apis, Bell., Con., Cupr., Glon., Gels., Merc.-cor., Stram., Tereb., Veratr.-vir.

(Uraemia) Iodum - chronic congestive headache in old people.

(Urinary difficulties) Lilium tig. - if desire is not attended to, feeling of **congestion** to chest.

(Uterus complaints) Abies can. - prolapsus from general defective nutrition, with little or no local **congestion**.

(Uterus complaints) Aloe - uterine **congestion** and prolapsus, with fulness and heaviness and labor-like pains in loins and groins, < standing.

(Uterus complaints) Apis-mel. - menses suppressed or diminished, with **congestion** to head.

(Uterus complaints) Aur-met. - uterus prolapsed from its great hyperaemic weight, backache, < during menses, with heat in vagina, < from straining or lifting, ischuria and constipation.

(Uterus complaints) Belladonna - cervical mucous membrane very much congested and reddened (Uterus complaints) Convallaria - diabetes, with intense itching at introitus and **hyperaemia**, > by cold water.

(Uterus complaints) Gelsemium - neuralgic and congestive dysmenorrhoea, with frontal headache and dim vision.

(Uterus complaints) Kali mur. - chronic **congestion** of uterus.

(Uterus complaints) Lac can. - congested condition of uterus, with extreme soreness and tenderness, making every motion, position, even breathing painful.

(Uterus complaints) Sepia - venous passive **congestion**, chronic metritis, displacements, especially retroversion.

(Uterus complaints) Tarentula hisp. - **hyperaemia** and hyperaesthesia of sexual organs.

(Uterus, subinvolution after childbirth) Sepia - venous **congestion** of uterus, stitching pains felt mostly in neck of uterus or extending to abdominal cavity.

(Uvula, affections of) Baryta mur - elongated uvula, with **hyperaemia** and blennorrhoea.

(Vertigo, dizziness) - from **rush of blood**: Eug., Glon., Grat.

(Vertigo, dizziness) Aesculus hip. - derangement of the portal system, producing nervous **congestion** in the brain.

(Vertigo, dizziness) Alumen - **rush of blood** to head.

(Vertigo, dizziness) Artemisia - great heaviness of head and **congestion** of all cerebro-spinal vessels.

(Vertigo, dizziness) Asafoetida - **congestion** of the portal system and pulsation of the veins.

(Vertigo, dizziness) Belladonna - epileptiform vertigo, often reflex from **congestion** of sexual organs or spinal cord.

(Vertigo, dizziness) Cactus - vertigo from sanguineous **congestion** to the head, frequently caused by derangement of the heart. Great nervous excitability, < from physical exertion, turning in bed, stooping, rising from recumbent position or deep breathing.

(Vertigo, dizziness) Causticum - **congestion** of the blood to the head, with heat and dimness of sight.

(Vertigo, dizziness) Ferr-phos. - **congestion** to parts of brain.

(Vertigo, dizziness) Moschus - **congestion** of blood to the head -vertigo, with violent **rush of blood** to the head, relieved in the open air.

(Vertigo, dizziness) Nux vomica - **congestion** of blood, with heat and redness of the face, also with violent pains in the forehead, with vertigo and fainting.

(Vertigo, dizziness) Psorinum - **congestion** of blood to the head, with red, hot cheeks and nose, redness of the eruption on the face, with great anxiety, every afternoon after dinner.

(Vertigo, dizziness) Salicylic acid. - **rush of blood** to head, excited mood.

(Vertigo, dizziness) Veratrum vir. - **congestion** of the brain from vascular irritation.

(Vision complaints) Arg-nit. - marked **hyperaemia** of conjunctiva with mucous discharge and redness of inner canthi.

(Vision complaints) Asarum europa asthenopia accompanied by congestive headaches (Vision complaints) Cactus - **hyperaemia** of fundus, sight blurred, cannot see at a distance. (Vision complaints) Gelsemium - after apoplexy, **congestion** of the head. (Visioncomplaints) - if **congestion** of blood to the head: Aur., Bell., Calc., Chin., Gels., Hyosc., Nux-v., Op., Phos., Sil., Sulph., etc. (Vision complaints) Phosphorus - retinal **hyperaemia**.

(Vision complaints) Sulphur - retinitis caused by overuse of eyes, **congestion** of optic nerve.

Cachexia, Cachectic, Dyscrasia

Acute and sub-acute diseases, which are long standing and not cured despite the best treatment, and where patient is much affected with disturbed day to day activity. For such long standing acute diseases we must think of the term '**Cachexia**'.

Acute diseases such as cough, cold, diarrhoea, skin rash etc. normally do not last long. When you find a patient with these complaints standing long for years and bothering him much, you may use the term '**Cachexia**'. We may otherwise call this as weakness of the system or of a part of body.

Dyscrasia: an abnormal state of the body or part of the body, especially one due to abnormal development or metabolism. In classical medicine the term was used for the imbalance of the four humours (blood, phlegm, yellow bile, black bile), which was believed to be the basic cause of all diseases.

Analogous to the above is another term. It is called 'lack of reaction'. (Also see page - 159: Lack of reaction)

Cachexia (in general): Ars., Badiag., Caps., Chim-umb., Clem., Coccus, Cund., Form., Iod., Kali-bi., Natr-m., Nitr-ac., Seneg.; Africana, Caps.; **bronchitis**, subacute attacks, Phos.; bronchial catarrh of old people, Hydras.; Cinchona, Ferr.; condylomata, of long standing, Kali iod.; catarrhal, or nerve deafness, Syph.; chronic disease, deep-seated progressive, Lyc.; with cough, Nitr.-ac.; debility and emaciation, Iod.; deep-seated, child weak and exhausted, with no other symptoms, Sul-ac.; dry habit, Nux-v.; dysentery, or gout, Colch.; long-lasting cases of intermittent fever when liver is involved and blood is anaemic, Nitr-ac.; disturbance of gastric and hepatic functions, Hydras.; glands enlarged and tender, Kali m.; helminthiasis, Cina; low state, Iod.; mercurial, Aur. met., Ferr. iod., Iod., Kali-m.; nosebleed, Sul-ac.; from faulty nutrition and assimilation, Ferr.; with oedema, Ol. jec.; nervous palpitation, Natr-m.; phosphatic, Calc-p.; purpura, rheumatism, Sec.; quinine, Eucal., Natr-m., Phos.; with stomach and liver troubles, Hydras.; loss of strength, Arg. nit.; caused by a suppression of habitual secretions, and excretions, Graph.; syphilitic eruption, pustular, or squamons, Kali-iod.; weakened by loss of blood, Chin-s.; vomiting, Sul-ac.; ordinary wounds and ulcers tend to take on a bad appearance, Cund.; remains long impressed by slight mechanical injuries, Arn.;

Remedies containing the symptom **cachexia**, dyscrasia among other symptoms are given below:

Top-grade remedies for weakly, cachectic individuals: 1, Arn., Calc., Chin., Natr-m., Nux-v., Phos. ac., Sulph., Veratr.; 2, Ars., Carb-v., Lach., Merc., Phos., Sec., Sep., etc.

Alumen - chronic, non-stopping haemorrhage, particularly bleeding from gums or continuous bleeding from uterus for months and years without a break.

Aranea diadema - scorbutic dyscrasia.

Aranea diadema - suitable to those who cannot live in damp places or on the water; ague dyscrasia, dyspeptics.

Arg-nit. - cachectic states, with loss of strength.

Arg-nit. (Hepatic derangements) - cirrhosis from malaria cachexia

Arnica - malarial cachexia. - swollen, pale, yellow, cachectic, sunken, cold, and covered with sweat. - chronic and dyscratic skin diseases, chorea minor and spasms in scrofulous and anaemic children.

Ars-alb. (Blepharophthalmia, blepharitis) - cachexia, with great restlessness, aggravation after midnight.

Ars-alb. (Haemorrhage from uterus) - tedious, long-continued flooding in feeble cachectic women afflicted with rheumatism, disorganization of uterus or ovaries, with great debility, restlessness and lancinating burning pains.

Ars-alb. (Heart diseases) - cardiac cachexia irritable heart, trembling, irregular action of the heart, intermitting.

Arsenic alb. - man, aged 40, lean, cachectic; drinking spirituous liquors - quotidian for a week.

Asarum europ. (Tuberculosis of lungs) - thin, scrawny, cachectic persons.

Aurum met. (Albuminuria) - mercurial and syphilitic cachexia, swelling of liver, caries. Renal troubles secondary to cardiac affections, causing a decided albinous crasis, passing over into hydraemia.

Aurum met. (Orchitis, and other affections of the testicles) - mercurial cachexia.

Badiaga - general cachectic appearance.

Badiaga (Exophthalmic goitre) - general cachectic appearance.

Badiaga (Syphilis and sycosis) - general cachectic appearance and rhagades here and there.

Baryta carb. - old cachectic people of scrofulous habit, especially when they suffer with gouty complaints.

Borax (Cough) - dry, cachectic cough, especially mornings when rising and in the evening when lying down.

Calc-carb. (Cornea, diseases of) - particularly valuable for corneal ulceration in fat, unhealthy children with a large abdomen who sweat much, especially about the head, and are very susceptible to cold air, also in deep, sloughing ulcers, found in weak, cachectic persons. pains, redness, photophobia, lachrymation are variable with no characteristic eye symptoms.

Capsicum - sea sickness; cholera; cachexia africana; yellow fever; typhus ictorodes.

Carbo-an. (Cancer) - cachexia fully developed. Scirrhous cancer on the forehead.

Carbo-an. (Haemorrhage from uterus) - menorrhagia from chronic induration of uterus, also in cachectic women with glandular affections, cancer, etc.

Carbo-veg. - gangrene: humid; senile; in cachectic persons; when vital powers have become weakened; great foulness of secretions; great prostration.

Carbo-veg. (Gangrene) - senile gangrene humid gangrene in cachectic persons whose vital powers are exhausted.

Carbo-veg. (Jaundice) - jaundice in cachectic or old people.

Carbon-sul. - gout, but not gouty dyscrasia.

Carbon-sul. - herpetic dyscrasia.

Carcinosinum - indigestion, accumulation of gas in stomach and bowels; rheumatism - cancerous cachexia.

Carduus mar. (Asthma) - cachexia of tunnel laborers.

Carduus mar. (Hepatic derangements) - cachexia of miners working deep under ground.

Chimaphila umb. - cachectic and scrofulous individuals.

Chimaphila umb. - woman, aged 26; in a cachectic condition, menses always scanty; scirrhous tumor of breast; the mother of patient had also had scirrhous tumor of breast, necessitating extirpation of gland.

China - young man, pale, cachectic appearance, suffered for ten weeks from quartan ague; enlarged spleen.

China (Morbus addisonii) - yellow, cachectic color of skin, debility., prostration of mind and body.

China-sulph. - cachectic persons weakened by loss of blood.

China-sulph. - intermittent fever in cachectic persons by loss of blood or from continued and long prostration.

Cina - cachexia of helminthiasis.

Cinnamomum - lymphatic, feeble, cachectic women, with lax tissues and languid circulation.

Clematis - torpid, cachectic conditions; swelling and induration of glandular system; syphilitic taint.

Cocculus - man, aged 30, cachectic appearance; colic.

Coffea cruda (Cough) - feels exhausted after coughing, with emaciation and cachectic appearance.

Colchicum - cachectic appearance —dysentery —gout.

Condurango - cachectic state of system, ordinary wounds and ulcers tend to take on a bad appearance.

Corydalis formosa - cancer cachexia pronounced.

Cundurango (Cancer) - hard, knobby, large swelling in pylorus, complete loss of appetite, emaciation, cachectic look, constipation.

Cundurango (Eczema) - cachectic or syphilitic dyscrasia.

Cundurango (Eczema) - chiefly when rhagades are present, oozing out a foetid fluid; cachectic or syphilitic dyscrasia.

Dulcamara - we are indebted to the eclectic school for this remarkable medicine as a "corrector of blood dyscrasia".

Eucalyptus - quinine cachexia.

Eupatorium perf. - cachectic condition of system from long continued or frequent attacks of bilious and intermittent fevers.

Eupatorium perfoliatum - cachexia from old chronic, bilious intermittents.

Ferrum iod. - mercurial cachexia.

Ferr-met. (Chlorosis) - animal food not desired by the appetite and not well borne by the stomach if taken into it; great paleness of face which is very apt to turn suddenly red; dyspnoea, palpitation and blowing murmurs in blood vessels, > by moderate exercise; muscles feeble and easily exhausted; desire for sour or piquant food; mucous membranes very pale; chilly during the day with bright red flushing of the cheeks in the evening; frequent and easy vomiting of ingesta, after eating and from motion which relieves gastrodynia; menses suppressed or profuse, watery, lumpy with labor-pains in abdomen. Indicated also for plump fat women suffering from false plethora, migraine (headache), anaemia, headaches; bruit de diable, paleness of mucous membranes, oedema. Diminution of haemoglobin, no dyscrasia.

Ferrum met. - a cachectic state from faulty nutrition and assimilation.

Fluoric-acid. (Hepatic derangements) - ulceration of liver; ascites from hepatic induration and portal congestion; craves refreshing drinks and is continually hungry; dropsy with feeling of fulness and pressure in epigastrium; ascites from enlarged and indurated liver, in consequence of alcoholic drinks; constipation with haemorrhoids; urine scanty, dark, pungent and foetid; restless sleep; sallow skin; complaints of premature old age, of bummers, in consequence of syphilo-mercurial dyscrasia.

Fluoric-acid. - complaints of old age, also premature old age, in consequence of syphilitic-mercurial dyscrasia.

Formica - watery swellings; dropsy; cachexies.

Graphites (Tumors) - tumors in persons with herpetic dyscrasia; wens, smooth and shining, on scalp; sebaceous cysts, particularly when atheromatous; pus scanty, and smelling like herring brine; sclerosis of connective tissue.

Graphites - dyscrasia, especially when caused by a suppression of habitual secretions and excretions. - Tumors in persons of herpetic dyscrasia; wens, smooth and shining, on scalp; sebaceous cysts, particularly when atheromatous; pus scanty and smelling like herring-brine.

Guaicum (Rheumatism) - follows well after caust. When there are contractions of tendons, drawing the limbs out of shape, < by any attempt at motion, in daytime, > by warmth, particularly where there are well-developed gouty nodosities on the joints; pains in all joints, even in chest; tearing, drawing lancinations; followed by exhaustion; syphilitic and mercurial dyscrasia.

Hydrastis - cachectic persons, with marked disturbance of gastric and hepatic functions. - catarrhal affections: in patients of a cachectic habit. - Emaciation; scrofula; cancer cachexia.

Hydrastis - man, aged 18, cachectic, consumptive appearance; scrofulous ulcers on leg.

Hydrastis (Anaemia) - atony, weakness, faintness and prostration from dyscrasic disorders injuring normal blood-formation; cancer, etc.; emaciation; expression dull; skin sallow, yellowish-white; bad effects from merc.

Hydrastis (Bronchitis chronica) - bronchitis of old people, with great debility, loss of appetite, cachectic state, great weakness.

Hydrastis (Scrofulosis) - cancerous cachexia.

Hydrastis - hydrastis is especially active in old, easily-tired people, cachectic individuals, with great debility.

Iodum - low cachectic condition with profound debility and great emaciation, with feeble pulse; - syphilis: mercurial cachexia; salivation; ulcers in throat; skin and muscles lax; nightly bone pain; very hard chronic buboes.

Iodum (Coryza, snuffles of children) - chronic coryza in cachectic, emaciated children, with enlarged and indurated glands.

Iodum (Jaundice) - dirty, yellowish skin; great emaciation; downcast, irritable mood; yellow, almost dark-brown color of the face; thick coating of the tongue; much thirst; intense canine hunger, with vomiting after eating; frequent eructations; gastralgia; white diarrhoeic stools alternating with constipation; dark, yellowish-green, corroding urine; organic lesions of liver; dyscrasia with hectic fever.

Iodum (Metritis) - low cachectic state of the system, with feeble pulse.

Iodum (Pruritus) - irresistible nocturnal itching, compelling one to scratch and thus causing insomnia, cachectic appearance, emaciation and dyspepsia.

Kali-carb. (Coryza, snuffles of children) - Anaemic in children of cachectic appearance, with puffy swelling over upper eyelids, especially mornings.

Kali-mur. (Cancer) - scurvy in cachectic people.

Kali-bich. - emaciation; anemia; general cachexia.

Kali-carb. (Diarrhoea) - chronic cases in cachectic, dyspeptic persons, with the characteristic puffiness under the eyebrows. Stools light-gray or brownish, corrosive, sometimes painless, < towards morning, with rumbling in bowels, acid eructations and irritable disposition.

Kali-iod. - condylomata of long standing in cachectic subjects.

Kali-nit. - non-stopping coryza from nose or chest catarrh, without intermission.

Kreosotum (Dentition, morbid) - suitable to delicate, cachectic children.

Kreosotum (Hearing, defective) - deafness of children from hereditary syphilitic dyscrasia, hard hearing during menses; stitches and itching in ears; humid tetters in and around ears, swelling of cervical glands; livid gray complexion.

Kreosotum (Leucorrhoea) - especially adapted to a cachectic state during and after climaxis or to blonde, overgrown girls of a sad, irritable disposition.

Kreosotum - girl, aged 9, had snuffles when she was a baby, teeth wedge shaped, very old looking, syphilitic dyscrasia; deafness.

Lachesis - elderly woman, thin and cachectic; phthisis pulmonalis.

Lachesis - lady, aged 43, slim, large, cachectic, scrofulous; intestinal croup.

Lactuca vir. - man, had suffered from blood dyscrasia and affection of brain for years; hydrothorax.

Lycopodium - man, aged 50, thin, cachectic, musician; cramps in stomach.

Lycopodium - woman, aged 50, weak, cachectic, formerly troubled with abdominal complaints and itch, has not menstruated for five years; impairment of hearing.

Lycopodium (Bronchitis chronica) - congestion of liver, flatulency, constipation, cachectic complexion, red gravel, acid dyspepsia.

Manganum oxydatum (Dropsy) - cachexia.

Merc-sol. (Cornea, diseases of) - deep or superficial ulcers or abscesses in pale, flabby, strumous children, with enlarged glands and general scrofulous cachexia.

Merc-sol. (Coxalgia, hip-disease) - cachectic children, sweating from least exertion and pains < after getting warm in bed. First sleep may be easy and quiet, but in a short time the child will wake up crying and unable to go to sleep again for some time.

Merc-sol. - woman, aged 36, no children, two years ago had inflammatory affection of chest, after nursing a cachectic husband; phthisis.

Merc-sol. (Scrofulosis) - cachexia and emaciation.

Mezereum - man, aged 43, nervo-bilious constitution, cachectic habit, leaden colored face, had lived the life of a tramp and had been several times syphilitic; pain and swelling in tibiae.

Mezereum (Scrofulosis) - herpetic dyscrasia; favus, pityriasis, tinea capitis; excoriations in throat and nose; joints feel bruised, weary, as if they would give way; engorged glands; abscesses of fibrous parts or of tendons; bones inflamed, swollen, especially shafts of cylindrical bones, which may feel distended.

Muriatic acid - woman, aged 60, unmarried, cachectic, has an eruption on lower limbs; typhoid fever.

Natrum mur. - adapted to cachectic persons and to those who have lost animal fluids; quinine cachexia. - cachexia from ague plus quinine.

Natrum mur. (Anaemia) - malarious cachexia.

Natrum mur. (Chlorosis) - chronic malaria in cachectic persons with dead, dirty, withered skin.

Natrum mur. (Hepatic derangements) - malarial cachexia.

Natrum mur. (Rheumatism) - chronic articular rheumatism, based on some dyscrasia (malaria); symptoms < forenoon; intermittent irregular heart's action and pulse; copious sweat with great relief; pains fixed (Sep., wandering and no thirst); sleeplessness; peevishness > towards evening; paralytic-like weakness of legs; tingling in limbs, especially on tips of fingers and toes, emaciation even while living well.

Natrum sulph. - man, aged 43, middle height, father of two healthy children, blonde hair, grey eyes, gonorrhoeal cachexia, hydrogenoid constitution; diabetes.

Nitric-acid. (Dyspepsia, weakness of stomach) - intestinal dyspepsia based upon mercurial or syphilitic cachexia.

Nitric-acid. (Haemorrhage from uterus) - absence of pain, copious flooding kept up by ulcers on os uteri, especially in cachectic women.

Nitric-acid. - diseases depending upon presence of syphilitic, scrofulous or mercurial poison; broken down, cachectic constitutions. - Due to syphilis, scrofula, intermittent fever with liver involvement and anaemia, etc.

Nux vom. - man, aged 48, yellow skin, cachectic appearance, small stature, suffering three years; cardialgia.

Nux vom. - man, aged 75; sickly, cachectic; extravasation of blood into conjunctiva.

Nux vom. - mania puerperalis from excitement, sleeplessness and prostration; had menorrhagia, and for the subsequent weakness drank much whisky and strong coffee; cachectic appearance.

Oleum jec. - rheumatism of long standing; patient confined to bed or room, and only in warm summer months experienced a slight alleviation of her sufferings; nearly whole body was attacked, but principally inferior extremities, sacrum, back and shoulders; walking was entirely prevented by the insupportable pains, stiffness and swelling of joints; a kind of hectic fever and constant nightly exacerbations destroyed all repose; patient was wasted, of a bleachy whiteness, of a cachetic appearance and habit, and had lost all hope of relief. - Scrofulosis: diseases of joints; in pale, thin cachectic subjects.

Phosphoric acid. (Albuminuria) - great torpor, melanotic dyscrasia, similar to scurvy and stupid typhoids; the heart relaxed, dilated, with thin walls; atheroma of the arteries, petechiae; insidious appearance of the renal degeneration, carelessness and apathy, perfect prostration, with low delirium, neither hunger nor thirst, nausea and vomiting, bleeding gums; urine contains much phosphates, fibrinous casts and epithelial cells, fatty corpuscles, rarely carbonate of ammonia, and never much alben; costiveness or light-yellow diarrhoea, no fever or heat; cool wrinkled skin, cool breath, cool sweat.

Phosphorus - glands enlarged, especially after contusions; glandular affections in weak cachectic individuals suffering from diarrhoea and colliquative sweats. - Suitable to young people with blonde hair, blue eyes, delicate skin, slender stature, with cachectic cough, diarrhoea, frequent exhausting sweats, great debility, with orgasm of blood; palpitation of heart or oppression of chest after exercise; copious stools, pouring away like water from a hydrant, with great exhaustion; glandular swellings, suppuration; appetite good; craves cold food, ice cream, etc

Phosphorus (Atrophy of children) - even thus early diarrhoea associated with dry cough, hence suitable to young girls with blonde hair, blue eyes, delicate skin, slender stature, with cachectic cough, diarrhoea.

Phosphorus (Bronchitis chronica) - subacute attacks of bronchitis in emaciated, cachectic, or young overgrown invalids.

Platina - woman, aged 38, cachectic appearance, suffering for two years; dysmenorrhoea.

Plumb-met. - deep melancholy, with timidity and restlessness; anxiety at heart, with sighing and trembling; dislikes to talk or work; maniacal rage, with cries and convulsions; absence of mind; stupidity; pale, miserable, cachectic appearance; somnolency; colic.

Plumbum met. (Insanity) - pale, miserable, cachectic appearance, colic, dry skin, dry short cough, sleeplessness or somnolency. Cirrhosis renalis.

Plumbum met. - Pale and cachetic.

Podophyllum - man, aged 33, cachectic appearance, liver or spleen or both disordered; asthma.

Prunus-sp. - dropsy caused by defective heart; abdominal dropsy; anasarca after any debilitating, chronic diseases, and particularly in those connected with cachectic affections.

Pulsatilla - woman, aged 26, yellow, cachectic appearance, suffering six months; vertigo.

Sarsaparilla (Albuminuria) - syphilitic taint, mercurial poisoning, scrofula, cachectic states from hepatic diseases or rheumatism.

Secale - feeble, cachectic women; thin, scrawny. - passive hemorrhage; blood dark and red, in feeble and cachectic persons, accompanied by tingling in limbs and prostration; desire for air; does not like to be covered; wishes to have limbs extended; skin cold.

Secale - rheumatism (peliosis rheumatica of schoenlein) generally is found in cachectic individuals, with purpura; affects joints, especially of lower extremities; thrombosis of abdominal vessels.

Secale - woman, aged 40, mother of seven children, weak, cachectic looking, suffering from prolapsus uteri; hysteria.

Secale (Ecthyma) - cachectic females with rough skin.

Secale (Haemorrhage from uterus) - painless flooding in feeble, cachectic, dyscratic women, or who have long resided in tropical climates.

Secale (Haemorrhage from uterus) - painless flooding in feeble, cachectic, dyscratic women, or who have long resided in tropical climates; general coldness, while the patient feels too warm and does not wish to be covered; feverish pulse; haemorrhage passive, dark-colored and continuous, seldom clotted, sometimes offensive, and the slightest motion aggravates the flow, particularly where the weakness is not caused by loss of blood. Haemorrhage, with strong and spasmodic contraction of the uterus, every flow preceded by strong, bearing-down pains; haemorrhage from atony of the uterus, especially after protracted labor or miscarriage, aggravated by the slightest motion; menses usually too profuse and too long-lasting, with spasms and mental depression or melancholy.

Secale - passive haemorrhages in feeble cachectic women.

Senega - subacute or chronic exudations of pleura, catarrhal pleuropneumonia (after bry) in cachectic pleuritis, in hydrothorax, oedema pulmonum, in diseases of heart, primary and secondary anasarca; in dropsies after albuminuria; hydrophthalmia with intraocular compression; in ascites accompanying hepatic diseases, peritonitis and abdominal tumors; in lymphatic constitutions with tendency to mucous and serous exudations.

Silicea - n, aged 12, cachectic and anemic; fistulae of thigh.

Silicea (Asthma) - asthma on a cachectic base, after its removal gummatous nodes on skull, clavicles and ribs.

Silicea (Prosopalgia) - face pale, cachectic.

Silicea-tumors in persons with herpetic dyscrasia; wens smooth and shining on scalp; sebaceous cysts, particularly when atheromatous; pus scanty and smelling like herringbrine.

Spongia - boy, aged 4, scrofulous, cachectic-looking; croup.

Squilla (Bedwetting in children) - especially for strumous or cachectic children who are troubled with worms.

Squilla (Urinary difficulties) - especially for strumous and cachectic children who are troubled with worms.

Sulphur - girl, aged 12, delicate, cachectic; vaginitis.

Sulphur - girl, aged 8, cachectic-looking; coxalgia of spine.

Sulphur (Epilepsy) - whenever some dyscrasia lurks in the system, or its outward symptoms were suppressed; chronic epilepsy; before the spell crawling and running as from a mouse down the back and arms, or up the leg to the right side of the abdomen; after the convulsions soporous sleep and great exhaustion; onanism.

Sulphur (Laryngitis and laryngeal phthisis) - arterial and venous vascular irritability; great impressionability of the skin and for diverse dyscrasiae as an interpolating remedy; hoarseness, voice very deep or aphonia, < mornings.

Sulphur (Sciatica) - neuralgia cruralis; subacute sciatica from some dyscrasia in organism; pain in small of back, stitching-drawing on rising from a seat; tensive pain in hip-joint, especially left one; drawing down the limb, accompanied by a bruised sensation; heavy feeling of affected limb and numbness as if paralyzed, < when walking; increase of pain at night from the warmth of bed; more or less rigidity of the knees; swelling of feet in chronic cases.

Sulphuric acid. (Dyspepsia, weakness of stomach) - vomiting of drunkards, of cachectic persons, going into steady decline.

Sulphuric acid. (Haemophilic, bleeders) - haemorrhages of black blood from all the outlets of the body; great exhaustion and debility from deep-seated dyscrasia.

Sulphuric acid. (Lienitis) - spleen enlarged, hard and painful, when coughing; diarrhoea with great debility, haemorrhage of black blood from all outlets of body (Crotal.); weak and exhausted from some deep-seated dyscrasia.

Sulphuric acid. - weak and exhausted from deep-seated dyscrasia. when some deep-seated dyscrasia prevails, the child weak and exhausted, with no other symptoms.

Thuja occidentalis - the main action of thuja is on the skin and genitourinary organs producing conditions that correspond with hahnemann's sycotic dyscrasia whose chief manifestation is the formation of wart-like excrescences upon mucous and cutaneous surfaces-fig-warts and condylomata.

Zincum met. - syphilitic-mercurial-scrofulous dyscrasia.

Diseases associated with 'cachexia' or 'dyscrasia'

(Albuminuria) Aur-met. - interstitial nephritis; contracted kidney, marked cardiac hypertrophy; mercurial and syphilitic cachexia, swelling of liver, caries. Renal troubles secondary to cardiac affections, causing a decided albinous crasis, passing over into hydraemia; at first the urine is increased in quantity, later it becomes scanty and albinous; bloated, shining face; vertigo as if he would fall to the left side; bruised pain in head and confusion in thinking, dyspnoea, palpitations.

(Albuminuria) Phosphoric acid. - great torpor, melanotic dyscrasia, similar to scurvy and stupid typhoids; the heart relaxed, dilated, with thin walls; atheroma of the arteries, petechiae; insidious appearance of the renal degeneration, carelessness and apathy, perfect prostration, with low delirium, neither hunger nor thirst, nausea and vomiting, bleeding gums; urine contains much phosphates, fibrinous casts and epithelial cells, fatty corpuscles, rarely carbonate of ammonia, and never much alben; costiveness or light-yellow diarrhoea, no fever or heat; cool wrinkled skin, cool breath, cool sweat.

(Albuminuria) Sarsaparilla - syphilitic taint, mercurial poisoning, scrofula, cachectic states from hepatic diseases or rheumatism; cloudiness of head; dim sight, as if looking through a mist; aphthae; frequent and copious micturition of pale urine, depositing a sediment; frequent desire, but scanty urination; foetid breath; dyspnoea; tearing in almost all the joints and limbs; great weakness; languid feeling; emaciation.

(Amenorrhoea.) For debilitated or cachectic individuals - Alet., Ars., Chin., Cyprip., Con., Graph., Helon., Iod., Natr-m., Puls., Polyg., Sep., Sulph.

(Anaemia) Hydrastis - atony, weakness, faintness and prostration from dyscrasic disorders of normal blood-formation; cancer, etc.

Emaciation; expression dull; skin sallow, yellowish-white; bad effects from Merc.

(Anaemia.) Natrum mur. - blood impoverished; anaemia from loss of fluids; malarious cachexia; emaciation; skin harsh, dry, yellow; great exhaustion from any little exertion of mind or body; palpitation, with sensation as if a bird's wing were fluttering in left chest; pressure and distension of stomach; constipation, with contraction of anus; terrible sadness.

(Asthma) Carduus mar. - nervous asthma of miners; cachexia of tunnel laborers; frequent urging to deep breathing, followed by painful sensations in abdomen; great debility; loss of appetite; empty eructations; restless, dreamy sleep; fulness of hypochondria which are painful to pressure.

(Asthma) Silicea - asthma on a cachectic base, after its removal gummatous nodes on skull, clavicles and ribs; shortness of breath and panting from walking fast and from manual labor; dyspnoea when at rest or when lying on back; oppression of chest, cannot take a long breath, cannot bear the slightest draught on the back of his neck, spasmodic cough, with spasm of larynx; catarrh of aged people.

(Atrophy of children) Phosphorus - emaciation combined with nervous debility; brain and spine suffered severely; child over tall, but slender, emaciated but big-bellied; face pale, almost waxen. Delicate eyelashes, soft hair, rapid breathing hint to sequelae; even thus early diarrhoea associated with dry cough, hence suitable to young girls with blonde hair, blue eyes, delicate skin, slender stature, with cachectic cough, diarrhoea; frequent exhausting sweats; great debility, with orgasm of the blood; palpitation of the heart or oppression of the chest after exercise. Copious stools, pouring away like water from a hydrant, with great exhaustion; glandular swellings, suppuration and caries (Sil.); appetite good; he craves cold food, ice cream; often awakens at night, hot and restless, and will drop off to sleep if fed; child irascible, vehement, susceptible to external impressions and to electric changes in atmosphere.

(Bedwetting in children) Squilla - especially for strumous or cachectic children who are troubled with worms; inability to retain the urine on account of abnormal irritation of the lining membrane of the bladder, often of rheumatic origin.

(Blepharophthalmia, blepharitis) Ars-alb. - burning in the oedematous swollen lids; lachrymation profuse, hot and acrid, excoriating the lids and cheek; cachexia, with great restlessness, aggravation after midnight; thirst, etc.

(Bronchitis chronica) Hydrastis - bronchitis of old people, with great debility, loss of appetite, cachectic state, great weakness; chronic cough, accompanied by febrile paroxysms evenings and night, and excessive prostration; sputa thick, yellowish, very tenacious, stringy and profuse; dry, hard cough with much laryngeal irritation, or loose but hard cough with much nasopharyngeal catarrh and marked prostration.

(Bronchitis chronica) Lycopodium - distressing, fatiguing, tickling cough, < afternoon, and evening, and on going to sleep and in the morning; chronic bronchitis, with copious muco-serous or mucopurulent sputa; congestion of liver, flatulency, constipation, cachectic complexion, red gravel, acid dyspepsia; dry cough, day and night, in feeble emaciated boys (florid scrofula); emphysema, dilation of air-tubes and senile catarrh; respiration short before and during cough, ending with loud belching; salty expectoration; emaciation of upper part of body; great fear of solitude.

(Bronchitis chronica) Phosphorus - subacute attacks of bronchitis in emaciated, cachectic, or young overgrown invalids; bronchopulmonary catarrhs from dilatation or fatty degeneration of the heart. Cough abrupt, rough, sharp, dry;

between each coughing spell a short interval; dry, tickling cough in the evening, with tightness across the chest and expectoration in the morning; pain in chest when coughing, relieved by external pressure; trembling of the whole body while coughing; cough gets worse when other people come into the room; tingling, soreness and rawness in the air-passages; dry cough, with expectoration of viscid or bloody mucus. Dilatation of the bronchi.

(Cancer) Carbo an. - cachexia fully developed. Scirrhous cancer on the forehead; sudden and short aching from colloid cancer in the pit of the stomach, on taking a deep inspiration, clawing and griping in stomach; violent pressing in loins, small of back and thighs during menses, with chilliness and yawning; weak, empty feeling in the pit of the stomach; it checks the putrid taste, the waterbrash, and contracting, spasmodic burning; scirrhus mammae with dirty bluish, loose skin or red spots on skin, burning and drawing towards axilla; axillary glands indurated.

(Cancer) Cundurango - most efficacious in open cancer or cancerous ulcers, where it effectually moderates the severity of the pain; epithelial cancer on lower eyelid, on left side of nose; cancer of lip, an unclean and sinuous ulcer, with surrounding hardness and swelling, burning pains, lip inverted; painful cracks at the angle of the mouth; ulcer on chin, perforating the gums; lumps on chin; cancer of tongue; cancer of stomach, severe pains, vomiting of coffee-ground masses; hard, knobby, large swelling in pylorus, complete loss of appetite, emaciation, cachectic look, constipation; scirrhus mammae, whole breast, skin and axillary glands; tumor hard, immovable, with severe lancinating pains, nipple retracted; skin purple in spots and wrinkled: ulceration with foetid sanious discharge and much sloughing.

(Cancer) Kali mur. - epithelioma of lip; ulceration of mouth has perforated cheeks and threatens to become cancer of the face; discharge ichorous and foetid; scurvy in cachectic people.

(Chlorosis) Ferr-met. - animal food not desired by the appetite and not well borne by the stomach if taken into it; great paleness of face which is very apt to turn suddenly red; dyspnoea, palpitation and blowing murmurs in bloodvessels, > by moderate exercise; muscles feeble and easily exhausted; desire for sour or piquant food; mucous membranes very pale; chilly during the day with bright red flushing of the cheeks in the evening; frequent and easy vomiting of ingesta, after eating and from motion which relieves gastrodynia; menses suppressed or profuse, watery, lumpy with labor-pains in abdomen. Indicated also for plump fat women suffering from false plethora, migraine (headache), anaemia, headaches; bruit de diable, paleness of mucous membranes, oedema. Diminution of haemoglobin, no dyscrasia.

(Chlorosis) Natrum mur. - chronic malaria in cachectic persons with dead, dirty, withered skin; palpitation and fluttering of heart; dyspnoea; splenitic stitches; suppressed menses, leucorrhoea; diminished sexual desire; sadness; gets easily tired, > towards evening; sad and tearful disposition.

(Cornea, diseases of) Calc-carb - particularly valuable for corneal ulceration in fat, unhealthy children with a large abdomen who sweat much, especially about the head, and are very susceptible to cold air, also in deep, sloughing ulcers, found in weak, cachectic persons. Pains, redness, photophobia, lachrymation are variable with no characteristic eye symptoms; pus is mostly bland and the opacity of cornea milky white or bluish. Calc-ars. Ought to be remembered.

(Cornea, diseases of) Merc-dulcis - deep or superficial ulcers or abscesses in pale, flabby, strumous children, with enlarged glands and general scrofulous cachexia.

(Coryza, snuffles of children) Iodum - chronic coryza in cachectic, emaciated children, with enlarged and indurated glands; nose painful and swollen, with foetid secretions, which at times become a clear and continuous stream; discharge hot.

(Coryza, snuffles of children) Kali-carb. Anaemic children of cachectic appearance, with puffy swelling over upper eyelids, especially mornings; cannot breathe through nostrils in a warm room, > in open air; nostrils raw and bleeding; profuse, foetid, yellow-green discharge.

(Cough) Borax - dry, cachectic cough, especially mornings when rising and in the evening when lying down; with stitching pain in upper part of right chest and right flank, > by pressure; washing the chest with cold water affords most relief; pains < after wine; violent dry cough with sticking pain in region of right nipple, has to press the chest with both hands, occasionally raises small white or yellow lumps of a mouldy odor. Cough after cold bathing.

(Cough) Coffea cruda - dry, hacking cough, like whooping-cough, but spasms are more felt during inspirations; short, dry cough, as from constriction of larynx; during cough stitches in side, anxiety, dimness before eyes and vertigo; < during evening to midnight, when falling asleep or soon after; during measles; irritation to cough, out-doors; feels exhausted after coughing, with emaciation and cachectic appearance.

(Coxalgia, hip-disease) Merc. - first and second stage, worse at night, restlessness and inclination to sweat; sharp stitching flashes through the joint, acute stitches in right ileum, boring pain in glutei; burning of nates; tearing pain in hip-joint, knee and femur, worse during motion; limbs feel stiff when walking; involuntary twitching of limbs; pain in right thigh as if bruised, worse after walking, suppuration seems inevitable; cachectic children, sweating from least exertion and pains < after getting warm in bed. first sleep may be easy and quiet, but in a short time the child will wake up crying and unable to go to sleep again for some time; eruptions on different parts of body.

(Dentition, morbid) Kreosotum - suitable to delicate, cachectic children; very painful, difficult dentition, < during whole night, so that the child gets little sleep and wants to be petted all the time; protruding gums filled with a dark, watery fluid, bluish-red, very painful and bleed easily; swelling of gum over a tooth which is not quite through causes convulsions; teeth, as seen through the gums, dark and show specks of decay down to the gums; teeth decay almost as soon as they appear; constipation, stools very hard and dry, or diarrhoea with dark-brown, watery, very offensive stools, very exhausting, excoriating, containing sometimes portions of undigested food; > after a good sleep.

(Diarrhoea) Kali-carb. - chronic cases in cachectic, dyspeptic persons, with the characteristic puffiness under the eyebrows. Stools light-gray or brownish, corrosive, sometimes painless, < towards morning, with rumbling in bowels, acid eructations and irritable disposition; colicky pains before and during stool, and burning at anus after. Desire for acids and sugar; aversion to rye-bread; much weariness with a desire to lie down.

(Dropsy) Manganum oxydatum - ascites from intermittent fever; cachexia; strong, irregular, trembling palpitation of the heart, without abnormal sounds.

(Dyspepsia, weakness of stomach) Nitric-acid. - intestinal dyspepsia based upon mercurial or syphilitic cachexia;

cadaverous smell from mouth; ulcers on tongue, with tough, ropy mucus; saliva foetid, acrid, corroding lips; longing for fat, herrings, chalk, lime, aversion to meat and drink; milk disagrees; nausea better from moving about or carriage-riding; bitter and sour vomiting, with much eructation; pain in cardiac orifice on swallowing food; abdomen distended with flatulence, very tender; painless constipation for several days, stools hard, preceded by great pressure and followed by mucous discharges; lancinating pains in rectum after stool, following even a soft stool; painful haemorrhoids, prolapsing with every stool, with loss of blood.

(Dyspepsia, weakness of stomach) Sulphuric-acid. - stomach rejects water, unless it is mixed with brandy; craving for alcoholic stimulants; vomiting of drunkards, of cachectic persons, going into steady decline; stomach feels relaxed and cold; excessive secretion of gastric mucosities rising up into the mouth, rendering teeth dull by their acidity; sour vomit, first water, then food; debilitating diarrhoea, yellow stringy stools, having a chopped appearance.

(Ecthyma) Secale cornutum - cachectic females with rough skin; black pustules with tendency to gangrene; < in warmth, > in cold weather.

(Eczema) Cundurango - chiefly when rhagades are present, oozing out a foetid fluid; cachectic or syphilitic dyscrasia.

(Epilepsy) Sulphur - whenever some dyscrasia lurks in the system, or its outward symptoms were suppressed; chronic epilepsy; before the spell crawling and running as from a mouse down the back and arms, or up the leg to the right side of the abdomen; after the convulsions soporous sleep and great exhaustion; onanism.

(Gangrene) Carbo-veg. - senile gangrene humid gangrene in cachectic persons whose vital powers are exhausted; great foulness of the secretions; great prostration; sepsis;

indifference; fainting after sleep, while yet in bed, morning; no restlessness.

(Haemophillic, bleeders) Sulphuric-acid. - haemorrhages of black blood from all the outlets of the body; great exhaustion and debility from deep-seated dyscrasia.

(Haemorrhage from uterus) Carbo-an. - menses too early, not too profuse, but last too long; great weakness of the thighs. After the appearance of the menses she feels so tired she is scarcely able to speak; menorrhagia from chronic induration of uterus, also in cachectic women with glandular affections, cancer, etc.; blood black, clotted, putrid.

(Haemorrhage from uterus) Ars-alb. - tedious, long-continued flooding in feeble cachectic women afflicted with rheumatism, disorganization of uterus or ovaries, with great debility, restlessness and lancinating burning pains; uterus larger and softer than usual, with dilated capillaries; aphthae in mouth indicate the low state of the system, the least effort exhausts her; chronic endometritis and passive hyperaemia, based on atony.

(Haemorrhage from uterus) For passive haemorrhage in debilitated cachectic subjects: 1, Chin., Croc., Puls., Sec., Sep., Sulph.; 2, Capsella, Bursa Pastoris, Carb-v., Nux-v., Ipec., Phos., Ruta, Veratr.; 3, Alet., Cauloph., Cimicif., Trill., Ust.

(Haemorrhage from uterus) Nitric-acid - uterine haemorrhage from overexertion of body; long-lasting cases; absence of pain, copious flooding kept up by ulcers on os uteri, especially in cachectic women; blood rather fluid from loss of plasticity; asthenia. After miscarriage or confinement, with violent pressure, as if everything would come out of the vulva, with pain in small of back and down through the hips to thighs.

(Haemorrhage from uterus) Secale - painless flooding in feeble, cachectic, dyscratic women, or who have long resided in tropical climates; general coldness, while the patient feels too warm and does not wish to be covered; feverish pulse; haemorrhage passive, dark-colored and continuous, seldom clotted, sometimes offensive, and the slightest motion aggravates the flow, particularly where the weakness is not caused by loss of blood. Haemorrhage, with strong and spasmodic contraction of the uterus, every flow preceded by strong, bearing-down pains; haemorrhage from atony of the uterus, especially after protracted labor or miscarriage, aggravated by the slightest motion; menses usually too profuse and too long-lasting, with spasms and mental depression or melancholy.

(Hearing, defective) Kreosotum - deafness of children from hereditary syphilitic dyscrasia, hard hearing during menses; stitches and itching in ears; humid tetters in and around ears, swelling of cervical glands; livid gray complexion.

(Heart diseases) Ars-alb. - cardiac cachexia irritable heart.

(Hepatic derangements) Arg-nit. - cirrhosis from malaria cachexia; stitches in liver, coming on as with a jerk; peculiar fulness in liver, painful, with occasional drawing and stinging, especially when walking, sometimes reaching into the chest; periodical dull stitches in the anterior surface of the liver; hepatic affection, ending in fatal dropsy; pigmentary degeneration, the fever may be stopped but the degeneration remains.

(Hepatic derangements) Carduus mar. - cachexia of miners working deep under ground; portal hyperaemia; gall-stones; catarrh of the biliary ducts; hepatic region sensitive to pressure, stitching, drawing pain in liver, < by pressure and lying on left side. Dropsical diseases, depending on organic affections of liver, frequently of long standing; jaundice, with dull headache, bitter taste, tongue white in centre, tips and edges red; nausea with vomiting of an acrid green fluid, stools pasty, clayey, urine golden-yellow. Implication of the lungs, showing itself by haemoptysis; vomiting of blood.

(Hepatic derangements) Fluoric-acid. - ulceration of liver; ascites from hepatic induration and portal congestion; craves refreshing drinks and is continually hungry; dropsy with feeling of fullness and pressure in epigastrium; ascites from enlarged and indurated liver, in consequence of alcoholic drinks; constipation with haemorrhoids; urine scanty, dark, pungent and foetid; restless sleep; sallow skin; complaints of premature old age, of bummers, in consequence of syphilo-mercurial dyscrasia.

(Hepatic derangements) Natrum mur. - malarial cachexia; dull, heavy aching and distention about liver after eating, > as digestion advances; stitches and tension in liver, skin yellow, earthy; obstinate constipation; short breathing, palpitations; stitches in spleen, < with every motion; paretic feeling in upper and lower extremities; < in summer and in thunderstorms.

(Insanity) Plumbum met. - deep melancholy, with timidity, restlessness, anxiety at the heart, with sighing and trembling; imagines he hears voices and thinks he is to be shot or poisoned (Lach., Rhus, Veratr vir., fear of being poisoned), sees frightful things which chase him out of bed; dislike to talk or to work; maniacal rage with cries, brawling and convulsions; absence of mind, stupidity; pale, miserable, cachectic appearance, colic, dry skin, dry short cough, sleeplessness or somnolency. Cirrhosis renalis.

(Jaundice) Carbo-veg. - hepatic region very sensitive and painful to touch, clothing unendurable, pain and tenseness in hypochondria; flatulent colic < from least food; stools of ashy-gray color; dark-red, bloody-looking urine; loathing of meat, butter, fat; jaundice in cachectic or old people

(Jaundice) Iodum - dirty, yellowish skin; great emaciation; downcast, irritable mood; yellow, almost dark-brown color of the face; thick coating of the tongue; much thirst; intense canine hunger, with vomiting after eating; frequent eructations; gastralgia; white diarrhoeic stools alternating with constipation; dark, yellowish-green, corroding urine; organic lesions of liver; dyscrasia with hectic fever

(Laryngitis and laryngeal phthisis) Sulphur - arterial and venous vascular irritability; great impressionability of the skin and for diverse dyscrasiae as an interpolating remedy; hoarseness, voice very deep or aphonia, < mornings.

(Leucorrhoea) - With cachectic appearance, and organic diseases of uterus and neighboring organs: Ars., Ars.-iod., Carb.-v., Graph., Kreos., Merc., Sulph.

(Leucorrhoea) Kreosotum - leucorrhoea, like menses, inclined to be intermittent, discharge nearly ceases, when, without cause, it reappears as bad as ever; discharge bland or acrid; before and after menses, especially when standing, hardly any when sitting or lying down; discharge of blood and mucus in the morning when getting up; acrid, yellowish-white leucorrhoea, with great itching at vulva; milky leucorrhoea, acrid leucorrhoea, leaving yellow spots on linen and stiffening it like starch, flesh-colored discharge, having a foul smell; yellow, offensive and acrid discharge with itching, biting, smarting and burning in pudendum, between labia and thighs; stitches in vagina from above downward, causing her to start; frequent urging to urinate, preceded by a white discharge from vagina, which colors her clothes yellow; ineffectual urging to urinate, and when accomplished is accompanied by chilliness and milky leucorrhoea; great debility, every little exertion throws her into a profuse sweat; white, painless leucorrhoea, smelling like fresh green corn, flowing like the menses, with pain in back and flushes of heat in face; especially adapted to a cachectic state during and after climaxis or to blonde, overgrown girls of a sad, irritable disposition.

(Lienitis) Sulphuric-acid. - spleen enlarged, hard and painful, when coughing; diarrhoea with great debility, haemorrhage of black blood from all outlets of body (Crotal.); weak and exhausted from some deep-seated dyscrasia.

(Mercury, ill effects of) The ill effects of mercury and sulphur together require: Bell., Puls., or even Merc. - antidotes to mercurial cachexia: Asa., Aur., Chin., Chionanth., Hep., Iod., Kali iod., Mez.

(Metritis) Iodum - acute pain in mammae, developed by the metritis; the mammae very sore; low cachectic state of the system, with feeble pulse.

(Morbus addisonii) China - yellow, cachectic color of skin, debility, prostration of mind and body; aversion to labor; irritability with excessive debility of nervous system; coldness and trembling and extremities, dimness of sight and surring in ears, fainting, restless sleep, nausea, anorexia, vomiting, gastric and abdominal pains with constipation or diarrhoea; dull, stitching pains in renal region; hydraemia (Chin. ars. and Chin. Sulph. or Mur.).

(Morbus basedowi) Badiaga - eyeballs tender, felt even when closing lids firmly; tremulous, vibrating palpitation upon slightest mental emotion; lying on right side heart is heard and felt to pulsate from chest up to neck; indurated and enlarged glands; general cachectic appearance; dullness and dizziness of head; restless at night, must often change position, body feels so sore.

(Orchitis, and other affections of the testicles) Aur-met. - atrophy, testes mere pendent shreds, especially in pining boys; chronic induration of testes, especially of right one; sensation as if a knife were drawn through the swollen testicle; pressive pain when touched or rubbed, as from a bruise; itching of scrotum; mercurial cachexia.

(Pemphigus) - a cachexia, with bullae on shin: Ars., Bell., Calc., Canth., Caust., Chin., Dulc., Gamb., Hep., Hydrocot., Jugl., Lach., Merc., Nitr-ac., Phos., Ran., Rhus, Sep., Sulph., Sulph-ac., Thuj.; Ars. and Lach. in chronic cases, the latter especially in old people; Ars. and Hydrocot. Sometimes in weekly alternation.

(Phthisis pulmonum) Asarum europ. - constant short, hacking cough; always sick, always cold, and shrinking from the cold; < in dry, cold weather, > in damp weather, frequent dull stitches in both lungs; thin, scrawny, cachectic persons.

(Prosopalgia) Silicea - dental nerves especially affected, pains more in jawbones than teeth; jaw swollen; toothache, < after being a short time in bed; gums very sore, inflamed; face pale, cachectic; restless and fidgety, starting at least noise; inveterate intermitting neuralgia.

(Pruritus) Iodum - papules that are very apt to run together or around which the skin is brownish and covered with scales; irresistible nocturnal itching, compelling one to scratch and thus causing insomnia, cachectic appearance, emaciation and dyspepsia.

(Rheumatism) Guaicum - follows well after Caust. when there are contractions of tendons, drawing the limbs out of shape, < by any attempt at motion, in daytime, > by warmth, particularly where there are well-developed gouty nodosities on the joints; pains in all joints, even in chest; tearing, drawing lancinating; followed by exhaustion; syphilitic and mercurial dyscrasia.

(Rheumatism) Natrum mur. - chronic articular rheumatism, based on some dyscrasia (malaria); symptoms < forenoon;

intermittent irregular heart's action and pulse; copious sweat with great relief; pains fixed (Sep., wandering and no thirst); sleeplessness; peevishness > towards evening; paralytic-like weakness of legs; tingling in limbs, especially on tips of fingers and toes, emaciation even while living well.

(Sciatica) Sulphur - neuralgia cruralis; subacute sciatica from some dyscrasia in organism; pain in small of back, stitching-drawing on rising from a seat; tensive pain in hip-joint, especially left one; drawing down the limb, accompanied by a bruised sensation; heavy feeling of affected limb and numbness as if paralyzed, < when walking; increase of pain at night from the warmth of bed; more or less rigidity of the knees; swelling of feet in chronic cases.

(Scrofulosis) Hydrastis - chronic catarrhs of mucous membranes wherever situated; constipation from weakened and congestive state of the lower bowel; cancerous cachexia; cancers hard, adherent; skin mottled, puckered, with lancinating cutting pains; atony of muscles.

(Scrofulosis) Merc-sol. - scrofulosis in children with unusually large heads and open fontanelles, particularly anterior ones; child is slow in learning to walk, teeth form imperfectly and slowly, and a damp, clammy feeling about limbs; offensive, oily perspiration on head; enlarged glands, with or without suppuration; cachexia and emaciation; exostosis, curvature, caries and other affections of bones; eruptions and corrosive herpes with crusts; tinea capitis; crusts in the face; ophthalmia, otitis, otorrhoea, coryza; slimy diarrhoea; suppuration, especially if too profuse; grayish ulcers on mouth and fauces; ulceration of tonsils; false membranes grayish, thick, with shredlike borders, adherent or free, but of marked consistence.

(Scrofulosis) Mezereum - herpetic dyscrasia; favus, pityriasis, tinea capitis; excoriations in throat and nose; joints feel bruised, weary, as if they would give way; engorged glands; abscesses of fibrous parts or of tendons; bones inflamed, swollen, especially shafts of cylindrical bones, which may feel distended.

(Syphilis and sycosis) Bądiaga - syphilis of infants, whole convolutes of hard, glandular swellings; bubo, left groin, hard, unequal, like scirrhus, violent burning stitches during night; chancres suppressed by cautery or mercurial ointment, leaving elevated, discolored cicatrices; general cachectic appearance and rhagades here and there; indurated, maltreated buboes.

(Tumors) Graphites - tumors in persons with herpetic dyscrasia; wens, smooth and shining, on scalp; sebaceous cysts, particularly when atheromatous; pus scanty, and smelling like herring brine; sclerosis of connective tissue.

(Ulcers) For atonic ulcers, as we find them among old, feeble, and cachectic persons, especially on the legs, ulcera atonica pedum: 1, Ars., Lach., Sil., Sulph.; 2, Calc., Carb-v., Graph., Ipec., Lyc., Mur-ac., Natr., Phos-ac., Puls., Ruta; 3, Amm., Amm-m., Fluor-ac., Nux-j.; 4, Aral., Bapt., Lycopus, Polyg.

(Urinary difficulties) Squilla - especially for strumous and cachectic children who are troubled with worms; inability to retain the urine on account of an abnormal irritation of the lining membrane of bladder, often of rheumatic origin; frequent urging to urinate, with profuse discharge of pale, limpid urine; continuous painful pressure on bladder.

Lack of reaction—Low vitality—When the indicated remedy fails to act

'When the indicated remedy fails' shakes the very foundation of homoeopathy and confidence of homeopath as well.

It is quite often when an indicated remedy fails and the homeopaths gives another constitutional or antimiasmatic drug, they profess that the later drug enhanced the action of the previous remedy. However this is not applicable all the time. Moreover, this is not at all 'lack of reaction'.

Most homoeopaths prescribe Aloe/Podophyllum for diarrhoea in a routine way and in most cases it acts, though may not be the correctly indicated remedy—the *similimum*. We do give wrong remedies (thinking it to be the similimum) and it gives relief to the patient, but we do come across case where routinism fails—that is the real challenge to learn homoeopathy in a better way.

In the remedy Amm-carb. (Boericke's Materia Medica) under the section skin we read "faintly developed eruptions with defective vitality". The correct meaning for this is: If a skin patient needs Amm-carb. no other homoeo remedy, nor best allopathic, ayurvedic drugs etc. can make any change in the patient. In other words Amm-carb. alone is the only hope for that patient.

'Lack of reaction' means no other method can cure the patient excepting that remedy. For example there was a skin specialist (using native herbs) and he was known not to have failed in any skin case. But he too came across a case where his herbals failed to effect any changes. Amm-carb. 10M single dose cured the patient.

That doesn't mean that when the routine remedy fails I must give Amm-carb. That idea is totally wrong. If you carefully examine that case, there too you would find the symptoms of Amm-carb.

A child of ten months was having chicken-pox and temperature was shooting up and allopathic drugs could not bring down the fever. We routinely give Bryonia-30 (3 doses every four hours) and it had never failed to subside the fever and bring out the eruption). In this case Bryonia failed. One thing I noticed was that when I tried to put the pills into the mouth of the child, he spit it out. (On earlier occasions when he was under my treatment he would ask for the sweet pills. This changed attitude made me to think). Under the section Mind in Boericke's Materia Medica, we find the word 'unreasonable'. I gave a dose of Amm-carb. and the child recovered in twenty-four hours.

One should read the remedy Tuberculinum in Kent's Lectures on Homoeopathic Materia Medica.

Tuberculinum is needed when the deep acting remedies acts for a short time, say a few hours or one day where they ought to act for weeks/months. So far I had two cases in my practice. The first case was headache. Even when I carefully select the remedy it acted for a day only; next day the modality of headache alone changed and the patient would be back in my office. On the prevailing symptoms I gave a second remedy and that too acted for one day only. Third day, again as per prevailing symptoms I selected the remedy and gave it to her. Soon she got relief. After she got total relief I gave her Tuberculinum 10M one single dose and there was relief for six months. When she came after six months, I gave one dose of a certain remedy as per indications. As soon as she got relief I gave one dose of Tuberculinum 50M. After eighteen months she reported with headache; and after giving the indicated remedy for the prevailing symptoms, as soon as she got relief I gave her Tuberculinum-CM. This stopped her headache permanently.

When the blood pressure does not come down even with the best allopathic drugs I think of Laurocerasus. ("Lack of reaction in heart and chest troubles" Boericke's Materia Medica) or Capsicum.

In cardialgia and dyspeptic troubles when even the best painkillers in allopathy fail to relieve you must think of Capsicum. That is the best way to learn homoeopathy. Think of Baptisia and Laurocerasus in mental cases. You must get rid of the notion that Baptisia is good for typhoid.

Remedies for 'Lack of reaction'.

Adonis vernalis - **low vitality,** with weak heart and slow, weak pulse.

Amm-carb. - the diseased conditions met by this remedy are such as we find often in rather stout women who are always tired and weary, take cold easily, suffer from cholera-like symptoms before menses, lead a sedentary life, have a **slow reaction** generally, and are disposed to frequent use of the smelling-bottle.

Amm-carb. (Hiccough, singultus) - hiccough in the morning after the chill; imperfect eructations, tasting after the food; exhaustion with **defective reaction.**

Amm-carb. (Menstruation and its ailments) - before: pale face, pain in belly and small of back, no appetite; at commencement cholera-like symptoms; during: very sad and fatigued, especially in thighs, with yawning, toothache, pain in small of back and chilliness; flow more abundant at night, blackish, in clots, passing off with spasmodic pains in belly and hard stools; menses copious, acrid, it makes the thighs sore and causes a burning pain; too late, scanty and short, always accompanied by frontal headache; very nervous and restless; exhaustion with **defective reaction;** during menses sleeplessness (Ign., Sep., Natr-m.); diarrhoea before and during; blood from rectum during menses (Amm-m.).

Ant-c. (Aphonia, loss of voice) - loss of voice on becoming heated by exertion; the voice returns by resting. Extreme feebleness of voice. Deficient muscular tonicity of the organs of speech, either from faulty assimilation or deficient innervation. Much hawking and expectoration of phlegm and **depressed vitality of the laryngeal mucous membrane;** sensation as of a foreign body in the throat.

Ant-c. (Cough) - **depressed vitality of the mucous membranes** (Amm-m.), cough shaking the whole body, with involuntary escape of copious urine; cough after rising in the morning, as if arising from the abdomen; first attack the most severe, subsequent ones weaker and weaker, until the last resembles only a hacking cough; cough in the hot sun, or when looking into a fire, coming into a warm room from the cold air; loss of voice when overheated.

Ars-alb. (Anaemia.) - disintegration of the blood-corpuscles; rapid, excessive prostration, with **sinking of the vital forces;** oedema; violent and irregular palpitations, with marked appetite for acids or brandy, emaciation, wants to be in a warm room; debility from overtaxing muscular tissues by prolonged exertion; extreme restlessness and fear of death; gastro-ataxia; pernicious anaemia.

Ars-iod. (Atrophy of children) - peaked, cadaverous face, with a purple, livid hue of skin; intense thirst with uncontrollable desire for cold water, which is almost immediately ejected; almost constant copious watery diarrhoea, and distressing nausea and vomiting; stools foul, irritating, excoriating the parts around anus; heaviness of the cold limbs, with weariness of the whole body and great vital prostration; rapid emaciation.

Aur-met. (Sexual instinct, morbid condition of) - testes mere pendent shreds; frequent nightly emissions or nightly erections without emission, or nightly erections and pollutions, without subsequent weakness; discharge of prostatic fluid from a relaxed penis, with settled suicidal melancholia; **sterility from lowered vitality of the parts with great mental depression.**

Aur-mur. (Syphilis and sycosis) - syphilitic gonorrhoea; chancres on prepuce and scrotum; bubo in left groin; condylomata on prepuce, anus and tongue; secondary syphilis, with exostoses and bone-pains in both shin-bones; snuffles in children suffering from hereditary syphilis; flat ulcers on scrotum secreting a foetid ichor; **diminished vitality;** melancholy; vaginitis and gonorrhoeal discharge, with swelling of both groins.

Calcarea hypophos. (ophthalmia neonatorum) - purulent conjunctivitis in **babes of little vitality.**

Caps. (Convalescence, hints upon) - want of reaction in persons of lax fibre.

Caps. (Dyspepsia, weakness of stomach) - dipsomania; morning vomiting, sinking at stomach; stomach icy cold or burning in it; dyspepsia from torpor, particularly in old people; flatulence and wind colic; heartburn, waterbrash; food tastes sour, bitter while eating, worse afterwards; water causes shuddering; purging, tenesmus and thin stools; anxiety and fear of dying; peevish, irritable, angry; foul breath;

haemorrhoids, **lack of reaction**; very offensive breath when coughing

Caps. (Haemorrhoids) - piles burning, swollen, cutting and smarting during defaecation, even when the stool is liquid; itching, throbbing, with sore feeling in anus; large piles, discharging blood or bloody mucus; blind piles with mucous discharge. Urinary troubles, tenesmus, frequent and futile urging to urinate, smarting and burning in urethra, during and after micturition; tenesmus ani, only relieved by squatting down on his heels; suppressed haemorrhoidal flow, causing melancholy; **lack of reactive power,** especially in fat, lazy people, easily exhausted and want to lie down constantly.

Caps. (Heart diseases) - fatty degeneration of heart and atheroma in fat people; clucking, rapid pulsations in some of larger arteries; pectoral anxiety; great desire to lie down and sleep; **vital forces below par.**

Caps. (Uvula, affections of) - elongated, flabby uvula, enlarged and painful cervical glands; **lack of reactive force;** mouth pasty, gums flabby, foetid breath; haemorrhoids and fissure ani.

Caps. - phlegmatic, awkward, easily offended; indolent, melancholic; **lack of reaction.** Gastric troubles.

Caps. - older people who have exhausted their vitality, especially by mental work, and poor living; blear-eyed appearance; **who do not react.**

Carb-v. (Atrophy of children) - **vital powers failing,** and no reaction to well chosen remedies; skin cold, pale or blue, the face having a greenish hue; feet and legs to the knees cold; anxious look, but too lifeless to move or to exhibit much restlessness; breath cold, pulse weak and rapid; stools dark, thin, cadaverous-looking; useful also in protracted sultry weather, when the days are hot and damp.

Carb-v. (Debility) - debility from defective circulation and imperfect oxidation of the blood; **vital forces nearly exhausted;** cold surface, especially from knees to feet; breath cool, pulse intermittent, thready; cold sweat on limbs; after a spree.

Carb-v. (Heart diseases) - carditis, visible palpitations, internal heat, especially when sitting; anguish and great thirst; pulse very irregular, intermittent, frequent; excessive palpitations for days, after eating, when sitting. Aneurisms, blue varicosities, fine capillary network having a marbled appearance. Praecordial anguish as if he would die. Impending paralysis of heart, **complete loss of vitality,** cyanosis, blood stagnates in capillaries, cold face and limbs, cold sweat, filiform pulse.

Carb-v. (Laryngitis and laryngeal phthisis) - long-standing catarrhs of elderly people or in persons **whose vitality is reduced to the lowest ebb** by insufficient nourishment rather than by disease, with venous capillary dilatation of the pharyngo-laryngeal parts and prevailing torpor of all the functions (Phos.); ulcerative pain in larynx, with scraping and titillation; putrid sputa. Complaints from revelling.

Carb-v. - (Gangrene): humid; senile; in cachectic persons; **when vital powers have become weakened;** great foulness of secretions; great prostration.

Carb-v. - organic detrition **without reaction. vital powers low,** venous system predominant.

Causticum (Cough) - catarrhal aphonia, or weakness of voice from overexertion; cough, after getting better, comes to a standstill, and there remains a dry, hollow cough; sore sensation in a streak down trachea and under sternum in chest when coughing, with tightly adhering mucus in the chest, with pain in the hip and involuntary passage of urine;

hacking cough from creeping and rawness in throat; cough relieved by a swallow of cold water; worse from exhaling cold air, from evening till midnight, when awaking; the quantity of mucus in the throat and chest produces spells of coughing, he cannot expectorate the acrid fatty-tasting mucus, but is obliged to swallow it (Arn.); he cannot cough deep enough to get relief, especially when lying down, from **diminished vitality,** > mornings.

China (Anthrax) - **exhaustion of vital power,** with excessive sensitiveness and irritability of the nerves, deficiency of animal heat; decomposition of animal matter with symptoms of putrid fever; malaria.

China (Cholera infantum) - collapse after violent, long-lasting cholera; breathing rapid; surface cool, **hardly any vitality left.**

Cochlearia - raises vital forces.

Crot-h. (Angina pectoris) - sudden and **great prostration of the vital forces;** frequent fainting spells, with imperceptible pulse and inclination to vomit; sudden breathing with open mouth and distortion of the eyes outward.

Crot-h. (Haematemesis, gastrorrhagia) - **low vital force** and decomposition of blood, which fails to coagulate; deathly nausea, jaundiced complexion, faintness, cold sweat, insatiable thirst, great prostration; weight, soreness and tenderness in stomach which ejects everything.

Cup-m. (Chlorosis) - after abuse of iron; symptoms in warm weather; **lack of reaction** in persons who are thoroughly run down by overtaxing mind and body.

Cup-m. (Colic) - cramps in the abdomen; violent, colicky, drawing-cutting pain in the abdomen; abdomen drawn in; colic not increased by pressure; violent spasms in abdomen and upper and lower limbs, with penetrating distressing screams; intussusception of the bowels, with singultus, violent colic, stercoraceous vomiting, and great agony; spasmodic movements of the abdominal muscles; cramps of the stomach and bowels, with vomiting and purging, and cutting pains in umbilical region as if a knife were thrust through to the back, with piercing screams; abdomen hard as a stone; constipation succeeded by watery, greenish or bloody stool; spasmodic vomiting > by a drink of cold water; collapse with great prostration and **lack of reaction**;

Digitalis (Meningitis, cerebro-spinalis) - heart's action irregular and labored; delirium like mania a potu; great pressure and weight in head; violent lancinating pains, especially in vertex and occiput; when sitting or walking the head falls backward, as if anterior cervical muscles were paralyzed; convulsive efforts to vomit; vomiting, with coldness, prostration and fainting; stiffness in the nape and side of neck; tearing sharp stitches, aching and cutting pains in nape of neck; convulsions, with retraction of the head, syncope, and **collapse of vital powers.**

Guarana (Headache) - migraine in persons who used tea and coffee in excess or in whom nervous headaches, followed by vomiting, are excited by any error in diet or depression of mind; neuralgia, nervousness and weariness, **reduced vitality,** weak beat of heart; drowsiness and heaviness of head, with flushed face, in persons of sedentary habits, after eating > after sleep.

Helleborus - a remedy in **low states of vitality and serious disease.**

Hydrocyanic acid. (Vertigo, dizziness) - insufficiency of arterial contraction, with frequent headaches, stupefaction and falling down; vertigo, with reeling; cloudiness of the senses, the objects seem to move; he sees through a gauze; is scarcely able to keep on his feet after raising the head when stooping, on rising from one's seat, worse in the open air; **no reactive power,** face pale, blue and cold.

Hypericum - preserves vitality of torn and lacerated members when almost entirely separated from the body.

Kali-iod. - tea-taster's cough due to inhaling the fungus; also brings about often favorable reaction in many chronic ailments even when not clearly symptomatically indicated.

Laurocerasus (Convalescence, hints upon) - **lack of reaction** in chest complaints.

Laur. (Insanity, mental derangement) - extreme despondency or lively, joyous mood; forgets very easily from the constant confusion in his head; fear and anxiety about imaginary evils; nervous agitation; rotary vertigo; sensation of coldness in forehead and vertex; want of energy of the vital powers and **want of reaction.**

Laur. (Mind symptoms) - indolence and indisposition to either physical or intellectual labor, so that patient becomes disgusted and tired of his life; fear and anxiety about imaginary evils; disposition to sleep; titillation in face, as if flies and spiders were crawling over face; want of energy of vital powers, **no reaction,** a paralytic weakness.

Laur. (See also Hydr-ac) (Syncope) - long-lasting faints, **no reactive power;** face pale-blue; surface cold; fluids, forced down the throat, roll audibly into the stomach; if the syncope is attendant upon some poison in the system, the symptoms are similar, the eruption being livid, and, when pressed, regains its color very slowly; fainting from cardiac weakness.

Laur. - **lack of reaction,** especially in chest and heart affections.

Ledum (Synovitis) - diseases of joints; but especially of knee; effusion, with sensitiveness of the parts to pressure; aching, tearing pains; great coldness; **want of vitality.**

Nat-c. (Anaemia.) - Pallid anaemia, with great debility, milky-white skin; **vitality below par;** emaciation; nervousness and anxiety,

Nicotine (Uraemia) - paralysis of diaphragm; indifference, want of reaction; cold forehead; thirstlessness; serous transfusions in intestines, without diarrhoea; want of secretion in liver and kidneys.

Opium (Drunkards, diseases of) - mania a potu, with dullness of the senses, and at intervals sopor, with snoring; sees animals; affrighted expression of the face; delirious talking; eyes wide open; face red, puffed up; fear; desire to escape, or dreams from which the patient wakes as soon as he is spoken to in a loud voice; dry, tickling, paroxysmal cough, with spasm of lungs and blue face when drinking; troublesome breathing; general sweat; epileptic convulsions; trembling of the extremities; lock-jaw; twitching of the muscles of the face and mouth; staring look; **want of vital reaction in old sinners whose many excesses destroyed their constitution.**

Opium (Paralysis) - paralysis, with insensibility after apoplexy, in drunkards or old people; weakness, numbness and paralysis of the legs and arms; stupefying sleep; the patient is dull, stupid, as if drunk; retained stool and urine; **want of vital reaction,** body cold, stupor.

Opium (Uterus, diseases of) - prolapsus uteri from fright; foetid discharge from uterus after fright; softness of uterus; **want of vital reaction.**

Opium - the effects of opium as shown in the insensibility of the nervous system, the depression, drowsy stupor, painlessness, and torpor, the general sluggishness and **lack of vital reaction,** constitute the main indications for the drug when used homoeopathically.

Phell. - adapted to persons of a feeble, irritable, lymphatic constitution, with **weak and defective reaction.**

Phos. (Gastritis) - cutting burning pains in the stomach; severe pressure in the stomach after eating, with vomiting of food; unquenchable thirst; cramps in stomach, radiating to the liver; goneness in gastric region; haematemesis, better from drinking cold water; great heat of the body, with cold extremities; frequent shudderings; convulsions; **sinking of the reactive power.**

Psor. (Cyanosis cardiaca, neonatorum) - **to increase vitality and circulation,** where other remedies failed.

Psor. - psoric constitutions; especially when other remedies fail to permanently improve; **lack of reaction** after severe diseases.

Psor. - **lack of reaction,** i.e., phagocytes defective; when well-chosen remedies fail to act.

Sulphur - when carefully-selected remedies fail to act, especially in acute diseases it frequently arouses the reactionary powers of the organism.

Sulphur (Aphonia, loss of voice) - chronic aphonia on a psoric basis; **when well-indicated remedies fail** it will rouse the slumbering vitality or excite the animal electricity,

Sulphur (Cyanosis cardiaca, in the new-born) - to increase vitality and circulation, **where other remedies failed.**

Tabacum (Uraemia) - paralysis of diaphragm; indifference, **want of reaction**; cold forehead; thirstlessness; serous transfusions in intestines, without diarrhoea; want of secretion in liver and kidneys.

Ver-alb. - rapid sinking of **vital forces;** collapse.

Ver-alb. - young people and women of a sanguine or nervo-sanguine temperament; also people who are habitually cold and **deficient in vital reaction;** gay dispositions; fitful mood.

Ver-alb. (Constipation) - constipation of infants; chronic constipation; inertia of rectum (Op.), **general depression of vitality;** predominant coldness of the body; first portion of stool is large and the latter part consists of thin strings; stools very large and very hard; very weak after stool; or strains at stool until he is covered with cold sweat and then gives up exhausted, tired of life and afraid to die; craves cool and refreshing things.

Ver-alb. (Headache, cephalalgia) - neuralgia in the head, with indigestion, features sunken; paroxysms in various parts of the brain, partly as if bruised; violent pains drive to despair, great prostration, fainting, with cold sweat and great thirst; cold sensation and pressure on vertex, generally attended by pain in stomach, relieved by pressing on vertex with hand (Meny.); nausea, vomiting and diarrhoea; habitual coldness and **deficiency of vital reaction.**

Ver-alb. (Hydrocephaloid) - sinking of the fontanelles, vision obscure, pulse filiform, **complete extinction of vital power;** cold, collapsed face; nausea and vomiting from least motion; tongue cold, and unquenchable thirst for very cold water or ice.

Xanth. - acts upon nervous system, mostly upon sensory nerves, but causes a marked **depression of vitality, a non-reactive state;** hence its use in chlorosis, measles, neuralgia, etc., when there is sensorial and bodily depression.

Zinc-met. - a state of the blood which in its qualitative analysis approaches chlorosis; **want of vitality,** as we find it after physical and psychical depression; heaviness and weakness in all organs, as we see in suppressed catamenia, but when menses flow it relieves all her sufferings.

Zinc-met. (dentition, morbid) - coma interrupted by piercing screams; slow development of teeth from **lack of vitality;** slow pulse in long waves; child drowsy and lies with its head pressed deeply into the pillow, eyes half open and squinting; face pale and rather cool or alternately red and pale; trembling all over, boring fingers into nose or pulling nervously at the dry, parched lips; automatic motions at different parts of the body, and restless, fidgety movements of feet; child excessively cross and irritable, especially at night, while the eruption of several teeth at once undermines his strength.

Zinc-met. (Meningitis basilaris) - **child has not vitality** enough to develop the eruption, or it was checked in its appearance; feet are in constant motion; distention of abdomen; constipation with hard and dry faeces; eyes sensitive to light; nose dry; appetite voracious, with gagging and vomiting; on awaking child shows signs of fear and rolls its head from side to side; cries out, starts and jumps during sleep.

Zinc-met. (Neuralgia) - neuralgic pains between skin and muscle in subcutaneous cellular tissue; great weakness of all the limbs; **deficiency of vital power.**

Diseases in which 'Lack of reaction' was found and their respective remedies are given below

(Anaemia) Ars-alb. - disintegration of the blood-corpuscles; rapid, excessive prostration, with sinking of the vital forces; oedema; violent and irregular palpitations, with marked appetite for acids or brandy, emaciation, wants to be in a warm room; debility from overtaxing muscular tissues by prolonged exertion; extreme restlessness and fear of death; gastro-ataxia; pernicious anaemia.

(Anaemia) Natrum carb. - pallid anaemia, with great debility, milky-white skin; vitality below par; emaciation; nervousness and anxiety, < during a thunderstorm; playing on piano or hearing music makes her nervous; inertia in psoric, phlegmatic persons.

(Angina pectoris) Crotalus hor. - sudden and great prostration of the vital forces; frequent fainting spells, with imperceptible pulse and inclination to vomit; sudden breathing with open mouth and distortion of the eyes outward.

(Anthrax) China - exhaustion of vital power, with excessive sensitiveness and irritability of the nerves, deficiency of animal heat; decomposition of animal matter with symptoms of putrid fever; malaria.

(Aphonia, loss of voice) Ant-crud. - loss of voice on becoming heated by exertion; the voice returns by resting. extreme feebleness of voice. deficient muscular tonicity of the organs of speech, either from faulty assimilation or deficient innervation. much hawking and expectoration of phlegm and depressed vitality of the laryngeal mucous membrane; sensation as if a foreign body is in the throat.

(Aphonia, loss of voice) Sulphur - chronic aphonia on a psoric basis; when well-indicated remedies fail it will rouse the slumbering vitality or excite the animal electricity, < in the morning.

(Atrophy of children) Ars-iod. - peaked, cadaverous face, with a purple, livid hue of skin; intense thirst with uncontrollable desire for cold water, which is almost immediately ejected; almost constant copious watery diarrhoea, and distressing nausea and vomiting; stools foul, irritating, excoriating the parts around anus; heaviness of the cold limbs, with weariness of the whole body and great vital prostration; rapid emaciation.

(Atrophy of children) Carbo-veg. - vital powers failing, and no reaction to well-chosen remedies; skin cold, pale or blue, the face having a greenish hue; feet and legs to the knees cold; anxious look, but too lifeless to move or to exhibit much restlessness; breath cold, pulse weak and rapid; stools dark, thin, cadaverous-looking; useful also in protracted sultry weather, when the days are hot and damp.

(Bronchitis chronica) Amm-carb. - bronchitis of the aged copious bronchial secretion, with great difficulty of expectoration and bronchial dilatation. Numerous coarse rattles, and yet he experiences no necessity to clear his chest. Cough in the morning or at night, disturbing sleep, with spasmodic oppression; incessant cough, excited by a sensation as if down in the larynx; < after eating, talking, in the open air, and on lying down, followed by exhaustion. Low vitality, and atony of the bronchial tubes, favoring emphysema. Catarrh of old people, beginning with the setting in of winter and continuing till summer heat prevails, < 3 to 4 a.m.

Cerebral anaemia and vital exhaustion, as in the last stage of phthisis: Amm-Carb., Mosch. and Phos. ign. acts well in children who may be overgrown.

(Chlorosis) Cuprum met. - after abuse of iron; symptoms < in warm weather; lack of reaction in persons who are thoroughly run down by overtaxing mind and body.

(Cholera infantum) China - collapse after violent, long-lasting cholera; breathing rapid; surface cool, hardly any vitality left.

(Colic) Cuprum met. - cramps in the abdomen; violent, colicky, drawing-cutting pain in the abdomen; abdomen drawn in; colic not increased by pressure; violent spasms in abdomen and upper and lower limbs, with penetrating distressing screams; intussusception of the bowels, with singultus, violent colic, stercoraceous vomiting, and great agony; spasmodic movements of the abdominal muscles; cramps of the stomach and bowels, with vomiting and purging, and cutting pains in umbilical region as if a knife were thrust through to the back, with piercing screams; abdomen hard as a stone; constipation succeeded by watery, greenish or bloody stool; spasmodic vomiting > by a drink of cold water; collapse with great prostration and lack of reaction; pulse soft, moderately frequent; skin warm and dry.

(Constipation in children) Veratrum alb. - faeces cannot be passed, from inertia of rectum, but a healthy stool can be procured at any time by an injection; pallor and cold sweat from the exertion, with exhaustion after stool; general depression of vitality.

(Constipation) Veratrum alb. - constipation of infants; chronic constipation; inertia of rectum (Op.), general depression of vitality; predominant coldness of the body; first portion of stool is large and the latter part consists of thin strings; stools very large and very hard; very weak after stool; or strains at stool until he is covered with cold sweat and then gives up exhausted, tired of life and afraid to die; craves cool and refreshing things.

(Convalescence, hints upon) Caps. - want of reaction in persons of lax fibre.

(Convalescence, hints upon) Laur. - lack of reaction in chest complaints.

(Cough) Ant-crud. - depressed vitality of the mucous membranes (Amm-m.), cough shaking the whole body, with involuntary escape of copious urine; cough after rising in the morning, as if arising from the abdomen; first attack the most severe, subsequent ones weaker and weaker, until the last resembles only a hacking cough; cough in the hot sun, or when looking into a fire, coming into a warm room from the cold air; loss of voice when overheated.

(Cough) Causticum - catarrhal aphonia, or weakness of voice from overexertion; cough, after getting better, comes to a standstill, and there remains a dry, hollow cough; sore sensation in a streak down trachea and under sternum in chest when coughing, with tightly adhering mucus in the chest, with pain in the hip and involuntary passage of urine; hacking cough from creeping and rawness in throat; cough relieved by a swallow of cold water; worse from exhaling cold air, from evening till midnight, when awaking; the quantity of mucus in the throat and chest produces spells of coughing, he cannot expectorate the acrid fatty-tasting mucus, but is obliged to swallow it (Arn.); he cannot cough deep enough to get relief, especially when lying down, from diminished vitality, > mornings.

(Debility) Carbo-veg. - debility from defective circulation and imperfect oxidation of blood; vital forces nearly exhausted; cold surface, especially from knees to feet; breath cool, pulse intermittent, thready; cold sweat on limbs; after a spree.

(Dentition, morbid) Zincum met. - coma interrupted by piercing screams; slow development of teeth from lack of vitality; slow pulse in long waves; child drowsy and lies with its head pressed deeply into the pillow, eyes half open and squinting; face pale and rather cool or alternately red and pale; trembling all over, boring fingers into nose or pulling nervously at the dry, parched lips; automatic motions at different parts of the body, and restless, fidgety movements of feet; child excessively cross and irritable, especially at night, while the eruption of several teeth at once undermines his strength.

(Diaphragm, diseases of) In coaffection of heart compare: Spig., Laur., Cann-sat., Ars., Veratr. - singultus in nervous persons: Bell., Hyosc., Ign., Mosch., Natr-m., Nux-m., Nux-v.; gastric and hepatic troubles: Bry., Chel., Natr-m., Nux-v., Puls., Sulph.; painful from inflammation of neighboring organs: Atrop., Bell., Hyosc., Op.; cerebral anaemia and vital exhaustion, as in the last stage of phthisis: Amm-carb., Mosch. and Phos. ign. acts well in children who may be livergrown.

(Drunkards, diseases of) Opium - mania? Potu, with dullness of the senses, and at intervals sopor, with snoring; sees animals; affrighted expression of the face; delirious talking; eyes wide open; face red, puffed up; fear; desire to escape, or dreams from which the patient wakes as soon as he is spoken to in a loud voice; dry, tickling, paroxysmal cough, with spasm of lungs and blue face when drinking; troublesome breathing; general sweat; epileptic convulsions; trembling of the extremities; lockjaw; twitching of the muscles of the face and mouth; staring look; want of vital reaction in old sinners whose many excesses destroyed their constitution.

(Dyspepsia, weakness of stomach) Abies nigra - total loss of appetite in the morning, craving for food at noon, and exceedingly hungry and wakeful at night; pain after a hearty meal, but abstinence from any particular food does not relieve the dyspepsia; belching and acid eructations, frequent vomiting; sensation as if some indigestible substance had stuck in the cardiac end of the stomach (Lact-ac.: sensation as if all food lodged under upper end of stomach); continual distressing constriction just above the pit of stomach, as if everything were knotted up, or as if a hard lump of undigested food remained there, < whenever his vital energy is below par; hypochondriasis; constipation.

(Dyspepsia, weakness of stomach) Capsicum - dipsomania; morning vomiting, sinking at stomach; stomach icy cold or burning in it; dyspepsia from torpor, particularly in old people; flatulence and wind colic; heartburn, waterbrash; food tastes sour, bitter while eating, worse afterwards; water causes shuddering; purging, tenesmus and thin stools; anxiety and fear of dying; peevish, irritable, angry; foul breath; haemorrhoids, lack of reaction; very offensive breath when coughing.

(Dyspepsia, weakness of stomach) Kali-carb. - dyspepsia of aged persons rather inclined to obesity, or after great loss of vitality;

(Fainting) Hydrocyanic acid. - long-lasting faints, no reactive power; face pale-blue; surface cold; fluids, forced down the throat, roll audibly into the stomach; if the syncope is attendant upon some poison in the system, the symptoms are similar, the eruption being livid, and, when pressed, regains its color very slowly; fainting from cardiac weakness.

(Gangrene) Carbo-veg. - humid; senile; in cachectic persons whose vital powers are exhausted; great foulness of the secretions; great prostration; sepsis; indifference; fainting after sleep, while yet in bed, morning; no restlessness.

(Gastritis) Phosphorus - cutting burning pains in the stomach; severe pressure in the stomach after eating, with vomiting of food; unquenchable thirst; cramps in stomach, radiating to the liver; goneness in gastric region; haematemesis, better from drinking cold water; great heat of the body, with cold extremities; frequent shudderings; convulsions; sinking of the reactive power.

(Glaucoma) Arnica - tongue coated and swollen; foetid, putrid smell from mouth; general sinking of vital power.

(Haematemesis, gastrorrhagia) Crotalus hor. - low vital force and decomposition of blood, which fails to coagulate; deathly nausea, jaundiced complexion, faintness, cold sweat, insatiable thirst, great prostration; weight, soreness and tenderness in stomach which ejects everything.

(Haemorrhoids) Capsicum - piles burning, swollen, cutting and smarting during defaecation, even when the stool is liquid; itching, throbbing, with sore feeling in anus; large piles, discharging blood or bloody mucus; blind piles with mucous discharge. Urinary troubles, tenesmus, frequent and futile urging to urinate, smarting and burning in urethra, during and after micturition; tenesmus ani, only relieved by squatting down on his heels; suppressed haemorrhoidal flow, causing melancholy; lack of reactive power, especially in fat, lazy people, easily exhausted and want to lie down constantly.

(Headache) Guarana - migraine (headache) in persons who used tea and coffee in excess or in whom nervous headaches, followed by vomiting, are excited by any error in diet or depression of mind; neuralgia, nervousness and weariness, reduced vitality, weak beat of heart; drowsiness and heaviness of head, with flushed face, in persons of sedentary habits, after eating > after sleep, < from study or mental exertion.

(Headache) Veratrum alb. - neuralgia in the head, with indigestion, features sunken; paroxysms in various parts of the brain, partly as if bruised, partly pressure; violent pains drive to despair, great prostration, fainting, with cold sweat and great thirst; cold sensation and pressure on vertex, generally attended by pain in stomach, relieved by pressing on vertex with hand (Meny.); nausea, vomiting and diarrhoea; habitual coldness and deficiency of vital reaction.

(Heart diseases) Capsicum - fatty degeneration of heart and atheroma in fat people; clucking, rapid pulsations in some of larger arteries; pectoral anxiety; great desire to lie down and sleep; vital forces below par.

(Heart diseases) Carbo-veg. - carditis, visible palpitations, internal heat, especially when sitting; anguish and great thirst; pulse very irregular, intermittent, frequent; excessive palpitations for days, after eating, when sitting. aneurisms, blue varicosities, fine capillary network having a marbled appearance. praecordial anguish as if he would die. impending paralysis of heart, complete loss of vitality, cyanosis, blood stagnates in capillaries, cold face and limbs, cold sweat, filiform pulse.

(Hepatic derangements) Laurocerasus - wasting away of liver (Phos.), nutmeg liver; sticking pain in liver, with pressure; distention of liver, pain as if an abscess would burst; burning or coldness in stomach and abdomen; constipation or diarrhoea; rapid sinking of the vital forces.

(Hiccough) Amm-carb. - hiccough in the morning after the chill; imperfect eructations, tasting after the food; exhaustion with defective reaction.

(Hydrocephaloid) Veratrum alb. - sinking of the fontanelles, vision obscure, pulse filiform, complete extinction of vital power; cold, collapsed face; nausea and vomiting from least motion; tongue cold, and unquenchable thirst for very cold water or ice.

(Hydrophobia) Scutellaria - depression of the nervous and vital powers; spasmodic or constricting closing of the jaws, tightness of the muscles of face; nervous agitation from pain; sleeplessness; frightful dreams; tremulousness and twitching of muscles (hale).

(Insanity) Helleborus - acute idiocy as well as chronic idiocy and cretinismus; diminished power of mind over body, cannot fix ideas, slow in answering, stares unintelligently; muscles fail to act properly if will is not strongly fixed upon their action; depression of sensory and obtuseness of intellectual faculties; stubborn silence; fixed delusions and hallucinations, especially towards morning; demoniac melancholy, sees spirits at night; woeful despairing mood, with tendency to drown himself; irritable, easily made angry, < from consolation; homesickness; anxiousness about heart, which prevents him from resting anywhere; want of bodily irritability; cold hands and feet, coldness of whole body, can bear neither heat nor cold; pale, sallow complexion.

(Insanity) Laurocerasus - extreme despondency or lively, joyous mood; forgets very easily from the constant confusion in his head; fear and anxiety about imaginary evils; nervous agitation; rotary vertigo; sensation of coldness in forehead and vertex; want of energy of the vital powers and want of reaction.

(Laryngitis and laryngeal phthisis) Carbo-veg. - long-standing catarrhs of elderly people or in persons whose vitality is reduced to the lowest ebb by insufficient nourishment rather than by disease, with venous capillary dilatation of the pharyngo-laryngeal parts and prevailing torpor of all the functions (Phos.); ulcerative pain in larynx, with scraping and titillation; putrid sputa.

(Leucaemia) Crotalus hor. - sudden and great prostration of vital forces; general excessive adynamia; idiopathic pernicious anaemia from mental shock or in constitutions broken down by gonorrhoea, syphilis, alcohol, etc.; petechiae? Haemorrhagic tendency.

(Lienitis) Psorinum - stinging sharp pain in region of liver and spleen; stitches in spleen, > when standing, < moving and continuing when again at rest; dyspnoea; dropsy; pain in abdomen while riding; psoric constitutions with lack of reaction after severe diseases.

(Mind symptoms) China - mental depression as a reflex of general lowered vitality; low-spirited, despondent and tired of life, with suicidal tendencies; great sensitiveness; easily moved to tears by the least contradiction; indifference and apathy with obstinate taciturnity; weakness and exhaustion after the least exertion, > in the evening and at night; nocturnal dread of dogs and other animals; desire for solitude.

(Mind symptoms) Laurocerasus - indolence and indisposition to either physical or intellectual labor, so that patient becomes disgusted and tired of his life; fear and anxiety about imaginary evils; disposition to sleep; titillation in face, as if flies and spiders were crawling over face; want of energy of vital powers, no reaction, a paralytic weakness.

(Meningitis basilaris) Ars-alb. - great depression of the vital forces, manifested by great prostration; emaciation; pallor; thirst; sometimes the child strikes its head with its fists, as if for temporary relief.

(Meningitis basilaris) Zincum met. - child does not have enough vitality to develop the eruption, or it was checked in its appearance; feet are in constant motion; distention of abdomen; constipation with hard and dry faeces; eyes sensitive to light; nose dry; appetite voracious, with gagging and vomiting; on awaking child shows signs of fear and rolls its head from side to side; cries out, starts and jumps during sleep.

(Meningitis, cerebro-spinalis) Digitalis - heart's action irregular and labored; delirium like mania a potu; great pressure and weight in head; violent lancinating pains, especially in vertex and occiput; when sitting or walking the head falls backward, as if anterior cervical muscles were paralyzed; convulsive efforts to vomit; vomiting, with coldness, prostration and fainting; stiffness in the nape and side of neck; tearing sharp stitches, aching and cutting pains in nape of neck; convulsions, with retraction of the head, syncope, and collapse of vital powers.

(Meningitis, encephalitis) Zincum met. - sharp, lancinating pains through head, < from wine and stimulants; pressing, tearing pains in occiput, particularly at base of brain, shooting through eyes and into teeth; distressing cramplike pains at glabella; meningitis from non-development of an eruption from lack of vital power.

(Menses complaints) Amm-carb. - before: pale face, pain in belly and small of back, no appetite; at commencement cholera-like symptoms; during: very sad and fatigued, especially in thighs, with yawning, toothache, pain in small of back and chilliness; flow more abundant at night, blackish, in clots, passing off with spasmodic pains in belly and hard stools; menses copious, acrid, it makes the thighs sore and causes a burning pain; too late, scanty and short, always accompanied by frontal headache; very nervous and restless; exhaustion with defective reaction; during menses sleeplessness (Ign., Sep., Natr-m.); diarrhoea before and during; blood from rectum during menses (Amm-m.).

(Neuralgia) Zincum met. - neuralgic pains between skin and muscle in subcutaneous cellular tissue; great weakness of all the limbs; deficiency of vital power.

(Ophthalmia neonatorum) Calc-hypophos. - purulent conjunctivitis in babies of little vitality.

(Paralysis) Opium - paralysis, with insensibility after apoplexy, in drunkards or old people; weakness, numbness and paralysis of the legs and arms; stupefying sleep; the patient is dull, stupid, as if drunk; retained stool and urine; want of vital reaction, body cold, stupor.

(Sexual complaints) Aurum-met. - testes mere pendent shreds; frequent nightly emissions or nightly erections without emission, or nightly erections and pollutions, without subsequent weakness; discharge of prostatic fluid from a relaxed penis, with settled suicidal melancholia; sterility from lowered vitality of the parts with great mental depression.

(Spasms) Spasms from lowered vitality: Lach.

(Sunstroke) Camphor - severe headache, congestion of brain, fainting, delirium, convulsions; skin icy-cold, covered with cold sweat; sinking of vital force; embarrassed respiration and circulation, with coldness of surface and extremities, tremors and cramps in muscles, cold sweat, especially about head and neck.

(Syncope) Laur (See also Hydr-ac.) - long-lasting faints, no reactive power; face pale-blue; surface cold; fluids, forced down the throat, roll audibly into the stomach; if the syncope is attendant upon some poison in the system, the symptoms are similar, the eruption being livid, and, when pressed, regains its color very slowly; fainting from cardiac weakness.

(Synovitis) Ledum - diseases of joints; but especially of knee; effusion, with sensitiveness of the parts to pressure; aching, tearing pains; great coldness; want of vitality.

(Syphilis and sycosis) Aur-mur. - syphilitic gonorrhoea; chancres on prepuce and scrotum; bubo in left groin; condylomata on prepuce, anus and tongue; secondary syphilis, with exostoses and bone-pains in both shin-bones; snuffles in children suffering from hereditary syphilis; flat ulcers on scrotum secreting a foetid ichor; diminished vitality; melancholy; vaginitis and gonorrhoeal discharge, with swelling of both groins.

(Uraemia) Nicotine. - paralysis of diaphragm; indifference, want of reaction; cold forehead; thirstlessness; serous transfusions in intestines, without diarrhoea; want of secretion in liver and kidneys.

(Uterus complaints) Ledum - fibrous tumors with menorrhagia; displacement of the uterus; abundant metrorrhagia and leucorrhoea; pale face, copious urination, even at night; < by warmth, as in bed or over a register; great sensation of coldness all through her, she cannot keep warm from deficiency of vital heat.

(Uterus complaints) Lilium-tig. - uterine symptoms following pregnancy and labor; subinvolution, uterus does not regain its normal size after confinement, when rising to walk, uterus falls by its own weight; heavy dragging sensation, principally in hypogastric region; she feels the need of some support to hold the abdominal organs up, sensation of dragging down from shoulders and chest, > by supporting abdomen with her hand (Sep., woman sits with legs crossed); watery, yellowish or yellowish-brown excoriating leucorrhoea; sharp pains across abdomen from one ilium to the other, marked bearing-down pains, so that she puts her hand over vulva to support it; prolapsus and retroversion; urging to urinate, urine smarting and burning; urging to stool, morning diarrhoea, hurrying her out of bed, stool yellow, papescent, excoriating feeling at anus; oppression of chest, with taste of blood in mouth and a feeling of a bullet in mammary region. Impairment of vitality in organism, no organic lesions or abnormal deposits; pruritus of genitals; uterine neuralgia; heaviness of head with staggering faint feeling, nervous palpitations or coldness about heart; oppressed breathing; nervous trembling; low-spirited, weeping, apprehensive; opposite and contradictory mental states. Suicidal disposition by poison.

(Uterus complaints) Opium - prolapsus uteri from fright; foetid discharge from uterus after fright; softness of uterus; want of vital reaction.

(Uvula, affections of) Capsicum - elongated, flabby uvula, enlarged and painful cervical glands; lack of reactive force; mouth pasty, gums flabby, foetid breath; haemorrhoids and fissura ani.

(Vertigo, dizziness) Camphor - vanishing of the senses; loss of consciousness; when walking he staggers to and fro; vertigo with heaviness of the head, which inclines backward; sudden and complete prostration of the vital forces, with great coldness of the external surface; great cardiac weakness.

(Vertigo, dizziness) Hydrocyanic acid. - insufficiency of arterial contraction, with frequent headaches, stupefaction and falling down; vertigo, with reeling; cloudiness of the senses, the objects seem to move; he sees through a gauze; is scarcely able to keep on his feet after raising the head when stooping, on rising from one's seat, worse in the open air; no reactive power, face pale, blue and cold.

Causations*

After a thorough case taking when we are ready with so many remedies and we want to select and confirm the similimum then 'causations' sometimes acts as a helpful tool.

Abies-n: Tea. Tobacco.

Acon.: Fear. Fright. Chill. Cold, dry winds. Heat; especially of sun. Injury. Surgical operation. Shock.

Actaea racemosa: Anxiety. Fright. Disappointed love. Business failure. Over-exertion. Child-bearing.

Act-sp.: Fright. Fatigue.

Agar.: Coitus, subjective symptoms arising after. Frost. Sun. Fright. Mental application or excitement. Over-exertion. Sexual excess. Alcoholism. Blood poisoning.

Agn.: Sexual excesses. Gonorrhœa or gleet, repeated attacks of. Sprains or over-lifting.

All-c.: Effects of exposure to damp cold winds and weather. Colds of spring; hay-fever of August; epidemics of spasmodic cough in autumn. Wet feet. Eating spoiled fish. Injuries. Surgical operations (fine shooting pains after), otherwise called 'ghost pain'.

---

*Compiled from Dictionary of Practical Materia Medica by Dr Clarke.

All-s.: Drinking bad water. Gluttony.

Aloe: Sedentary habits.

Alumen: Bad news. Operations on eyes; on teeth.

Alum.: Anger. Disappointments. Lifting. Bodily exertion.

Anac-or.: Checked eruptions. Examinations.

Ant-c.: Gluttony. Hot weather. Heat of sun. Getting over-heated. Disappointed love. Suppressed eruptions.

Ant-t.: Effects of anger (cough) or vexation.

Apis.: Grief. Fright. Rage. Vexation. Jealousy. (The queen bee is the most jealous thing in nature). Hearing bad news, mental shock. Suppressed eruptions.

Arg-m.: Onanism. Sunstroke.

Arg-n.: Apprehension, fear or fright. Eating ices. Intemperate habits. Mental strain and worry. Onanism and venery. Sugar. Tobacco (boys).

Armor.: Checked foot-sweat. Nervous excitement. Cold.

Arn.: Mechanical injuries. Fright or anger. Excessive venery (vaginitis in the female, impotence in the male).

Ars.: Chill in the water. Eating ices. Poor diet. Fruits, ailments from. Drunkenness. Effects of tobacco; of quinine; of iodine. Sea-bathing and sea-travelling. Climbing mountains. Strains. Fit of passion. Care. Grief. Fright. Chronic effects of food poisoning.

Ars-i.: Study (headache).

Ars-m.: Laughing (headache). Thinking (headache).

Art-v.: Blow on head. Fright or grief or bad news.

Asaf.: Checked skin affections.

Aur.: Mercury. Alcohol. Iodide of Potassium. Effects of grief; fright; anger; disappointed love; contradiction; reserved displeasure.

Aur-m-n.: Vexation (Jaundice).
Aur-mur.: Chagrin. Fright. Vexation.
Bar-c.: Checked foot-sweat.
Bell.: Hair-cutting. Head, getting wet. Sausages. Sun. Wind, walking in.
Bellis.: Injuries. Effects of cold drinks when overheated. Wetting when overheated.
Bism.: Abdominal operations.
Bry.: Anger; fright; chagrin. Suppressed eruptions and discharges. Alcohol. Gluttony. Wounds. Cold winds.
Cact.: Sun. Damp. Love disappointment.
Cadm-s.: Sun. Draught of air. Cold wind. Alcohol.
Cain.: Fatigue.
Caj.: Effects of checked perspiration.
Calc.: Alcohol. Cold, moist winds. Excessive venery. Self-abuse. Injury to lower spine. Over-lifting. Strains. Mental strain. Losses of fluids. Suppressed sweat. Suppressed eruption. Suppressed menses. Fright.
Calc-p.: Over-growth. Lifting. Ascending. Over-study. Sexual excesses. Sexual irregularities. Grief. Disappointed love. Unpleasant news. Operation for fistula. Getting wet.
Camph.: Shock from injury. Eruptions, suppressed. Cold air. Sunstroke. Vexation.
Carb-a.: Loss of fluids. Lifting. Strain. Eating. Eating spoiled fish. Eating decayed vegetables. Quinine.
Carb-v.: Alcohol. Bad food: eggs, wines, liquors, fish. Fat food. Butter. Salt or salt food. Poultry. Ice-water. Debauchery. Strains. Lifting. Over-work (asthenopia). Change of weather. Warm, damp weather. Hot air inhaled from fire. Overheating.

Caust.: Burns or scalds. Fright. Grief or sorrow. Night-watching. Suppressed eruptions. Ulcers maltreated with lead.

Cham.: Dentition. Anger. Indigestion. Pain.

Cheir.: Cutting wisdom teeth.

China-a.: Fluids, loss of. Onanism. Chill. Anger. Coryza, suppressed. Tea. Alcohol. Mercury.

Chininum Arsenicosum: Tobacco.

Cimic.: (See Actaea Racemosa)

Cina: Worms. Yawning.

Cocc.: Anger. Fright. Noise. Sleep, loss of. Seasickness. Travelling. Overstrain, mental or bodily. Sun. Tea-drinking.

Cod.: Fatigue and excessive mental excitement = headache.

Coff.: Effects of sudden emotion, especially pleasurable ones. Fear or fright. Wine (wine-drinkers should take coffee; beer-drinkers should take tea). Over-fatigue and long journeys.

Colch.: Grief. Misbehaviour of others. Wetting. Checked perspiration.

Coloc.: Anger. Indignation. Chagrin. Grief. Catching cold.

Con.: Contusions. Blows. Grief. Sexual excess. Sexual abstinence. Excitement. Over-work. Snowy air. Spring.

Crot-h.: Fright. Sun. Lightning. Alcohol. Foul water. Noxious effluvia.

Cup-ac.: Overworked brain. Repelled eruptions.

Cup-m.: Suppressions. Fright.

Dig.: High living. Sexual abuse, or sexual excess. Alcohol.

Dios.: Tea-drinking. Excess in eating. Fasting. Errors in diet. Onanism.

Dulc.: Damp with cold. Wading. Washing. Injuries. Checked eruptions. Checked perspiration.

Epip.: Physical or nervous over-strain. Any unusual exertion or excitement, as going on a visit, or doing a day's shopping.

Fer-p.: Checked perspiration on a warm summer's day. Mechanical injuries.

Ferr-pic.: Fatigue.

Form.: Checked foot-sweat.

Gels.: Depressing emotions. Fright. Anger. Bad news. Sun. Heat. Damp weather, warm or cold. Thunderstorms. Alcohol. Self-abuse.

Glon.: Sun. Bright snow. Fire-heat. Fear or fright. Jarring. Injuries.

Graph.: Grief. Fear. Overlifting.

Grat.: Abuse of coffee.

Gunpowder: Blood-poisoning.

Ham.: Injuries.

Hekla: Injury to bone.

Hell.: Checked exanthemata. Blows. Disappointed love.

Hep.: Cold, dry winds. Injuries.

Mercury: Suppressed eruptions.

Homarus: Milk, effects of.

Hydrophob. (Lyssinum) : Dog-bites.

Hyos.: Jealousy. Lochia, suppressed. Milk, suppressed.

Hyp.: Fright. Bites. Wounds. Shock.

Ign.: Grief. Fright. Worry. Disappointed love. Jealousy. Old spinal injuries.

Iod.: Nervous shock. Disappointed love.

Ipec.: Vexation and reserved displeasure. Injuries. Suppressed eruptions. Quinine. Morphia. Indigestible foods.

Kali-bi.: Indulgence in beer and malt liquors. Hot weather. Autumn. Spring.

Kali-br.: Anger. Fright. Emotional disturbance. Worry. Business losses and embarrassments. Sexual excess. Sexual abuse.

Kali-c.: Catching cold. Overstrain.

Kali-i.: Drinking cold milk.

Kali-m.: Vaccination. Sprains. Burns. Blows. Cuts. Rich food. Deranged internal functions.

Kali-n.: Eating veal.

Kali-p.: Mechanical injuries. Blows. Sexual excitement, indulged or suppressed.

Kali-s.: Chill when over-heated. Injury.

Kalm.: Chill. Exposure. Wind. Sun.

Kreo.: Bad smells. Sprains.

Lac-c.: Result of fall.

Lac-d.: Injuries.

Lach.: Injuries. Punctured wounds. Poisoned wounds. Grief. Vexation. Anger. Fright. Jealousy. Disappointed love. Alcohol. Masturbation. Sprain (bluish swelling of joints). Sun. Warm weather. Draught of air.

Lathyrus.: Cold and damp weather.

Laur.: Fright.

Led.: Alcohol, abuse of. Hair-cutting. Suppressed discharges. Wounds: Bruises; Bites; Punctured wounds; Stings.

Lith-c.: Bruises. Falls.

Lob-i.: Alcohol. Tea. Tobacco. Wetting feet. Suppressions. Foreign bodies.

Lob-p.: Snake-bites. Blood poisoning.

Lob-s.: Grief. Suppressions.

Lycopodium: Fear. Fright. Chagrin. Anger. Vexation. Anxiety. Fevers. Over-lifting. Masturbation. Riding in carriage. Tobacco-chewing. Wine.

Lycopus vir.: Suppressed haemorrhoidal flow.

Lyssin.: See Hydrophobinum.

Mag-c.: Vexation. Fit of passion. Mental distress. Shocks, blows. Pregnancy. Dentition. Cutting wisdom teeth. Injudicious feeding. Milk.

Mag-m.: Sea-bathing.

Mag-p.: Dentition. Cold winds. Cold bathing. Standing in cold water. Working with cold clay. Study. Catheterism.

Maland.: Vaccination.

Malar.: Wetting. Camp life.

Menth-p.: Early rising.

Meny.: Injuries to nerves (tooth broken in). Quinine.

Mer-per.: Blow on head.

Mer-bin.: Wetting. Washing floor. Weather changes.

Mer-pro.: Cold draught when perspiring. Cold, damp weather. Spring.

Merc.: Fright. Suppressed gonorrhoea. Suppressed foot-sweat.

Mez.: Anger. Mercury. Vaccination.

Mill.: Falls (from height). Over-exertion. Lifting. Suppressed lochia. Suppressed menses. Suppressed milk.

Morph.: Electric shock. Lightning-stroke. Thunderstorms.

Moschus: Chill.

Mur-ac.: Sun.

Naja: Grief.

Nat-c.: Cold drink when over-heated. Milk. Sun's rays (chronic effects). Gaslight. Heat. Change of temperature. Storms. Electric states. Over-study. Strains. Sweat, suppression of.

Nat-m.: Disappointment. Fright. Fit of passion. Loss of fluids. Masturbation. Injury to head. Quinine. Lunar caustic. Bread. Fat. Wine. Acid food. Salt.

Nat-p.: Sugar. Milk. Fat food. Bitter foods. Thunderstorms.

Nat-s.: Anger. Injury to head (fall). Suppressed gonorrhoea.

Nitric-acid: (deafness from). Cabbage. Suppressed eruptions. Sprains.

Nit-s-d.: Cheese. Salt. Stormy weather.

Nux-m.: Fright. Mental exertion. Suppressed eruption. Bath (suppressed menses). Over-eating. Milk. Bad beer. Alcohol.

Nux-v.: Anger. Coffee. Alcohol. Debauchery. Masturbation. Sexual excess. Injury.

Oen.: Injuries.

Ol-an.: Suppressed foot-sweat.

Onos.: Eye-strain. Sexual excess.

Opi.: Fear. Fright. Anger. Shame. Sudden joy. Charcoal fumes. Alcohol. Lead. Sun.

Ovi-g-p.: Over-exertion. Strain.

Ox-ac.: Coffee.

Oxyg.: Morphia. Strychnine.

Paeon.: Bruises. Pressure (bed-sores, tight boots). Bad news.

Paris: Injury. Suppressions.

Pet.: Vexation. Riding in carriage or ship.

Ph-ac.: Bad news. Grief. Chagrin. Disappointed love. Separation from home. Loss of fluids. Sexual excesses. Injuries. Operations. Over-lifting. Over-study. Shock.

Phos.: Anger. Fear. Grief. Worry. Mental exertion. Strong emotions. Music. Strong odours. Gas. Flowers (fainting). Thunderstorms. Lightning (blindness). Sexual excesses.

Loss of fluids. Sprains. Lifting. Wounds. Exposure to drenching rains. Tobacco (amblyopia). Washing clothes. Having hair cut.

Phys.: Emotions. Grief. Bathing. Injuries. Blows.

Phyt.: Exposure to cold and damp.

Pic-ac.: Fatigue. Study. Mental exertion.

Plant.: Bruises. Burns. Cuts. Punctured wounds. Snake-bites.

Plat.: Fright. Vexation. Bereavement. Fit of passion. Sexual excess. Masturbation.

Plb.: Repelled eruptions. Sexual excess.

Pod.: Over-lifting or over-straining (prolapsus uteri). Summer (diarrhoea).

Polyg.: Cold. Damp. Sprains.

Prun-s.: Sun. Sprains. Over-lifting.

Psor.: Emotions. Over-lifting. Mental labour. Repelled eruptions. Stormy weather. Thunderstorm. Injuries. Blows. Sprains. Dislocations.

Ptel.: Repelled eruption (asthma).

Puls.: Chill. Wetting feet. Eating: Pork; Fats; Pastry; Ice-cream; Mixed diet. Thunderstorm. Tea.

Pyro.: Blood poisoning. Ptomaine poisoning. Sewer-gas poisoning. Typhoid fever (remote effects of). Dissecting wounds.

Quercus.: Alcohol.

Rad-br.: Effect of X-ray burns.

Ran-b.: Anger (slightest fit of, = trembling and dyspnoea). Change of temperature or weather. Injury. Alcohol. Rheum: Eating prunes. Eating unripe fruit. Dentition. Spasms. Dislocations.

Rhod.: Stormy weather. Thunder. Sprains. Eating fruit. Getting wet Catching cold.

Rhus-t.: Slightest anger. Cold. From wetting head. Damp sheets. Bathing, in fresh or salt water. Getting wet when heated. Strains. Over-exertion. Over-lifting. Raising arms high to lift things. Drinking ice-water. Beer (headache).

Rhus-v.: Sprains.

Ruta: Bones, injuries of. Bruises. Fractures. Sprains. Carrying heavy weights. Over-exertion of eyes.

Sabad.: Fright. Mental exertion. Thinking. Worms.

Sac-lac.: Mental excitement. Over-fatigue.

Sac-off.: Anger.

Sal-ac.: Suppression (foot-sweat).

Samb.: Fright. Grief. Anxiety. Injury (hydrocele) Excessive sexual indulgence.

Sang-n.: Driving in cold wind. Winter weather. Exposure.

Sanic.: Strains. Jarring.

Squil.: Blood-letting.

Scroph.: Vexation.

Scut.: Excitement. Influenza. Overwork (mental or physical). Tobacco (heart). Pain (causes nervous agitation).

Sec.: Lifting (= abortion). Injury (= gangrene). Sexual excess.

Sel.: Alcohol. Tea. Sugar. Salt. Lemonade. Debauchery. Walking. Exertion. Masturbation. Loss of fluids.

Senec.: Venesection. Suppressed menstruation. Wounds.

Seneg.: Bites, poisonous. Sprains.

Sep.: Anger and vexation. Blows. Falls. Jar. Injury. Overlifting (dyspepsia). Snowy air. Tobacco (neuralgia). Laundry work. Wetting. Alcohol. Milk, boiled (diarrhoea). Fat Pork.

Sil.: Vaccination. Stone-cutting. Loss of fluids. Injury. Strains. Splinters. Foreign bodies.

Causations

Sin-n.: Damp weather. Summer season.

Skook.: Vaccination.

Spigelia: Chill. Tobacco.

Stan.: Emotions. Fright. Masturbation. Dentition. Using voice.

Staph.: Anger. Anger suppressed or reserved. Injury; falls; clean-cut wounds; operations. Coitus. Masturbation. Sexual abuse. Sexual craving. Emissions. Dentition. Tobacco. Mercury.

Stict.: Fall. Haemorrhages.

Stram.: Shock. Fright. Sun. Childbirth. Suppressions.

Stront-c.: Operation (photopsia). Sprains. Haemorrhages (chronic sequelae).

Stroph.: Alcohol. Tea. Tobacco.

Sul.: Suppressions. Alcohol. Sun. Sprains. Chills. Over-exertion. Reaching high. Falls. Blows. Bed-sores.

Sul-ac.: Lifting arms. Falls. Bruises. Concussion (of brain). Chafing. Surgical operations. Sprains.

Symph.: Fractures. Injuries (to eye; bone; periosteum). Falls. Blows. Sexual excess.

Syph.: Sun. Damp weather. Thunderstorms.

Tar-h.: Fall. Unrequited love. Bad news. Scolding. Punishment. Sepsis.

Tell.: Falls. Rice (vomiting).

Ter.: Alcohol. Falls. Strains. Tooth extraction. Damp cellars.

Teuc.: Concussion (brain). Injuries likely to set up tetanus.

Ther.: Sea-travelling. Riding. Washing clothes.

Thuja: Vaccination. Gonorrhoea, badly treated or suppressed. Sunstroke. Sexual excess. Tea. Coffee. Beer. Sweets. Tobacco. Fat meat. Onions. Sulphur. Mercury.

Upas.: Sexual excess.

Urt-u.: Burns. Bee-stings. Blows. Suppressed milk. Suppressed nettle-rash.

Val.: Injuries (slightest injury = spasms. Bed-sores form soon in typhoid).

Variol.: Contusion (enlarged testicle).

Verat.: Fright. Shock of injury. Disappointed love. Injured pride or honour. Suppressed exanthema. Opium. Tobacco. Alcohol.

Verat-v.: Sun. Suppressed menses. Suppressed lochia.

Vinc.: Anger (red nose). Mental exertion (tremulousness and starting).

Viol-o.: Suppressed discharges.

Viol-t.: Suppressed milk-crust (nervous paroxysms).

Visc.: Chill. Wetting. Fright. Suppression of menses.

Xan.: Injury to nerve. Wetting (getting feet wet). Suppression of menses.

Zinc.: Grief. Anger. Fright. Night watching. Operations. Frost-bite. Suppressions: eruptions; otorrhoea; menses; lochia; milk.

Zinc-ac.: Night-watching.

Zing.: Melons. Bread.

Cross, Crossing

(THE UNMANAGEABLE PATIENT WHO CROSSES ARGUES OR QUARRELS WITH THE DOCTOR)

(A practitioner should not be upset or get offended if a patient talks in an unruly or insulting way. That in itself is a symptom!)

A patient is supposed to follow the instruction of his doctor: but suppose he challenges or argues with the doctor. He is crossing! Here two top-ranking remedies that should at once come to your mind are *Chamomilla* and *Nux-vomica*.

Rarely we come across patients who are unmanageable.* Under the remedy *Lycopodium* in Boericke Mat. Med. we find the symptom 'haughty and arrogant when sick'.

Cases with so-called unmanageable patients you should not quarrel or argue with them nor argue to say that their attitude is not justified.

The word *cross* should come to your mind while dealing with such harsh and unmanageable patients. Without keeping this word in mind mere repertorisation has led to failures. An allopath, in such cases, may simply write on the case sheet 'patient unmanageable and not cooperating'. But in homoeopathy "the high and only mission of the physician is to cure always..." (Section 1 of the *Organon*) following case will suffice to illustrate the crossness of the patient.

Case: A boy of twelve years was having unbearable muscular pain in abdomen/hip extending to knee and it was intermittent. This pain was started few months back after diving in a swimming pool. Later it went off. Now for the last few days the pain had been occurring intermittently but almost daily.

The mother gave me an important information i.e. seeing no improvement with various doctors of several systems of medicine, whenever a new doctor was proposed, the boy would tell that he would give only thirty days (one month) time. If not cured within this time, he would stop that doctor.

This patient is 'crossing' the doctor. No sane person would enter into argument or put conditions on the doctor.

'Crossness' (more often found in children and sometimes in adults) along with the symptoms and remedies are given below for ready reference:

(For the convenience of the eye and easy reference the word 'cross' is given in bold type).

Aesculus hip. - feels miserably **cross**.

Ars-sul-rub. - **crosser**, and also acts with more energy.

Benzoic acid. - child **cross**, wants to be nursed in arms.

Chamomilla - insulting, **cross** and uncivil in temper.

Chamomilla - she is sleepless and **cross**.

China-off. - ill humor; cheerful persons become **cross** and irritable.

Cina - the Cina patient is hungry, **cross**, ugly and wants to be rocked.

Cina - child exceedingly **cross**, cries and strikes at all around him.

Coffea cruda - child frets and worries in an innocent manner; is not **cross**, but sleepless; it laughs one moment and cries the next.

Crotalus-hor. - snappish temper; irritable, **cross**, infuriated by least annoyance.

Cuprum-met. - changeable mood; children **cross** and irritable, or indifferent and dull, in brain affections.

Dioscorea. - irritable; feels **cross** and troubled.

Hepar-sul. - strumous, outrageously **cross** children.

Hepar-sul. - temper obstinate and **cross**, a ferocious spleen which would lead to cold blooded murder even among those habitually gay and benevolent.

Ictodes - **cross**; impetuous; inclined to contradict.

Iodum - **cross**, with excessive nervous excitability.

Kalmia - toward evening and next forenoon very **cross**.

Lac-can. - very **cross** and irritable only while headache lasts.

Lycopodium - sensitive, irritable disposition; peevish and **cross** on getting awake; easily excited to anger; cannot endure slightest opposition, and is speedily beside herself. Dictatorial. Talks with an air of command. Peevish, dissatisfied. Talks imperious. Manner stiff and pretentious.

Lycopodium - suitable for: old women and children; persons of keen intellect, but feeble muscular development; upper part of body wasted, lower part semi-dropsical; lean and predisposed to lung and hepatic affections; herpetic and scrofulous constitutions; hypochondriacs subject to skin diseases; lithic acid diathesis, much red sediment in urine, urine itself transparent; sallow people with cold extremities, haughty disposition, when sick, mistrustful, slow of comprehension, weak memory; weak children with well developed heads but puny, sickly bodies, irritable, nervous and unmanageable.

When sick, after sleep **cross**, pushing every one away angrily.

Lyssin. - very **cross**, so much so that his children expressed great surprise; he took offense at veriest trifles, scolded his wife and children, felt wretched, could not concentrate his attention on anything; sullen, does not wish to see or speak to any one.

Medorrhin. - **cross** through day, exhilarated at night, wants to play.

Menyanthes - ill humored, **cross**.

Natrum mur. - great irritability; child irritable and **cross** when spoken to; crying from slightest cause.

Nux vomica - Fiery, zealous temperament. (A boy of eleven developed pain in hip and thigh after diving in a swimming pool. All tests and treatment having failed, the parents tried alternative medical doctors. To each doctor, the boy would say that he would give only one month time and if not cured within that period, he would stop that doctor's treatment Nux-vom-1m single dose cured him.

Sinapis nigra. - **cross**, dissatisfied without cause; must guard himself constantly or be uncivil and pettish.

Stramonium. - child is very **cross**, and strikes or bites.

Tarentula hisp. - **cross**, tendency to get angry and to speak abruptly; is obliged to move limbs.

Uran-nit. - great despondency; ill-temper; **cross**; disagreeable.

Zincum met. - child **cross** toward evening; brain affected.

Diseases in which 'crossness' were found

(Addison's disease) - Natrum mur. - prevailing depression of mind, with spells of irritableness and **crossness**.

(Arthritis, gout) Bryonia - patient unbearably **cross**.

(Asthma of children) Ignatia - a **cross** word or correcting the child may bring on the attack.

(Atrophy of children) Abrotanum - child is **cross** and depressed, < from mental exertion.

(Atrophy of children) Calc-carb. - child obstinate, self-willed, **cross** before stool and faint after.

(Atrophy of children) Cina - child picks nose, is restless, **cross** and unamiable.

(Atrophy of children) Lycopodium - child weak, with well-developed head, but puny, sickly body, is irritable, nervous and unmanageable when sick, after sleep **cross** and pushes every one away angrily.

(Atrophy of children) Sulphur - child **cross**, obstinate, cannot bear to be washed or bathed.

(Bedwetting in children) Chamomilla - child **cross**, has to be carried.

(Blepharophthalmia, blepharitis) Ant-crud. - especially in **cross** children.

(Blepharophthalmia, blepharitis) Sulphur - blepharitis after the suppression of an eruption or when the patient is covered by eczema, especially in strumous children, who are **cross** and irritable by day and feverish and restless at night.

(Bronchitis) - Cina - child, though weak, was **cross** and obstinate, and cried when his will was not humored.

(Chorea) Cina - child outrageously **cross** and peevish, does not wish to play.

(Chorea) Lycopodium - **cross**, kicks, scolds, or awakens terrified, as if dreaming

(Chronic intestinal catarrh) - Ars-alb. - very **cross** and despondent.

(Constipation) Aethusa - morose and **cross**.

(Convulsions in children) Cina - child **cross**, will not be pleased, strikes around him.

(Convulsions in children) Zincum met. - child has been **cross** and irritable for days previous, with hurried motions, distended abdomen and more frequent urination than usual.

(Cough) Lycopodium - children are **cross** and naughty when awaking from their nap

(Crying of children) Chamomilla - cries pitifully when refused the least thing, wants to be carried rapidly, is **cross** and fretful.

(Crying of children) Cina - exceedingly **cross**, cries and strikes at all around him.

(Dentition, morbid) Zincum met. - child excessively **cross** and irritable, especially at night, while the eruption of several teeth at once undermines his strength.

(Diarrhoea of infants) Chamomilla - child wants to be carried, is **cross**, feverish and very thirsty.

(Diarrhoea of infants) Gnaphalium - **cross** and irritable children.

(Diarrhoea of infants) Natrum mur. - child **cross** and irritable.

(Diseases of cornea) Chamomilla - ulceration in **cross**, peevish children during dentition.

(Diseases of cornea) Hepar sulph. - marked sensitiveness of the eye to touch. lids red, swollen, spasmodically closed and bleed easily upon opening them. general chilliness. strumous, very **cross** children.

(Dropsy) Lycopodium - very **cross** after getting awake. ascites from liver affections, abuse of alcoholic drinks.

(Drunkards, diseases of) Cimicifuga - no disposition to talk, **cross** and dissatisfied, very restless, cannot sit long in one place, as it makes him frantic.

(Drunkards, diseases of) Sulphuric acid - **cross** and irritable.

(Eczema) Staphisagria - skin peels off with itching, hair falls out. Sunken face, nose pointed, blue rings around eyes. **Cross** words injure feelings.

(Eyes, chronic spasms) - Agaricus. - **cross**, self-willed, stubborn.

(Gastric catarrh, febris mucosa, biliosa) Ant-crud. - gastric catarrh from pastry, from overloading stomach, after fat food, from excessive heat of summer. children **cross** and peevish.

(Head, periodical neuralgia, in) Syphilinum - **cross**, irritable, peevish.

(Headache) Lac-can. - has the "blues", is **cross** and irritable.

(Headache) Lyssin. (Hydrophinum) - is **cross** and annoyed by trifles.

(Hysteria) Iodum - patient irritable, **cross** and sulky, hates to be touched anywhere.

(Infantile remittent fever) Nux vomica - child **cross** and irritable.

(Influenza) Iodum - **cross** and sulky, hates to be touched.

(Irritation of brain,due to dentition) Cuprum acet. - restless, **cross** and full of fear; respiration, sobbing, short and anxious; face pale and bloated; when drinking, child bites into glass or spoon; strength gradually sinking.

(Keratitis) Calc-carb. - child restless and **cross** during day.

(Marasmus) Abrotanum - the child is **cross** and depressed.

(Mastitis, inflammation of breast) Chamomilla - mammae hard and tender to touch, with drawing pains, is fretful, sleepless and **cross**.

(Meningitis, encephalitis) Cina - child **cross** and peevish.

(Metritis) Chamomilla - irritable and **cross**, can hardly restrain herself to treat people decently.

(Morbus addisoni) Natrum-mur. - **cross** and irritable.

(Morbus brighti, albinuria) Uranium nit. - ill-tempered, **cross** and irritable.

(Mortification, insults:) Chamomilla - **cross** against others.

(Ophthalmia) Ant-crud. - pustules on cornea or conjunctiva, especially in **cross** children afflicted with pustules on face and moist eruptions behind ears.

(Ophthalmia) Sulphur - chronic blepharitis in strumous children who are irritable and **cross** by day and feverish and restless at night.

(Rachitis, rickets) Calc-carb. - child is **cross** before stool and faint afterwards.

(Respiratory affections in children) Chamomilla - cough awakens it from a sound sleep and makes it **cross** and fretful, or child may sleep through the cough without awaking.

(Scrofulosis) (cane sugar.) - **cross** and whining.

(Simple continued fever) Chamomilla - child is **cross** and irritable when feverish.

(Sleeplessness) Cuprum met. - child awakes **cross** and irritable, kicking the clothes off and striking every one about it (Bell.).

(Sleeplessness) Stramonium - child awakes **cross** and irritable, as if frightened, knows no one, shrinks away or jumps out of bed.

(Spasm of glottis or larynx) Ignatia - caused in children by a **cross** word or necessary correction.

(Urinary difficulties) Helleborus - retention of urine in children without any particular cause, child **cross** and fretful, will not allow anyone to touch it.

(Worms) Filix mas. - irritable and **cross**.

Plethora, Plethoric individuals, Precocity

This is a general symptom but when noticed in a patient you cannot ignore it.

You must keep the name of disease (pathology) away from your mind while trying to find a remedy for a patient. We do not merely prescribe on pathology alone. In allopathy no doctor would prescribe insulin for typhoid, or antibiotics for diabetes. This is because they treat diseases.

In homoeopathy we treat 'a patient with diabetes' or 'a patient with typhoid' and so on and so forth. What is the difference?

In homoeopathy one and the same remedy may be indicated for typhoid in one patient and for diabetes in another patient.

'Plethora' means 'excess or abundant energy in body'. These persons are called plethoric individuals.

The dictionary defines 'plethora' as over-fullness or excess in any way; [an excess of (bodily fluid, particularly blood.) Excessive fullness of blood.]

Plethoric persons can do the job of ten persons single-handedly, both quantitatively as well as qualitatively. Other examples of plethoric persons are those who have done several Ph.D.s or who does Ph.D. at their sixtieth year of age; also those who have done several postgraduate studies in many subjects; also those who start studying, learning and mastering a subject or art even at their forty-five years of age. 'Tiredness' is not in their vocabulary. Work for them is worship. They are workaholics. Old age is not a deterrent for them.

Therefore, in the absence of more valuable symptoms in a case, if you find the patient is of the above type you may use the term plethora. This is a general symptom.

We see a person drinking liquor daily morning till night with little or no food. In an average individual this would mean vomiting, headache etc. But there are persons who are not at all affected by drinking whole day even if this repeats day after day, we call this abdominal plethora. Also those who take food daily in enormous quantity without putting on weight or any after-effects; these persons are also known plethoric—excess energy in the body or mind.

Plethoric individual: 1, Acon., Aur-met., Bell., Cal-c., Lyc., Phos., Sep., Sulph.; 2, Arn., Bry., Chin., Ferr., Nat-m., Nux-v., Rhus-t, Thuj.

— Complaints of plethoric, debilitated, hypochondriac, or nervous individuals. The principal remedies are: Acon., Amb., Am-c., Arn., Aur-met., Bell., Bry., Cal-c., Carb-v., Caust., Chin., Croc., Fer., Hep., Iod., Kalm., Kreos., Lyc., Natr-m., Nux-v., Op., Petr., Phos., Phos-ac., Rhus., Samb., Sarsap., Senn., Sep., Sil., Stann., Sulph., Thuj.

— Nervous, very irritable individuals: Acon., Amb., Arn., Aur-met., Bell., Cal-c., Chin., Ferr., Lyc., Nux-v., Petr., Samb.

Remedies for 'plethora'

Arnica. - In cases of sanguine plethoric people with lively expression, nervous women, very red face, disposed to cerebral congestion. - prolapsus uteri.

Artemisia - girl, aged 18, strong, well developed, plethoric; epilepsy.

Asarum - plethoric young woman suffered for years from headaches.

Asterias - man, aged 56, plethoric constitution, sedentary since eight years; epilepsy.

Aurum met. - violent orgasm; plethora.

Bryonia - plethora.

Cactus - sanguineous congestions in persons of plethoric habit.

Calc-carb. - congestions: head; eyes; ears; nose; face; chest; abdomen, limbs; plethora.

Calc-carb. - girl, aged 20, small, plethoric and blonde. - chlorosis with hermicrania.

Calc-carb. - nervous, hemorrhoidal, plethoric and lymphatic constitutions; disposed to grow fat.

Calc-carb. - plethoric woman. - vulvar tumor.

Calc-carb. - puberty: girls who begin with menses too early and too profuse; fat, yet chlorotic; plethoric girls, amenorrhoea, etc.

Capsicum - a relaxed plethoric sluggish, cold remedy.

Carbo-an. - elderly persons, especially with venous plethora, blue cheeks, blue lips, debility, etc.

Carbo-an. - venous plethora; threatened stagnation of circulation, cyanosis, vital heat sinks to a minimum.

Chelidonium - distension of veins; abdominal plethora; haemorrhoids.

Chelidonium - suits every age, sex and temperament, but particularly spare subjects disposed to abdominal plethora, cutaneous diseases, catarrh or neuralgia.

Chimaphila umb. - plethoric, hysterical young woman; dysuria.

Chimaphila umb. - plethoric young women with dysuria.

China-sulph. – a man, of plethoric habit; intermittent prosopalgia.

China-sulph. - plethoric woman, aged 30; intermittent apoplexy.

Coca. - weakly, nervous, fat or plethoric persons and such as have disease of heart and lungs suffer more from veta.

Cocculus - chronic prosopalgia in ladies of high rank, of ages varying from 30 to 40 years; abdominal plethora, extreme irritability of nervous system, especially of spinal cord; wind in epigastrium; acidity; obstinate constipation; diarrhoea; menstrual colic; bland, thick leucorrhoea; spinal irritation, with nocturnal pains; temperament choleric; through long-continued suffering had been brought into a state of desperation, constantly changing, and that quickly, from pusillanimity and despondency to extreme gaiety.

Cocculus - miss h., aged 35, plethoric; headache for 15 years came shortly after appearance of menses.

Cocculus - woman, aged 26; plethoric constitution; menorrhagia.

Colocynth - neuralgia of the small branches of the infraorbital nerves, in plethoric, choleric, irritable men, from 40 to 50 years of age, and disposed to hemorrhoidal and gouty affections and to congestions towards head; most frequent cause was vexation, but sometimes too close application to business; but once produced, this neuralgia was apt to recur many days successively at same hour, in forenoon.

Conium. - woman, aged 54, plethoric; uterine polypi.

Ferrum-iod. - symptoms of plethora; general turgescence of peripheric capillary system.

Ferrum-met. - pseudo-plethora; congestions, etc., yet anemic; face is earthy, flushing easily.

Ferrum-met. - best adapted to young weakly persons, anaemic and chlorotic, with pseudo-plethora, who flush easily; cold extremities; oversensitiveness; worse after any active effort.

Ferrum-met. - states of debility where the blood is poor in hematin require material doses; plethoric, haemorrhagic conditions call for small doses, from the second to the sixth potency.

Ferrum-phos. - the typical Ferr. phos. subject is not full blooded and robust, but nervous, sensitive, anaemic with the false plethora and easy flushing of ferrum.

Ferrum picricum - acts best in dark-haired patients, plethoric, with sensitive livers.

Glonoine - florid, plethoric, sensitive women.

Glonoine - seeming plethora, rapid deviations in distribution of blood; useful as a substitute for bleeding.

Hamamelis - woman, plethoric habit; epistaxis.

Ignatia - plethoric lady, aged 35, mother of eleven children; prosopalgia.

Ipecac. - plethora, fat children.

Kali-bich. - officer, aged 24, strong, plethoric constitution, choleric temperament, 15 months ago had chancre; syphilis.

Lachesis - man, plethoric, tendency to hydrothorax; periodic asthma.

Lachesis - woman, aged 53, plethoric, robust, choleric; ulcer on leg.

Lilium-tig. - dysentery; mucus and blood, with tenesmus, especially in plethoric and nervous women at change of life.

Lycopodium - man, aged 76, strong, corpulent, plethoric, highly fed, fond of wine and tobacco, is affected several times every year with severe catarrh, for eight years has had ulcer on right ala nasi; ulcer on leg.

Merc-sol. - girl, aged 19, well nourished, plethoric; dysentery.

Merc-sol. - woman, aged 54, small, plethoric; glossitis.

Merc-sol. - woman, aged 70, plethoric habit, bilious diathesis, subject to fluent hemorrhoids; bilious diarrhoea.

Mezereum - man, abdominal plethoric constitution, dark skin, had several tumors on head removed several years ago, suffering one year; prosopalgia.

Muriatic-acid. - man, aged 65, corpulent, plethoric, indulging in much food and drink, suffering from chronic bronchial catarrh, complicated by slight emphysema which dulcam. removed; passage of feces while urinating.

Opium - plethora.

Petroleum - man, aged 50, plethoric, corpulent, suffering several months; mental disturbance.

Phosphorus - man, aged 32, large, plethoric, light hair and eyes, formerly had scrofulous affection, for which he took blue pill and later corrosive sublimate; fungus haematodes.

Phosphorus - man, very stout, plethoric, worker in a brewery, suffering three months; hepatic congestion.

Pulsatilla - man, plethoric habit, subject to attacks of rheumatic gout; rheumatism in hand.

Pulsatilla - Mrs. c., aged 37, large, plethoric, light hair, blue eyes, suffering for years; headaches.

Sabadilla - young man, aged 16, plethoric; taenia.

Secale - irritable plethoric subjects.

Senega - especially suitable for plethoric, phlegmatic persons.

Sepia - jewess, aged 38, blonde, plethoric, in poor circumstances, suffering since last childbirth three years ago; amenorrhoea.

Stannum-met. - mr. e. j., aged 38, fleshy, hearty, plethoric; solar neuralgia.

Stramonium - plethoric, especially young persons.

Sulphur - itching and burning of anus; piles dependent upon abdominal plethora.

Sulphur - persons of nervous temperament, quick-motioned, quick-tempered, plethoric, skin excessively sensitive to atmospheric changes.

Sulphuric acid. - veins (of feet) distended; venous plethora.

Tussilago - compare: tussilago fragrans (pylorus pain, plethora and corpulency); tussilago farfara (coughs); as an intercurrent medicine in phthisis pulmonalis. (see tuberculinum).

Verat-vir. - especially adapted to full-blooded plethoric persons.

Verat-vir. - young lady, strong and plethoric, after sweeping a cold, damp floor in her slippers; amenorrhoea.

Diseases in which the symptom 'plethora' was found and their respective remedies

Congestion - complained by plethoric, debilitated, hypochondriac, or nervous individuals. The principal remedies are: 1, Acon., Aur., Calc., Hep., Kalm., Kreos., Lyc., Phos., Sep., Sulph.; 2, Amb., Amm., Arn., Bell., Bry., Carb-v., Caust., Croc., Chin., Fer., Iod., Natr.-m., Nux-v., Op., Petr., Phos.-ac., Rhus, Samb., Sarsap., Senn., Sil., Stann., Thuj.

- rush of blood of plethoric individuals requires: 1, Acon., Aur., Bell., Calc., Lyc., Phos., Sep., Sulph.

(Amenorrhoea) - for anaemia of plethoric individuals use: Acon., Bell., Bry., Gels., Nux-v., Op., Plat., Sabin., Sulph.

(Anaemia) Ferr-met. - pure anaemia with appearance of false plethora.

(Apoplexy) Arnica - involuntary discharge of urine and faeces. Suits middle-aged, plethoric and stout constitutions.

(Asthma) Belladonna - asthma of plethoric persons (especially in hot damp climates), < afternoon and evening.

(Back pain–spinal irritation) Nux vomica - backache accompanying abdominal plethora, with piles, constipation and urging to urinate, must sit up in order to turn from one side to the other.

(Bone diseases, osteitis, periostitis, exostosis, caries, necrosis, etc.) Carbo an. - venous plethora.

(Chlorosis) Ferr-met. - menses suppressed or profuse, watery, lumpy with labor-pains in abdomen. indicated also for plump fat women suffering from false plethora, migraine, anaemia, headaches.

(Constipation) Aloe - constipation of old people with abdominal plethora.

(Constipation) Belladonna - plethora, abdominal and spasmodic.

(Constipation) Lycopodium - abdominal plethora, with constipation in elderly people of the higher classes, suffering from retarded defaecation.

(Debility) Acon. - suitable to young people, especially young girls, when plethoric and leading a sedentary life, or for extreme sensitiveness to pain

(Debility) Ferr-m. - pseudoplethora, even tendency to get fat.

(Diaphragm, diseases of) Bell. - in plethoric persons with sympathetic affection or inflammation of liver.

(Gastralgia) Lycopodium - abdominal plethora.

(Gastralgia) Sulphur - venous plethora, haemorrhoids.

(Haematemesis, gastrorrhagia) Aloe - abdominal plethora, hepatic complications.

(Haemorrhages) - For active haemorrhages of young plethoric subjects: 1, Acon., Bell.; 2, Croc., Fer., Hyosc., Puls.; 3, Arn., Calc., Cham., Chin., Erecht., Erig., Gels., Geran., Ipec., Kalm., Lyc., Lycopus, Merc., Nitr-ac., Nux-v., Phos., Rhus, Sab., Sang., Senec., Sep., Stram., Sulph., Trill., Veratr-vir.

(Haemorrhage from uterus) - for active haemorrhage in plethoric persons give: 1, Acon., Bell., Bry., Calc., Cham., Fer., Nux-V., Plat., Sab., Sulph. 2, Arn., Croc., Hyosc., Ign., Ipec., Phos., Sil., Veratr.; 3, Trill.

(Haemorrhage from uterus) Camphor - metrorrhagia some days after delivery, unaccompanied by plethora.

(Haemorrhage from uterus) Sabina - plethoric women with habitual menorrhagia, who began to menstruate very early in life, always menstruated freely, and showed more or less a tendency to miscarriage.

(Haemorrhages) Belladonna - in plethoric people with red faces.

(Haemorrhoids) Aesculus-hip. - depressed and irritable. angina granulosa, a dark-red congestion of fauces, with dryness and soreness, from abdominal plethora.

(Headache) Glonoine - bad sequelae of cutting hair. intense congestion of the brain in plethoric constitutions, with persistent sensation of pulsation, from sudden suppression of menses, after anxiety and worry with sleeplessness.

(Headache) Sepia - sudor hystericus. Arthritic headaches, < mornings, with nausea and vomiting, urine loaded with uric acid, from abdominal plethora or menstrual disturbances.

Brain-fag from one-sided mental strain, loss of animal fluids or other depressing causes, < from any mental exertion, > after meals and from sleep.

(Headache) Sulphur - headache from abdominal plethora, from suppressed skin diseases, or chronic gouty and rheumatic headaches, increased by mental exertion, motion, coughing, sneezing.

(Heart diseases) - palpitation from plethora: acon., aur., cact., coff., dig., gels., glon., lach., nux m., op., phos., sulph., veratr. vir.

(Heart diseases) Ferr-met. - anaemia masked behind plethora and congestions, pale color of mucous membranes, with nun's murmur.

(Heels, pains in) Sabina - plethoric women, suffering from rheumatic inflammation.

(Hepatic derangements) Carbo-an. - venous plethora (Hepatic derangements) Chelidon - abdominal plethora from simple congestion to positive inflammation (Insanity) Stramonium - mental and nervous troubles especially in children or in plethoric young persons. (Mind symptoms) Nux vomica - abdominal plethora and constipation. (Mind symptoms) Sulphur - abdominal venous plethora, venous lethargy (Menses complaints) Glonoine - plethora. (Migraine) Nux vomica - patient irritable with his abdominal plethora. (Neuralgia) - in plethoric persons: 1, Acon., Arn., Bell., Fer., Hyosc., Merc., Natr-m., Nux-v., Puls.; 2, Aur., Bry., Calc., Chin., Lyc., Nitr-ac., Phos., Sep., Sulph.; (Neuralgia) Gelsemium - hysterical palpitation in plethoric women.

(Neurasthenia) Graphites - rush of blood to chest and head, but not from true plethora (Neurasthenia) Sulphur - abdominal plethora, haemorrhoids. (Sexual complaints) Silicea - nymphomania with plethora.

(Sleeplessness) Belladonna - sleeplessness, especially of plethoric children, from nervous excitement, from local congestion, from irritation in various parts

(Sleeplessness) Ferr-met. - weak, nervous persons with false plethora. (Stomatitis, inflammation and ulceration of buccal cavity). Capsicum - or to phlegmatic, plethoric persons, who lead a sedentary life (Tonsillitis) Kali-nit. - tonsillitis in strong, plethoric persons.

(Vagina affections) Belladonna - plethoric persons disposed to phlegmonous inflammations.

(Vertigo, dizziness) Aloe - severe headache and vertigo from abdominal plethora. Vertigo in women of nervous, relaxed or phlegmatic habits during climaxis.

Precocious children

(Note: What we call plethora in adults is called precocity in case of children. It is otherwise also called as child prodigy.)

(Precocious = having developed certain abilities or an inclination at a certain early age than usual. Strikingly advanced or mature in mental development, speech, social behaviour etc. Developed in advance of the norm either mentally or physically or both).

Atrophy of precocious children: Calc., Lyc., Merc., Phos., Sulph.

Belladonna (Atrophy of children) - for precocious children, with blue eyes and fair hair. The child does not sleep much, though appearing to be drowsy; it lies half sleeping and half waking; moaning; jerking of the muscles.

Lycopodium - mild temperaments of lymphatic constitution, with catarrhal tendencies; older persons, where the skin shows yellowish spots, earthy complexion, uric acid diathesis, etc.; also precocious weakly children.

Merc-sol. (Atrophy of children) - emaciation; skin dry, rough; dirty yellow or clammy, especially that of the thighs; icy-cold sweat on forehead, sour or oily sweat on scalp; pustular or suppurating herpes; glands swollen and suppurating; skin chaps easily, becomes raw and sore; frequent attacks of jaundice; abdomen, especially right hypochondrium, swollen and sore to pressure; stool green, sour, watery, with emaciation; diarrhoea bloody, slimy, green, with tenesmus often continuing after stool; genitals sore and excoriated, urine causes pain; child pulls at penis; child pale, weak, and obtuse, or precocious and restless; fontanelles open, the head large and covered with offensive sweat; gums soft and bleed easily; sour night-sweats; blepharophthalmia suppurativa.

Nux vom. - boy, aged 9, precocious, intellect highly cultivated, allowed no associates; enuresis.

Phosphorus - chlorosis, anemia: with too rapid growth; with excessive muscular debility, but without loss of adipose tissue, in patients with precocious puberty; deep-seated chronic cases, with tubercular diathesis;

Old age, Senility, Presenility

Mind symptoms and rare-strange-peculiar symptoms may misguide us. But general symptoms never misguide us. Old age, senility, presenility is another general symptom.

(Senile = Related to the involutional changes associated with old age. Senile dementia = Deterioration of mental activity in the elderly associated with an impaired blood supply to the brain.

Senility = A state of mental and physical deterioration resulting from old age. Presenile = Prematurely aged in mind and body.) Senile decay: Agn., Arg-n., Ars., Bar-c., Can-i., Con., Fl-ac., Iod., Lyc., Oophor., Phos., Thiosin., Senile enlargement of prostate: Aloe., Bar-c., Bez-ac., Con., Dig., Iod., Nux-v., Sabal., Sel., Staph., Sul. Senile pruritus: Ars., Bar-c., Calc-p., Con., Cop., Crot-t., Dolichos., Fogop., Mez., Puls., Sulph., Senile gangrene: Oxygen, Amm-m., Ars., Carb-v., Chin., Con., Euphor., Phos-ac., Plumb., Sec., Solanum. Senile gangrene of toes: Carb-an., Carb-v., Cupr., Ph-ac., Sec. Senile uraemia: Iod., Lyc. Pre-senility: Bone and teeth affected: Selen.

While on this chapter, we must keep a remedy in mind as the foremost and it is our great Selenium. The key-words that should lead you to this remedy are bone and teeth.

Teeth decay (even since childhood); had been going to dentist several times; then he has bone complaints, mainly backache.

With the above two symptoms in a patient you may ask a question whether he has sun aggravation (headache or tiredness by going in the sun) and if the patient confirms, it is Selenium and Selenium alone. Let me explain you what is the kind of sun aggravation in a Selenium patient. If has to go in the hot sun (9 a.m. to 4 p.m.) even to cross the street to go to the opposite house, he will cover his head, at least even with a newspaper or hand bag. Such a short distance of hundred steps too he is intolerant of sun heat falling on his head. (For those people, you must advise wearing of white cotton cap in the hot summer while going out).

Whenever a patient complains of chronic bad teeth and you also find that he has back pain, in these cases your next question should be about intolerant of sun heat falling on his head, and if he affirms, it is Selenium.

Remember the first sentence in Boericke Materia Medica: Selenium is a constant constituent of bones and teeth. One more key-word in some Selenium patient is emaciation of thighs. If he is emaciated and is prematurely old-looking you cannot think of any other remedy than Selenium.

Selenium is one of the best remedies for senility and pre-senility provided the above three symptoms agree viz., early and frequent decay of teeth, backache and intolerant of sunlight falling on his head even for a minute.

Remedies for 'senility'

Agaricus (Paralysis) - sense of languor as if the body were bruised and the joints dislocated; sense of weariness and weakness all down the spine; paralysis of lower limbs, with slight spasms of arms; palsy of upper and lower limbs from incipient softening of spinal cord; paraplegia from congestion of lumbar cord; violent pains in all paralyzed parts; pain in lumbar region and sacrum, agg. while sitting or during exertion in daytime; formication in upper and lower limbs as if gone to sleep; limbs cold, blue; crosswise affections. Senile tremor.

Allium cepa - gangrene senilis, woman, aged 80 (externally as a salve). -woman, aged 80; senile gangrene.

Ambra (Asthma) - asthma senile et siccum; also suitable to children and scrofulous persons, with short, oppressed breathing, paroxysms of spasmodic cough, with expectoration of mucus, wheezing in the air-passages and pressure in the chest, followed by eructations of wind from stomach; asthma accompanied by cardiac symptoms, oppression of breathing and a feeling as of a load or lump in left chest and fluttering in the region of the heart, or palpitations, especially in nervous, thin, scrawny women; oppression in left chest through to the back and between the shoulders, as if emanating from the heart, with palpitations, anguish and loss of breath; asthma while attempting coition.

Ambra grisea - tearing pain in upper half of brain. Senile dizziness.

Anacardium orientale - senile dementia.

Ant-tart. (Asthma) - asthma senile; asthma of children; anxious oppression, difficulty of breathing and shortness of breath, with desire to sit erect; oppression and suffocative fits, coming on suddenly, agg. evening, morning, in bed; mucus and rattling in chest; suffocative cough or congestion of blood to chest and palpitation of heart; gasping inhalation, feeling of fulness and contraction of chest; the cough after having lasted some time becomes loose and relieves the contraction of chest.

Old age, Senility, Presenility 219

Ars-alb. (Asthma) - periodical asthma; asthma of senility, after suppressed coryza and coexistence of emphysema and cardiac affections; loss of breath immediately on lying down, in the evening, with whistling and constriction in the trachea, agg. from motion; must incline chest forward, must spring out of bed, especially about midnight, in order to breathe; chest feels as if too narrow; throat and chest feel as if bound together; increasing dyspnoea with despair and anxious sweat all over; asthma from fatigue, from emotions, from suppressed itch; agg. after coughing, with sensation of contraction of chest and stomach, abating as soon as he raises frothy saliva, thick mucus or streaked with blood; amel. From warmth, warm food, agg. from cold things.

Ars-alb. (Gangrene) - senile gangrene; ulcers extremely painful or entirely insensible, with elevated edges, secreting a bad, watery foetid ichor; hard, shining, burning swelling with bluish-black, burning vesicles, filled with acrid ichor, amel. from warmth, agg. from cold; extreme restlessness; gangrene accompanied by foetid diarrhoea; great weakness and emaciation; numbness, stiffness and insensibility of the feet; general coldness with parchment-like dryness of the skin, followed by heat.

Ars-alb. (Pruritus) - itching with burning or an eruption emitting watery fluid like sweat and attended with much constitutional weakness; chronic cases; senile pruritus in broken-down constitutions, agg. from cold applications, amel. from warmth; itching of genital organs.

Ars-alb. - gangrena senilis sicca, with coldness, desire for more covering; > from warmth.

Ars-iod. - arteriosclerosis, myocardial degeneration and senile heart. - myocarditis and fatty degeneration.

Asparagus off. (Dropsy) - old people with heart disease; weak action of heart; when urinating the last drops, constricting pain in cardiac region, turns blue in face, urine has an unpleasant odor; must sit up in bed to relieve dyspnoea. Hydrothorax in senility on a gouty diathesis.

Baryta carb. (Debility) - suits first childhood and senility (old age) with mental or physical debility; old people, especially when fat or when they suffered from gout; constantly weak and weary, wishes to lean on something, to sit or lie down, and still feels weak and weary; deficient memory, absent-mindedness.

Baryta carb. - emaciation senilis.

Baryta carb. (Asthma) - asthma senile (after Ant-tart.); suffocative catarrh of fleshy old people, with impending paralysis of lungs; cough and shortness of breath in old phlegmatic persons; night cough with asthmatic breathing, chest full of phlegm, want of clear consciousness; whining mood; circumscribed redness of cheeks; immovable pupils; cold hands and feet. Asthma of scrofulous children, with enlargement of tonsils and cervical glands; light hair; agg. from wet weather, warm air, and followed by frequent and copious urination.

Baryta carb. (Insanity) - senile dementia, mental and physical debility; mental weakness and timidity of dwarfish children with undeveloped brain, who learn with difficulty because they cannot remember; forgetful, in the midst of a speech the most familiar words fail him; loss of memory, especially for recent events, groaning and murmuring, pusillanimous; peculiar dread of men, imagines she is laughed at, which frightens her; full of anxiety and evil forebodings about the most trivial affairs; no self-confidence, fears to undertake anything; full of delusions, thinks his legs are cut off, and that he walks on his knees; aversion to strangers, fear of and in the presence of others.

Baryta carb. - affects glandular structures, and useful in general degenerative changes, especially in coats of arteries, aneurism, and senility. - senile dementia.

Baryta mur. - arterio-sclerosis of the lung, thus in senile asthma, modifies the arterial tension.

Benzoic acid. (Heart diseases) - gout or rheumatism affecting the heart and nodular swellings in the joints; pains change place incessantly, but are more constant about heart; awakens after midnight with violent palpitation of heart and temporal arteries; at times tearing rheumatic pains in extremities relieve the heart; palpitation and trembling while sitting, agg. after drinking, at night; undulating or intermitting beats of heart; dysuria senilis; urine dark and of an offensive odor.

Benzoic acid. (Kidney/bladder stone) - nephritic colic; morbid condition of urine in persons with calculous or gouty diathesis; urine containing urates of ammonia and having a strong ammoniacal smell. Dysuria senilis from irritability of the bladder and mucopurulent discharge.

Benzoic acid. (Prostate gland, diseases of) - enlargement of prostata; sensibility of bladder with muco-purulent discharge; dysuria senilis; weak loins, when the gravel is trifling; urine of a repulsive odor; formication at anus.

Benzoic acid. (Urinary difficulties) - vesicular catarrh; irritability of the bladder; nocturnal enuresis in children; too frequent desire to evacuate the bladder, urine being normal; decrease of the quantity of urine, which is thick and bloody; urine has strong odor like that of horses and contains excess of hippuric acid (Nitr-ac.); urine brownish, cloudy, alkaline or dark-reddish, high specific gravity and acid reaction, sometimes of a putrid, cadaverous smell; morbid condition of urine, as in persons with calculous or gouty diathesis; dysuria senilis, when gravel is trifling and the irritable state of bladder and pains are induced by other causes, with too frequent desire to urinate, though urine appears normal.

Bufo rana - prematurely senile.

Carbo veg. - (gangrene): humid; senile; in cachectic persons; when vital powers have become weakened; great foulness of secretions; great prostration. - sepsis; indifference; fainting after sleep, while yet in bed, morning; no restlessness. - moist skin; hot perspiration; senile gangrene beginning in toes; bed sores; bleed easily.

Causticum - broken down seniles.

Cocainum - chorea; paralysis agitans; alcoholic tremors and senile trembling.

Conium (Apoplexy) - the senile women's remedy; numbness, with sensation of coldness on one side of head; headache, as if head were too full and would burst, morning when awaking; hemiplegia, sweat as soon as he falls asleep and even with the closing of the eyes.

Conium (Asthma) - asthma senile; scrofulosis with enlarged and indurated glands; dry, nightly, tickling cough; evening dyspnoea, agg. in wet weather, in the morning when awaking; want of breath from slight exercise; copious mucous expectoration with the cough.

Conium (Insanity) - senile dementia, ailments of old maids and widows from ungratified sexual desire; folie circulaire, alternate excitement and depression; cannot endure any kind of excitement, it brings on physical and mental depression, weakness; inability to sustain any mental effort, excessive difficulty to recollect things, especially dates; desire for solitude and unsympathizing insensibility from indolence; aversion to company and yet averse to being alone, is inclined to abuse company, scolds and will not bear contradiction; chilliness, frequent spasmodic motions; weak sexual power and frequent pollutions; anaemia of brain.

Conium (Sexual complaints) - premature senility; atrophy of testicles, bad effects from suppressed sexual desire or from excessive indulgence; painful seminal emission instead of the normal pleasurable thrill; sexual desire without erection or with an insufficient one; pollutions, with subsequent excitement of the sexual desire, even when merely dallying with women; discharge of prostatic juice during every motion, without lascivious thoughts.

Crotalus hor. (Insanity) - incipient stage of senile dementia; mental delusions, such as mistakes in keeping accounts or writing letters, forgetfulness in figures, names and places; awaking at night struggling with imaginary foes; thinks he is the prey of enemies or of hideous animals; dislike to members of his own family; marked indifference and apathy, seems only half alive; fits of drowsiness or coma; apoplexy in broken-down constitutions or inebriates.

Crotalus hor. (Mind symptoms) - timidity, fear, anxiety; weeping or snappish temper, cross; irritable, infuriated by the least annoyance; sadness; her thoughts dwell on death continually; twitching and nervous agitation; lethargy, loss of co-ordination; incipient stage of senile dementia.

Crotalus hor. - hd., aged 69, during incipient stage of senile dementia, delusions, etc. - mental delusions, such as mistakes in keeping his accounts and in writing letters, forgetfulness of figures, names and places; awaking in the night struggling with imaginary foes; imagines himself surrounded by enemies or hideous animals; taking antipathies to members of family. - incipient stage of senile dementia.

Cuprum met. - gangrena senilis of foot in a man.

Digitalis (Prostate gland, diseases of) - senile hypertrophy of prostate, cardiac symptoms marked; dribbling discharge of urine and continued fulness after micturition or fruitless effort to urinate; throbbing pain in region of neck of bladder during the straining efforts to pass water; increased desire to urinate after a few drops have passed, causing the old man to walk about in distress, though motion increases desire to urinate; frequent desire to defaecate at the same time; very small, soft stool passed without relief; urine pale, slightly cloudy, looking smoky.

Digitalis - senile pneumonia.

Dolichos - senile pruritus.

Drosera - the attacks of cough are of a spastic character, depending on irritation of the vagus, and affect the bronchi; whooping cough, bronchial catarrh, bronchitis in senility, emphysema and bronchiectasis.

Euphorbium (Gangrene) - gangrene following gastritis or enteritis, temperature continually falling; inflammation and swelling, followed by cold gangrene; great torpor; insensibility of parts affected; chilliness and shuddering over whole body; gangraena senilis.

Fagopyrum - pruritus senilis.

Ferrum pic. - senile hypertrophy of the prostate. Epistaxis.

Ichthyolum - rectal suppositories for senile prostate.

Ictodes - spasmodic asthma; senile catarrh.

Iodum (Uraemia) - uraemia from senile hypertrophy and induration of prostata; urine dark, thick, ammoniacal; chronic congestive headache in old people.

Jaborandi - contra-indicated in heart failure, and in post-puerperal uraemia, and in senile cases.

Kreosotum - senile gangrene.

Lachesis - senile erysipelas. - senile gangrene.

Lobelia inflata - senile emphysema.

Lycopodium (Bronchitis chronica) - distressing, fatiguing, tickling cough, agg. afternoon, and evening, and on going to sleep and in the morning; chronic bronchitis, with copious muco-serous or mucopurulent sputa; congestion of liver, flatulency, constipation, cachectic complexion, red gravel, acid dyspepsia; dry cough, day and night, in feeble emaciated boys (florid scrofula); emphysema, dilation of air-tubes and senile catarrh; respiration short before and during cough, ending with loud belching; salty expectoration; emaciation of upper part of body; great fear of solitude.

Mezereum - man, aged 74, weak and dyspeptic, a subject of emaciation senilis; pruritus senilis.

Moschus - premature senility.

Phosphoric acid. (Gangrene) - senile gangrene. - external parts become black.

Phosphorus (Headache) senile cerebral atrophy; softening of brain with persistent headache, slow answering questions, vertigo, feet drag, formication and numbness of limbs; in washerwomen fear of washing, as it causes rush of blood to head, red face and eyes; weakness of memory and difficulty of thinking.

Phosphorus (Headache) - washerwomen's headache; senile cerebral atrophy; brain-fag from mental overwork and constant strain of eyes; salivation with headache (Epiph.).

Pulsatilla (Pruritus) - itching and burning on inner and upper side of prepuce; itching, agg. at night, from pastry or pork, from delayed menses, amel. from cold water. Pruritus senilis.

Rhus aromatica - enuresis due to vesical atony; senile incontinence.

Secale - woman, aged 80; senile gangrene. - incipient cataract, senile especially in women.

Secale (Insanity) - paralytic mental state; insanity with inclination to bite, with inclination to drown himself; impaired power of thinking; apathy and indifference; treats his family with contempt and sarcasm; wandering talk and hallucinations; great anguish, wild with anxiety; senile dementia, senile gangrene.

Selenium - Abject despair, uncompromising melancholy. Bone and teeth are affected.

Staphisagria (Vulva, pruritus and tumors) - prurigo senilis, or from parasites; stinging-itching of vulva.

Strophanthus - senile vertigo.

Tarentula cubensis - "senile" ulcers.

Thlaspi bursa pastoris (Urinary difficulties) - haematuria; dysuria and strangury, amel. after passing a quantity of renal sand; urine turbid, with deep-red sediment (needs proving); dysuria senilis.

Tuberculinum - as the surgeon before the anaesthetic, so must the physician know the heart before administering this drug, especially to children and seniles-and to young seniles.

Vipera (Dyspepsia, weakness of stomach) - nausea, vomiting, with vertigo and dyspnoea, syncope, jaundice, colliquative diarrhoea, palpitations; numbness and general lassitude; dyspepsia of old people, or of persons prematurely senile, suffering from spasmodic affections of throat and chest; periodical attacks of dyspepsia.

Remedies for presenility

Bufo rana - prematurely senile.

Vipera (Dyspepsia, weakness of stomach) - nausea, vomiting, with vertigo and dyspnoea, syncope, jaundice, colliquative diarrhoea, palpitations; numbness and general lassitude;

dyspepsia of old people, or of persons prematurely senile, suffering from spasmodic affections of throat and chest; periodical attacks of dyspepsia.

Complaints in old age, old people

Aethusa - old woman during cholera season. — cholerine.

Agaricus - difficult emission of urine in elderly persons, stream slow, feeble, intermitting, or only in drops; discharge viscid, tenacious; frequent urging to urinate and frequent erections; burning itching of skin; cramp like drawing in groin during micturition.

Agnus castus - old sinners, with impotence and gleet.

Agnus castus (Gonorrhoea) - yellow and purulent discharge after inflammation has subsided; excoriations about genitals; induration of testicles. helps the gleet of old sinners who cannot get up a decent erection and whose sexual desire is below par.

Agnus castus (Sexual complaints) - diminished sexual instinct; after an embrace he feels easy and light; complete prostration and impotence; semen watery and deficient; penis so relaxed that voluptuous fancies excite no erections; testes cold, swollen, hard and painful; impotence, with gleet, especially with those who frequently had gleet; pollutions from irritable weakness with prostatorrhoea; prostatic juice passes with hard stool. Premature old age in young persons from abuse of sexual functions, with melancholy, apathy, mental distraction, self-contempt, general debility, and spermatorrhoea of old sinners, though impotent.

Allium cepa - an old woman; whitlow.

Aloe - old men with enlarged prostate.

Aloe - colic, especially in elderly people, with intense griping pains across the lower portion of abdomen, with a preference for right side, before and during stool, which is windy and watery; after stool all pain ceases, leaving the patient bathed in sweat and extremely prostrated; painfulness over the whole abdomen, especially along both sides of the navel, which parts cannot endure being touched; on making a false step a pain in stomach; discharge of much flatus, burning, smelling offensive.

Ambra. - a very old man. - brittle finger nails. - asthma when attempting coition.

Ambra. - old persons and children. - asthma.

Ammoniac. - aged people suffering during cold weather. see bronchial affections.

Angustura. - old woman: loose cough every afternoon at 3 o' clock.

Ant-crud. - elderly persons with diarrhoea all at once get costive.

Apis - apoplexies in old persons.

Apis - old woman, light complexion, lymphatic temperament; with dropsical swellings.

Apocynum cannabinum - aralia hispida - wild elder - a valuable diuretic, useful in dropsy of the cavities, either due to hepatic or renal disease with constipation.

Argentum nitricum - old man's look; tight drawing of skin over bones.

Aurantium - diseases of old men, especially with coldness and chilliness.

Baptisia - old woman, aged 79; oedema.

Baryta carb. - especially adapted to diseases of old men.

Baryta carb. - many of symptoms suggest sclerosis of brain and spine, especially in children and the aged. Compare Bar.-m

Baryta mur. - complaints of elderly people, arising from chronic endoarteritis and atheromatous condition of arteries; pulse rapid and full, beating of heart irregular, pulse scarcely perceptible.

Bellis perennis - vertigo in elderly people.

Berberis vul. - an old woman, aged 70; heartburn of thirty years standing.

Bovista - adapted to stammering children, old maids with palpitation; and "tettery" patients.

Bovista. - old maids; palpitation.

Bryonia. - old women, accustomed to taking alcohol. asthma.

Calcarea-carb. - should not be repeated too frequently in elderly people.

Calc-carb. - more frequently indicated with the young; cannot be often repeated with the old, unless higher potencies are used.

Carbo-veg. - long-standing catarrhs of elderly people or in persons whose vitality is reduced to the lowest ebb by insufficient nourishment rather than by disease, with venous capillary dilatation of the pharyngo-laryngeal parts and prevailing torpor of all the functions (Phos.); ulcerative pain in larynx, with scraping and titillation; putrid sputa.

Carbo-an. - elderly persons, especially with venous plethora, blue cheeks, blue lips, debility, etc.

Causticum - old maid, aged 75, fond of coffee; chronic headache.

Causticum - old maid, weakly, pale; prosopalgia.

Chamomilla - adults, even aged persons with arthritic or rheumatic diathesis.

Chelidonium - an aged woman; pneumonia.

China - an old woman, reduced by care and poverty; pneumonia following intermittent.

China - old women after menopause; pleurisy, dropsy.

Citrus limonum. - diseases of old men, especially with coldness and chilliness.

Cocculus - old man, compelled to stand during his work; inguinal hernia.

Coffea tosta - coffee and tea are injurious to the young, but beneficial to the old, because they increase the nitrogenous bodies by diminishing tissue waste.

Conium - troubles at the change of life old maids and bachelors.

Conium (Insanity) - senile dementia, ailments of old maids and widows from ungratified sexual desire; folie circulaire, alternate excitement and depression; cannot endure any kind of excitement, it brings on physical and mental depression, weakness; inability to sustain any mental effort, excessive difficulty to recollect things, especially dates; desire for solitude and unsympathizing insensibility from indolence; aversion to company and yet averse to being alone, is inclined to abuse company, scolds and will not bear contradiction; chilliness, frequent spasmodic motions; weak sexual power and frequent pollutions; anaemia of brain.

Conium - hypochondriacal old maids; old, weak and feeble men.

Cyclamen - weakly old man, with pale, herpetic face and red nose; enteralgia.

Cypripedium - headaches of elderly people and during climacteric.

Digitalis (Prostate gland, diseases of) - senile hypertrophy of prostate, cardiac symptoms marked; dribbling discharge of urine and continued fulness after micturition or fruitless effort to urinate; throbbing pain in region of neck of bladder during the straining efforts to pass water; increased desire to urinate after a few drops have passed, causing the old man to walk about in distress, though motion increases desire to urinate; frequent desire to defaecate at the same time; very small, soft stool passed without relief; urine pale, slightly cloudy, looking smoky.

Euphrasia - old woman, gouty; obscuration of cornea.

Ferrum-phos. - old maid, aged 75; chronic diarrhoea.

Geranium - constant hawking and spitting in elderly people.

Grindelia - old man, broken down with years of sickness, with organic disease of heart, just rallying from an attack of pneumonia; paresis of pneumogastric.

Hamamelis - old man, hemiplegic; epistaxis.

Helleborus - an old woman having been accused of theft by the women around, took it so much to heart that she hanged herself. This suicide produced a profound effect upon the women of the village. One after another accused herself of having caused the death of the old woman by their insinuations; they wept and howled, ran about day and night wringing their hands and despairing of salvation on account of their sin; they became quite irrepressible and deranged. in this way twenty-four or twenty-five women were affected, every fresh case being followed by another. - hysterical mania.

Hyoscyamus. - hysterical women and young girls; old men; drunkards.

Hyoscyamus. - old man; diarrhoea.

Ictodes - catarrh of aged persons.

Ignatia - aged women, oversensitive to external impressions; spinal affection (paralysis, fixed pain in spine); habitual constipation; right half of body weakest; vertigo.

Iodum - a colored child, two years old, with the face of an old man, dry skin, large head and stomach, very large genitals, thin arms and legs, is hardly able to stand, sits by preference out doors in the burning sun of the tropics; is always hungry; has a blood boil on left forearm near the wrist; iodium was followed by a fine eruption, resembling itch when the child began to improve and got well.

Iodum - aged persons.

Kali-carb. - adapted to fleshy, aged people, and to complaints following parturition; diseases characterized by stitching pains.

Kali-carb. - dropsical affections and paralysis of old persons.

Kali-carb. - old woman; asthma.

Kreosotum - often indicated for old women.

Lachesis - elderly woman, thin and cachectic.

Lycopodium (Sexual complaints) - mental, nervous and bodily weakness; impotence; penis small, cold and relaxed; erections feeble; falls asleep during an embrace; excessive and exhausting pollutions; desponding, grieving, extremely sensitive; weakness of memory; pale, wretched complexion; weak digestion; the old man's balm; strong desire, but cannot get up an erection.

Lycopodium - depressed and imperfect digestion; constant sensation as if the bowels were loaded; torpor of bowels, faeces hard, scanty, passed with difficulty, from constriction of the sphincter ani, and feeling as if much remained behind; much loud flatus and croaking in left hypochondrium; obstructed flatus, with pains striking from right to left; itching and tension at anus in the evening in bed; itching eruptions at anus, painful to touch; sense of fulness after eating, even very little, with drowsiness, sour vomiting; nightly restlessness; agg. 4 to 8 p. m., from cold food, cabbage and vegetables with husks, oysters, from wrapping up, amel. in company, on getting cool, after loosening garments, discharge of flatus either way, from uncovering head or body, from warm food; abdominal plethora, with constipation in elderly people of the higher classes, suffering from retarded defaecation.

Lycopodium - suitable for: old women and children; persons of keen intellect, but feeble muscular development; upper part of body wasted, lower part semi-dropsical; lean and predisposed to lung and hepatic affections; herpetic and scrofulous constitutions; hypochondriacs subject to skin diseases; lithic acid diathesis, much red sediment in urine, urine itself transparent; sallow people with cold extremities, haughty disposition, when sick, mistrustful, slow of comprehension, weak memory; weak children with well developed heads but puny, sickly bodies, irritable, nervous and unmanageable when sick, after sleep cross, pushing every one away angrily.

Mag-mur. (Haemorrhage from uterus) - metrorrhagia of old maids, blood clotted; < at night in bed, causing hysteria; uterine diseases complicated with hysteria; after abuse of mercury.

Manganum acet. - old man; podagra.

Merc sol. - epistaxis; hemorrhages in old women after climacteric period; haematuria in typhoid fever; blonde hair, lax skin and muscles; tongue and mouth moist, with thirst; sweat of feet without odor; disposition earnest, anxious; blood light colored; scorbutic condition of gums. —hemorrhages.

Mezereum - old man; shingles.

Millefolium - for the aged, atonic; for children and women.

Natrum mur. - elderly lady, teacher, after loss of daughter; excessive grief.

Natrum mur. - old woman, from her youth up; hemicrania.

Nux vom. - elderly unmarried woman; disorder of stomach.

Nux vom. - lady, elderly, spare, suffering six weeks; ulcer on gums.

Oleum jec. - chronic gout and rheumatism of elderly persons, with rigidity of muscles and tendons, joint nearly inflexible.

Opium - congestive chills, especially in children and elderly people chill without thirst, followed by heat with deep soporous sleep, open mouth, twitching of limbs; spasmodic contraction of facial muscles, ending in hot profuse sweat, with desire to uncover; heat and sweat intermingle, sweat does not relieve. aversion to food; longing for spirituous liquors. apyrexia: cerebral congestion with profound stupor; complete indifference; suppression of secretions.

Opium (Atrophy of children) - child wrinkled, looks like a little dried-up old man; stupor.

Opium - elderly woman, robust, with rosy cheeks; vomiting.

Opium - emaciation; child wrinkled and looks like a little driedup old man; stupor.

Opium - especially suitable for children and old persons.

Opium - mania a potu: with dullness of senses, at intervals sopor, with snoring; in old, emaciated persons; sees animals coming towards him; people want to hurt him, execute him; creeping under covers or jumping out of bed; in old sinners whose long lives of excess have thoroughly destroyed their constitutions; in those who have had the disease repeatedly, it taking but a small quantity of liquor to throw them again into delirium; face wears a constant expression of fright and terror; preceded by epileptiform fits; imagine they see frightful objects and are in great fear; believe themselves to be murderers or criminals to be executed; want to run away; staring look; twitching of muscles of face and mouth; lockjaw; tremor.

Paeonia - a poor old man, suffering ten years; ulcer of leg.

Phosphorus (Heart diseases) - premature old age and overgrown adolescents.

Populus tremuloides - chronic catarrh; chronic gleet; elderly persons; ardor urinae or perfect retention; urine scanty, with large quantities of mucus or pus and severe tenesmus as soon as the last drops are voided, or a little before.

Pulsatilla - continued dull stitches in neck of bladder, with a pressure of urine, while lying upon his back; after micturition spasmodic pains in neck of bladder, extending to pelvis and thighs; prostatic troubles of elderly people, faeces flat, small in size.

Secale - gangrene: from anemia; external injuries, application of leeches or mustard; > from cold, < from heat; dry, of old people.

Selenium - marked effects on the genito-urinary organs, and often indicated in elderly men especially for prostatitis and sexual atony; abject despair, uncompromising melancholy.

Sulphur (Atrophy of children) - emaciation; skin dry, harsh and wrinkled, giving the child an "old man" look; offensive odor of body, not removable by washing; eczema (capitis) dry, easily bleeding, itching more at night, scratching relieves but causes bleeding; intertrigo, especially at anus; glands swollen, particularly cervical, axillary and inguinal; appetite voracious, child grasps at everything within reach and thrusts it into its mouth, or drinks much and eats little when the violent thirst is on.

Sulphuric acid. - bluish spots on forearm, as if ecchymosed; haemorrhage of black blood from all outlets; extreme weakness, exhaustion and tremor all over body, without trembling. Acts best on elderly people.

Sulphuric acid. - too early, too copious and too long. Before: nightmare with choking during: great haste, talks, eats and works in a hurry; trembling sensation without trembling; general debility. After: sexual excitement; climacteric spitting of blood; uterine diseases in elderly women.

Tarentula hisp. - mocks aged people with their old age, if restrained becomes violent.

Teucrium - old persons and children.

Teucrium - polypi in ear and nose, especially among old and middle.

Diseases of old age, prematurely old, senility or presenility

(Apoplexy) Baryta-carb. - general paralysis of old age (Apoplexy) Conium - the senile women's remedy (Asthma) Ambra - asthma senile et siccum (Asthma) Ant-tart. - asthma senile (Asthma) Baryta-carb. - asthma senile (after Ant.-tart.) (Asthma) Conium - asthma senile (Bronchitis chronica) Baryta-carb. - useful in infancy and in old age (Bronchitis chronica) Drosera - bronchitis of old age, in connection with emphysema or bronchiectasis.

(Bronchitis chronica) Lycopodium - emphysema, dilation of air-tubes and senile catarrh.

Cataract (Cataract) - for granular (fatty) cataract with arcus senilis: Phos., Sil.;

(Colic) Carbolic acid. - flatulence of old age, depending on imperfect digestion.

(Cystoplegia) Sec-cor. - ischuria paralytica. Enuresis of old age (Debility) Bar-c. - suits first childhood and senility (old age) with mental or physical debility.

(Debility) Conium - debility from old age or masturbation.

(Diarrhoea of infants) Arg-nit. - child looks prematurely old, feels and looks prostrated.

(Distension of abdomen and flatulence) Carbolic acid. - flatulence of old age, dependent on imperfect digestion.

(Dropsy) China - in old persons or people prematurely aged by excesses, and in drunkards, after excessive depletion. Skin waxy pale or yellow, cold and blue.

(Dyspepsia, weakness of stomach) Vipera torva - dyspepsia of old people, or of persons prematurely senile, suffering from spasmodic affections of throat and chest.

(Gangrene) Ars-alb. - senile gangrene.

(Gangrene) Carbo-veg. - senile gangrene humid gangrene in cachectic persons whose vital powers are exhausted

(Gangrene) - senile: Oxygen, Amm-m., Ars., Chin., Con., Euphor., Phos-ac., Plumb., Sec., Solanum.

(Gangrene) Phosphoric acid - senile gangrene.

(Headache) Phosphorus - senile cerebral atrophy.

(Heart diseases) Phosphorus - premature old age and overgrown adolescents.

(Hepatic derangements) Fluoric acid. - complaints of premature old age, of bummers, in consequence of syphilo-mercurial dyscrasia.

(Insanity) Baryta carb. - senile dementia, mental and physical debility (Insanity) Conium - senile dementia, ailments of old maids and widows from ungratified sexual desire.

(Insanity) Crotalus hor. - incipient stage of senile dementia.

(Insanity) Secale - senile dementia, senile gangrene.

(Mania) Selenium - complaints incident to old age, particularly at the critical age.

(Mind symptoms) Crotalus hor. - incipient stage of senile dementia.

(Ophthalmia) Baryta carb. - amylopia. of old age.

(Paralysis) Agaricus - crosswise affections. senile tremor.

(Prostate gland, diseases of) Digitalis - senile hypertrophy of prostate, cardiac symptoms marked.

(Prostate gland, diseases of) Secale - enuresis in old age, bloody urine.

(Pruritus) Ars alb. - senile pruritus in broken-down constitutions, < from cold applications, > from warmth (Rheumatism) Phosphorus - rheumatic stiffness with morning aggravation, especially when coming on in old age.

(Scrofulosis) Baryta carb. - suits the extremes of life, infancy and old age.

(Sexual complaints) Agnus castus - prostatic juice passes with hard stool. premature old age in young persons from abuse of sexual functions, with melancholy, apathy, mental distraction, self-contempt, general debility, and spermatorrhoea of old sinners, though impotent.

(Uraemia) Ars., Aur., Cann., Ind., Carbol-ac., Cupr., Hydr-ac., Iod., Nicotin, Phos., Tereb., where uraemic blood-poisoning complicates morbus Brightii; but we must not neglect to use the catheter twice or three times a day. - senile uraemia: Iod., Lyc.

(Uraemia) Iodum - uraemia from senile hypertrophy and induration of prostata (Urinary difficulties) Baryta carb - in old age frequent micturition

(Vision complaints) - in old age: Aur., Bar-c., Con., Op., Phos., Sec.

Diabetes mellitus—Glycosuria

This chapter does not ensure that after reading it, anybody can cure any diabetes case. It is just to provide some basic tools which can guide you to select the similimum.

Diabetes is a symptom of an organ – the pancreas.

If there are no 'general' or 'mind' or 'uncommon symptom' in a given case, you may, as a matter or exception, go through this chapter for finding the remedy. Thus, this work is not exhaustive to treat all cases of diabetes. Let us take an actual case.

Case: A 74-year old gentleman consulted me for diabetes. He *also* asked if I can do something for his overweight. Upon questioning, I found out that his diabetes is twenty-five year old. He started putting weight after the age of sixty year. He also asked me if I can give him some medicine for impotency. But we did not consider this for selecting the remedy at first because 'impotency' is a common symptom for a person with diabetes at the age of seventy four years.

'Obesity' has not much value in prescribing; so also 'diabetes'. But when these two symptoms are compared, obesity, being a general symptom (though of least value among general symptoms) has more value than diabetes.

When two or more symptoms are in a case, we must arrange them in order of their 'grade' or 'value'.

Kent's Repertory—GENERALITIES—OLD PEOPLE—Acon., Agar., Aloe, Alumn., Ambr., Am-c., Ammc., Anac., Ant-c., Ant-t., Ars., Aur., Bar-c., Bry., Calc-p., Camph., Carb-an., Carb-v., Caust., Cic., Coca., Colch., Con., Fl-ac., Iod., Kali-c., Lyc., Nat-m., Nit-ac., Op., Sabad., Sec., Sel., Seneg., Sulph., Sul-ac., Teucr. *(Let us call this as List 'A').*

Now, instead of looking for these six remedies under 'Diabetes' you must take another general symptom. Kent's Repertory—GENERALITIES—SYPHILIS: (several remedies) + List 'A' above = Ars., Aur., Carb-v., Caust., Con., Fl-ac., Nit-ac., Sul. Sexual symptoms are 'generals'.

The above eight remedies were studied in the chapter Sexual Instinct (p. 951-959) of Lilienthal's. HOMOEOPATHIC THERAPEUTICS.

In Fl-ac., we find the following: Increased sexual desire in old men.

Fluoric acid. - 1M single dose and placebo were given. (Patient is under treatment.)

By this the reader should not run to the hasty conclusion that the remedy Fluoric acid should be included under 'Diabetes' in our repertories.

"Give the remedy indicated by the totality of (general and/or uncommon and/or mind) symptoms irrespective of the fact whether such a remedy was ever given in that disease before".

Keep away from pathology. The more you do this the better will be your success.

This chapter is not totally useless. Apart from common symptoms of diabetes it gives symptoms not commonly found among diabetics e.g. *furunculosis* under the remedy Phos-ac. etc.

Remedies for diabetes

Diabetes due to diseases of pancreas: Ars., Phos., Uran. Nitr.

Epidemic or malignant diseases of pancreas causing epidemic diabetes: Calc-ars., Rhus-t.

Acetic-ac. (Debility, asthenia) - great debility, polyuria and glycosuria, intense thirst; sensation as if an ulcer were in stomach, giving great uneasiness.

Acetic-ac. - abundant sugar in urine, increased and light-colored, great thirst, but cold drink lies heavy on stomach; ascites and hydrothorax, oedema pedum; gangrenous ulcers; pale, waxen skin; extreme prostration; decomposition of animal matter.

Adrenalinum - slowing of pulse, (medullary vagus stimulation), and strengthening of heart beat (increased myocardial contractility), resembling digitalis; increased glandular activity, glycosuria; depression of respiratory center; contraction of muscular tissue of eye, uterus, vagina; relaxation of muscular tissue of stomach, intestines, bladder.

Arg-met. - profuse, turbid, sweetish urine; < at night, sometimes like whey, it distresses him at night, has to rise so often; emaciation and great weakness; face pale and sallow, scrotum and feet oedematous and itching; pruritus scroti seu vulvae; foetid taste in mouth; disposition to gangrene.

Arnica- diabetes.

Ars-alb. - tormenting hallucination, as if there was one by his side who did that entire he was doing, eating, washing, etc. diabetes. herpetic eruptions, syphilitic excrescences, glandular tumors and indurations, cancer, locomotor ataxia, and obstinate intermittents.

Ars-brom. - herpetic eruptions, syphilitic excrescences, glandular tumors and indurations, cancer, locomotor ataxia, and obstinate intermittents, and diabetes are all greatly influenced by this preparation.

Ars-brom. - mineral spring of Ashe Co., N. C. (Liquor Ars., Brom.) Needs proving, though highly recommended.

Asclepia vincet. - see Vincetoxicum.

Berb-v. - constant urging, with pain in neck of bladder, urine very slow to flow, with pain in lumbar and renal region, > by rest; after urinating sensation in bladder as if one must go again soon or as if some urine remained behind; pale-yellow urine, with a gelatinous sediment; weakness of sexual organs; pale, sallow face, sunken cheeks; sickly expression; dryness and sticky feeling in mouth and fauces; sticky, frothy saliva, like cotton; increased thirst and appetite, > by eating; pulse slow and weak; paralyzed, bruised sensation in back, < from slight exertion; skin sticky and scaling off; intense coldness of knees.

Bovista - frequent desire to urinate, even immediately after urination, with emission of a few drops; urine bright-red or yellowish-green, becomes turbid; bright yellow, with slowly forming cloud; turbid, like loam-water, with violet sediment; general languor and enervation, particularly in joints; visible palpitation after exertion, as if the heart were working in water; backache, with stiffness after stooping; urticaria.

Calc-phos. (Diabetes with menses complaints) - menses too early in young girls, with bright-red blood; too late, blood first bright, then dark, with women; dark blood in rheumatic women; menses during lactation. before: great sexual desire, followed by a copious flow, headache three to seven days before; griping and rumbling in bowels. during: vertigo and throbbing in forehead, pressure over os pubis, she feels pulse in all parts; want of appetite, diarrhoea, backache, shooting pains from left to right, lower limbs heavy, fatigued; great weakness and sinking sensation; leucorrhoea like albumen, < morning after rising, of a sweetish odor, for two weeks after menses. lack of development; stenosis in women about 25 or 30 years, their difficulties dating back to puberty; tuberculosis.

Calc-phos. - glycosuria when lungs are implicated, diminishing the quantity of urine and lowering its specific gravity; sore aching in bladder, < after urinating, involuntary sighing; chronic cough of consumptives, who suffer with cold feet; profuse sweat in phthisis.

Carbolic-acid. - short, dry, hacking cough; excessive urination, the urine containing sugar; copious flow of limpid, colorless urine; diarrhoea or torpor of intestines; unusual appetite and thirst for stimulants; languor and profound prostration; cold skin, horripilations; obesity.

Carlsbad. - famous for its action on the liver and in the treatment of obesity, diabetes, and gout.

Chelidonium - a man, aged 31; diabetes.

Chionanthus - large amount of high specific gravity; frequent urination; bile and sugar in urine.

Chionanthus - gallstones. (Berberis; Cholest.; Calc.) diabetes.

Coca - diabetes, with impotency.

Codein. - woman, aged 68; diabetes.

Conium - a man, aged 48; first threatened softening of brain, helped by laches., then right-sided paralysis, particularly facial, helped by caustic., afterwards diabetes of two years standing, with swelling and suppuration of left parotid and profuse sweat with insomnia.

Convallaria (Diabetes with diseases of uterus) - sore, aching pain in lower part of abdomen; feeling as if uterus had descended and pressed upon rectum, causing a hard, aching pain in rectum and anus; flatus become incarcerated in rectum; dull, aching or sore, bruised feeling in lumbar region; faintishness from slight cause, sleepy and tired out; great prostration and dull feeling in head; pelvic pains < from motion, sitting up straight or leaning back, > by bending forward when sitting, by lying on back; glycosuria, with intense itching at introitus and hyperaemia, > by cold water.

Crataegus - diabetes, especially in children.

Cuprum ars. - diabetes.

Cuprum met. - urine acid, straw-colored, turbid after standing, a reddish, thin sediment adhered to vessel, viscous, offensive, bloody, scanty or suppressed; great and slowly progressing emaciation; suppurating tuberculosis of lungs and evident signs of depression of brain; great thirst; increased hunger; sweetish taste of mouth; increased urination, especially at night; dry, very infrequent stool; decrease of sexual desire.

Curare - diabetes acutissimus, threatening life; clear and frequent urine, with digging, crampy pains in kidneys; shooting in stomach; dry mouth; great thirst, especially evenings and at night; sugar in urine; great emaciation. Glycosuria with motor paralysis. Emaciation.

Eup-pur. - albminuria, diabetes, strangury, irritable bladder, enlarged prostate are a special field for this remedy.

Glycerinum - deeply and long, building up tissue, hence of great use in marasmus, debility, mental and physical, diabetes, etc.

Grindelia robusta - sugar in urine.

Helon. (Diabetes with dyspepsia, weakness of stomach) - great prostration of nervous system; anaemia; pulse small and feeble; paleness and icteric color of skin; loss of appetite, bitter taste; constricting, pressing pain in stomach; empty eructations; vomiting, borborygmi and sensation as if diarrhoea would set in, but stools are regular; tongue red at tip and borders, white in centre; albuminuria, diabetes, sorrowfulness and melancholy; patient excitable and wishes to be let alone; renal and uterine troubles.

Helon. - (Diabetes with menses complaints) - too frequent, too profuse and too exhausting, blood dark and smelling badly, especially in women, feeble from loss of blood; flow passive, dark, clotted and offensive; profuse flooding during menopause. Before: pressing pain in sacrum and soreness of breasts. during: sharp, cutting and drawing pains from back to uterus; pruritus of vulva and vagina; albuminous urine; depressed, melancholy; breasts swollen, nipples tender, cannot bear pressure of clothing; sallow face with an expression of sorrow and suffering; backache, constant tenderness in renal region; great general languor; loss of sexual desire with or without sterility.

—— woman, aged 65; diabetes.

Hepar sulph. - the slightest contradiction makes him break out into the greatest violence, he could kill somebody without hesitation; sight gets dim when reading; heaviness and pressure in stomach after a moderate meal, unusual hunger, much thirst; desire for acids and wine; sexual desire increased, erections feeble; urine acrid, burning, making the inner surface of the prepuce or of the pudenda sore and ulcerated; emission of much pale urine, with pressure on bladder; emission of pale, clear urine, which on standing becomes turbid, thick, and deposits a white sediment.

Insulinum - besides the use of insulin in the treatment of diabetes, restoring the lost ability to oxidize carbohydrate and again storing glycogen in the liver, some use of it homoeopathically has been made by Dr. Wm. F. Baker, showing its applicability in acne, carbuncles, erythema with itching eczema. - in the gouty, transitory glycosuria. When skin manifestations are persistent give three times daily after eating.

Inula - diabetes.

Kali-br. - (Diabetes with urinary difficulties) - irresistible desire to urinate, but no flow except with urging and difficulty; glycosuria, urine loaded with sugar; dribbling of urine at beginning of stool.

Kali-br. - emaciation, paleness, skin cold and dry, pulse rapid and feeble, tongue red and tender, gums spongy and bleeding; thirst excessive; appetite voracious; bowels constipated; urine pale, frequent, of great density, and loaded with sugar; liver tumid and tender (Ars-brom.).

Kali-mur. - excessive and sugary urine; itching in urethra; stomach and liver deranged; dry and light-colored stools; pain in kidneys; great weakness and somnolence.

Kali-phos. - Nervous weakness; breath peculiar, of haylike odor; thirst, voracious hunger, emaciation; hepatic troubles.

Kreos. - perfect depression of the trophic nervous system. Heaviness all over, with drowsiness; depression of spirits; head feels confused and dull; dimsightedness; flat, bitter taste; appetite, with sensation of fulness; intermittent, hard, dry stool; frequent and copious emission of hot, clear urine; bruised sensation in chest and all along the back; physical exhaustion, worse from rest; great itching of genitals during and after micturition

Lac-def. - excessive aching of back; enormous quantities of urine voided daily, with excessive lassitude and prostration; intense throbbing headache, especially in forehead, with nausea, vomiting and most obstinate constipation.

Lachesis - despondency and peevishness; dimness of eyes; livid-grey complexion; readily bleeding gums; sweetish taste; constipation; violent urging to urinate, with copious discharge; impotence; difficult suffocative breathing; laming pain and weakness in back and extremities; gangrene; emaciation with muscular relaxation.

Lact-ac. - excessive thirst; frequent and copious micturition; urine contains sugar; skin rough and dry; obstinate constipation; tongue dry, sticky; gastric ailments; debility and emaciation; feels constantly tired and exhausted from slightest exertion; rheumatic pains with profuse urination.

Lact-ac. - morning sickness, diabetes, and rheumatism offer a field for this remedy.

—— boy, aged 16, suffering six months; diabetes. - man, aged 62, phlegmatic, dark complexion, dark hair and eyes, has had dropsy several times; diabetes.

Lith-c. - very frequent urination, disturbing sleep; turbid urine, with much mucous deposit; dark reddish-brown deposit in urine.

Lycopodium - peevish and depressed in mind; thirst and hunger constant, but worse at night; flatulence; faeces small in quantity; want of natural warmth; sexual desire and power gone; lithic acid gravel; pulmonary phthisis, pituitosa and purulenta, with hectic; great emaciation; mental, nervous and bodily exhaustion; gouty lithaemia.

Lycopus - diabetes mellitus and insipidus from some derangement of the central nervous system or sympatheticus; morbus Basedowii; copious flow of clear urine of great density, containing sugar; intense thirst; great emaciation, etc.; increased bronchial irritation, with sighing respiration; cardiac depression. Woman, mother of two children, suffering about a year with diabetes.

Magnesia usta - sad mood; dryness of the eyes; dullness of hearing; pale, earthy complexion; looseness of the teeth, with swelling and bleeding of the gums; dryness of the mouth, especially at night and in the morning; burning in the throat, with dryness and roughness; urine increased, pale, watery, with white sediment; itching and great dryness of the skin.

Mag-p. - child, teething, mother died of diabetes; profuse and frequent urination.

Mag-sulph. - gloominess, especially mornings, and disinclination for work; mouth and throat very dry, as if numb, with a sweetish-bitter taste, in the morning, disappearing after breakfast; aversion to all food; slight thirst which can be resisted; urine copious, light-yellow, soon becomes turbid and deposits copious red sediment; erections without desire for an embrace; exhaustion and prostration, > by rest momentarily.

Menyanth - diabetes.

Mineral waters - Carlsbad, Gastein, Vichy, Buffalo Lithia Springs, Bethesda, Gettysburg, Napa Soda, Cal., the Geysers, Brom. ars., water of Ashe Co., N. C. - clysmic water may be used with equal benefit in polyuria and glycosuria.

Moschus - unquenchable thirst; great emaciation; costiveness; impotence; frequent passage of large quantities of saccharine urine; paralytic condition of the brain; dimness of sight; earthy complexion; great dryness of the mouth and putrid taste; great thirst for stimulants and aversion to food; prickling in the skin; general exhaustion, with coldness all over.

―――― Man, aged 43; married; diabetes with impotency.

Nat-mur. - diabetes.

Nat-phos. - diabetes with hepatic derangements - Cirrhosis of liver; hepatic form of diabetes, especially when there is a succession of boils; intense pressure and heat on top of head as if it would open; yellow, creamy coating at the back part of tongue and roof of mouth; acidity and acid dyspepsia; weak feeling in back and limbs.

Nat-sul. - depressed, irritable, taciturn, tired of life; dullness in head and weakness of sight; dryness and burning in the eyes; nosebleed; dryness of mouth and throat; great thirst for very cold drinks; voracious appetite, with a boring pain; disgust while eating; foetid flatus; increased urination, especially at night; pains in small of back, with burning urine; haemoptoë; cough, with purulent expectoration.

—— Man, aged 43, middle height, father of two healthy children, blonde hair, grey eyes, gonorrhoeal cachexy, hydrogenoid constitution; diabetes.

Nux-v. - good livers and sedentary habits. Acidity, with dyspeptic troubles; constriction of the throat; dry cough; pains in the back; numbness; paretic condition of the lower extremities; after ineffectual desire to urinate, frequent and more copious urination than could be expected from the quantity of liquid taken; sexual desire strong; spinal lesions exciting cause.

Opium - After mental shocks or injuries. Dullness, sadness, weak memory; vision obscured as by a fog; face bloated, congested or sunken and pale; tongue thickly coated, dry mouth and oesophagus dry; frothy sputa; ravenous hunger and unquenchable thirst; constipation more than diarrhoea; great pain and difficulty in expelling urine; no passage of urine or faeces; urine turbid, brown, with an iridescent film, scanty; weariness and numbness all over.

Phaseola - diabetes.

Phos-acid. - neurogenic glycosuria. Debility from loss of animal fluids; bad effects from grief, anguish, sorrow and care; all the joints feel bruised; very sensitive to fresh air; lassitude and heaviness; weakness of mind; falling out of the hair; dimness of eyes; excessive thirst; eructations from acids;

pressure in stomach; hard, difficult stool; shortness of breathing; urine thick, like milk (chyluria) or lime-water, with whitish curds, with stringy, bloody lumps, or clear, limpid, and containing much sugar; pain in back and kidneys; dull pressure in bladder; great weakness and emaciation; furunculosis.

—— Man, aged 40; diabetes. - gentleman, aged 52, stout, well formed, of active habits, had myelitis; diabetes.

Phos-acid. - pyrosis, flatulence, diarrhoea, diabetes, rhachitis and periosteal inflammation.

Phosphorus (Diabetes with diseases of pancreas) - Tuberculosis and fatty degeneration in different organs, especially of heart, liver, pancreas or kidney; distressing burning pains in coeliac axis; stools undigested, containing particles of fat or looking like cooked sago; pale, yellow face; anaemia; atrophy of pancreas with diabetes; neuralgia of coeliac plexus; morbus brightii.

Phosphorus (Diabetes with duodenitis and duodenal catarrh) - tuberculosis; distressing, burning pain in coeliac axis; stools undigested, containing particles of fat; pale, yellow face; anaemia; atrophy of pancreas with diabetes.

Phosphorus - atrophy with diabetes. - Diabetes, with phthisis; urine profuse, pale, watery; or turbid, whitish, like curdled milk, with brickdust sediment and variegated cuticle on surface; gouty diathesis; cerebral disease; cheesy degeneration of lungs.

Picric-ac. - cortex of brain congested; urine contains sugar and albumen, dark red, of high specific gravity; great indifference, lack of will power to do anything; eyes feel dry, as if full of sand, sight dim and confused; saliva white, frothy and stringy; disgust for food; very great thirst for cold water; great sexual desire with emissions; excessive languor and prostration, it seemed difficult to move the limbs; feet cold, chilly, cannot get warm, followed by clammy sweat; chilly all over, except head and spine; throbbing, jerking of muscles with great pains between hips.

Plumbum met. - lowness of spirits, anguish and melancholy; diminution of sight; dryness of mouth; dry, cracked tongue; feeling of contraction and constriction in throat; fever with unquenchable thirst; dingy color of skin; gangrene; constipation; hectic fever with dry, hacking cough from suppuration of lungs; great exhaustion; impotence; excessive emaciation; great hunger; obstinate belching and vomiting. Chronic lead-poisoning produces a perfect picture of glycosuria and of morbus Brightii, and Hering considered it one of the most important drugs in this form of disease.

Podophyl. - chalky stools; profuse and frequent micturition immediately after drinking; excessive hepatic action; hot, sour flatus.

—— boy, aged 1; diabetes. - boy, aged 9; diabetes insipidus.

Ratanhia - considerable emaciation and weakness; limbs sore and aching; great appetite; insatiable thirst and constant dryness of the mouth; gums livid and swollen; soreness in the kidneys; severe pains in small of back, improved by motion; hard stool, with straining; frequent urging to urinate, with scanty discharge, or passes large quantities of light-colored urine.

Rhus aromatica - diabetes, large quantities of urine of low specific gravity. - renal and urinary affections, especially diabetes.

Secale - great general lassitude; heaviness of limbs; loss of strength; emaciation; gangrene; skin dry; and withered; furuncles;

petechiae; fever, with unquenchable thirst; diminished power of the senses; dryness of the mouth; morbidly great appetite; cardialgia; costiveness; diarrhoea; watery urine; increased quantity of urine. Diabetes with opthalmia.

Sulph-ac. - lassitude; debility; despondency; dimness of mind and sight; itching over the whole body; flatulency upward and downward; stitches in hepatic region; skin completely inactive, cold and dry; large quantities of sugar in urine; typhoid condition.

Syph. - Mrs. suffering from diabetes, subject to rheumatism in rainy weather; rheumatic ophthalmia.

Syzygium - if administered at suitable intervals in diabetes mellitus, the blood sugar is maintained at a normal level and the urine remains free of sugar. - a most useful remedy in diabetes. - has an immediate effect on blood sugar. - Diminishes the amount of urine secreted and causes sugar to disappear. No proving!

Tarent-hisp. - profound grief and anxiety; great prostration, and pain as if the whole body were bruised; loss of memory and dimness of sight; constant craving for raw articles; intense thirst; lips and mouth so dry that he wants to moisten them with his tongue; insatiable appetite; disgust for meat and general wasting away; constipation; polyuria, with violent pains in the lumbar region and paralysis of the lower extremities; miliary eruptions and furuncles.

Terebinth - inability to concentrate the mind; dull, languid mind, relieved by frequent micturition; despondency; wearied of life; obscuration of sight; sunken features; lips cracked and slightly bleeding; epistaxis; spongy gums; tongue dry and red; foul breath; hunger and thirst, with debility; aversion to meat; rancid or acrid eructations; burning in stomach and hypochondria; tympanitis; albuminuria, with frequent micturition; sugar is noticed in urine after large doses of Oil Tereb.

Thuja - glycosuria after a long-suppressed gonorrhoea, frequent desire to urinate day and night; craving alternates with want of appetite; longs for cold food and drink; urine contains sugar, foams, deposits a brown mucus; debility < mornings.

Uran-nit. - diabetes mellitus and insipidus. great emaciation; tendency to general dropsy; effusion of serum from all serous membranes, especially pleura and peritoneum; brights disease, and kindred renal maladies; contracted, gouty kidneys, with gastric disturbances; irritable condition of renal plexus, of sympathetic.

Uran-nit. - is known to produce nephritis, diabetes and increased urine, degeneration of the liver, high blood pressure and dropsy.

Uran-nit.(Diabetes with albuminuria) - patient is compelled to rise often during the night and urinate, which disturbs his sleep; ill-tempered, cross and irritable; pains over left eye; disturbed stomach, faintness of stomach, even after a hearty meal; cardiac complications; diabetes; pregnancy.

Uran-nit. (Diabetes with diseases of pancreas) - ulceration of duodenum and pyloric end of stomach; vomiting of a white fluid; putrid eructations, pains < from fasting; urine deposits a mucopurulent sediment, containing albumen, phosphates, lithic acid in excess; glycosuria.

Uran-nit. - great emaciation; diabetes; tendency to general dropsy; effusion of serum from all serous membranes, especially pleura and peritoneum.

Uran-nit. - defects of digestion and assimilation; hepatogenic diabetes. Causes sugar to be deposited in the urine. General languor; debility; cold feeling; vertigo; purulent discharges from eyelids and nostrils, with ulceration of cheeks from the acrid discharge; copious salivation; vomiting, with great thirst; putrid eructations; urgent desire to evacuate bladder and rectum; frequent micturition; cough, with purulent discharge from nostril; lung infiltrated with gray tubercles; stiffness in loins; languor on rising from bed, with fishy smell of urine; prostration, somnolence, and shivering during the day; restless at night.

- Boy, aged 3; diabetes. - man, aged 70, hale and hearty; diabetes.

Urea pura - albuminuria, diabetes; uraemia.

Vanadium - tuberculosis, chronic rheumatism; diabetes.

Vincetoxicum - arthritis, bleeding of gums, insatiable hunger; impotency; emaciation.

Malignant diseases

(Note: Life threatening complaints are general symptoms. These cannot be ignored.)

Homoeopathy vs allopathy: Regarding comparison of homoeopathy with allopathy, when we consulted *I-Ching*, the ancient book of wisdom of China, we got the following answer:

"What is easy for allopathy is difficult for homoeopathy; What is difficult for allopathy is easy for homoeopathy".

The aspiring homoeopath must note that Homoeopathy is Advanced Allopathy.

Therefore, you must attempt to treat only those patients who are having chronic illnesses, those who are not cured by the best doctors of other medical systems and, more particularly, only those patients with diseases for which allopathy has no cure and patient is condemned to death. If you do so, you not only get success but also you would be making the best use of homoeopathy; you get good name and soon gain popularity among patients.

In homoeopathic literature you may not find the terms 'renal failure' 'terminal cancer' etc. whenever you get a patient with unfavourable prognosis *i.e.,* it would soon end up in death, this chapter would be of excellent help.

If you completely cure malignant diseases, particular terminal cancer etc. that is the best job you would be doing in medical practice.

Thus, in this Chapter I am giving you remedies for malignant diseases; at the end, you would also see a list of remedies for malignant cancer.

Malignant = A term applied to any disease of a virulent and fatal nature. Virulent = extremely severe or harmful in its effects. Malignant pustule = Anthrax Malignant endocarditis.

Malignant exopthalmos = a condition seen in thyrotoxicosis where there is raised intraocular pressure causing pain and the threat of damage to the optic nerve.

Malignant growth or tumour = a tumour which has the properties of anaplasia, invasion and metastasization. Malignant hypertension.

Ailings of teething children. - complementary in malignant diseases: ars.; phos.; sulph.

In malignant diseases after Kreosotum, Ars., Phos., Sul. follow as complementary remedies.

(Jaundice) - malignant jaundice: Acon., Ars., Ars-i., Chin., Chin-mur., Chel, Crot-h., Elaps., Dig., Lach., Pic-ac, Vip.

Powerful adjuvants in treatment of malignant disease – compare: anti-vaccinal remedies - Vaccininum: Variolin; Malandrinum; Thuja.

(Pancreatitis) - malignant or epidemic form: Calc., Ars., Rhus-t.,

Suppuration, malignant: 1, Asa., Chin., Hep., Merc., Phos., Pyrogen., Sil.; 2, Ars., Calc., Carb-v., Caust., Kreos., Nitr-ac., Rhus, Sulph., Sulph. ac.

(Tumors) Semi-malignant fibroid: Bry., Con., Led., Sil.; enchondroma: Sil.; epulis: Sil.; lupus: Ars., Ars. Iod., Sil.; epithelioma: Acet-ac.,

Aur., Carb-an., Con., Hydrast., Kreos., Sil.; lymphoma: Ars., Phos.

Malignant scirrhus: Acet-ac., Arn., Ars. Iod., Brom., Carb-an., Carbol-ac., Con., Gal., Hydrast., Lap-alb., Merc-aur., Mur.-ac., Nitr-ac., Sil. encephaloma: Ars., Ars.-iod., Bell., Calc., Carbol.-ac., Croc., Gal., Hydrast., Kali-hydr., Lach., Nitr.-ac., Phos., Sil., Thuj.;

Melanosis: Phos., Sang.;

Colloid: Hydrast., Carbol-ac., Phos.;

Fungus haematodes: Ars., Phos., Sil., Staph., Sep., Carb-v., Nitr.-ac., Thuj.;

Medullary fungus: Carb-an., Nitr-ac., Phos., Sil., Thuj.

Remedies for malignant states

Abscesses, chronic: if there arises on any internal or external part a painful, red, inflamed swelling, which may point and form a suppurating swelling, bell., or if this does not succeed in twenty-four or forty-eight hours, Hep. will often disperse the whole swelling and keep suppuration off; but when once matter has formed, Merc. will bring on the discharge of the pus and frequently finish up the case, its chief indication being that suppuration must have already taken place should the open wound not heal under the continuation of Merc. give Hep. or Sil., which are the real specifics against all benign or **malignant** suppurations. if the abscess looks erysipelatous, Apis, Bell.; if bluish, Lach.

Anthrax - the **malignant** pustule generally yields to: 1, Ars., Bell., Sil., Rhus, or, perhaps, Chin., Hyosc., Mur.-ac., Sec., Sep.; 2, Anthrac., Apis, Carb.-v., Kreos., Hydr., Tarent. cubana.

Mumps: (Parotitis) - for **malignant** parotitis, passing over into ichoration.

Suppuration, **malignant**: 1, Asa., Chin., Hep., Merc., Phos., Pyrogen., sil.; 2, Ars., Calc., Carb-v., Caust., Kreos., Nitr.-ac., Rhus, Sulph., Sulph-ac.

Acetic acid. (Haemorrhoids) - **malignant** diseases of rectum; profuse haemorrhoidal **bleeding**; **haemorrhage** from bowels after checked metrorrhagia; obstinate constipation.

Aconite (Jaundice) - severe and constant pain in epigastrium, pressing outward; pain going to the navel or changing from stomach to liver; yellowish-white thick fur in mouth. jaundice from a cold with catarrh of the small intestines, after fright, during pregnancy, in newborn children. from atrophy of liver **malignant** jaundice (tincture according to jousset); constipation or diarrhoea.

Aethiops antimonialis (Scrofulosis) - scrofulous glandular and skin diseases; blepharitis, conjunctivitis and keratitis scrofulosa, even with a **malignant** tendency; boils and furuncles.

Ailanthus (Puerperal fever) - **malignant** puerperal fever; ichorous and foetid lochia; deliria; diarrhoea; eruption all over body; constant thirst, longing for brandy; soreness, irritability, pricking and tingling everywhere.

Ailanthus (Scarlatina) - adynamic **malignant** scarlatina from the start; general prostration and marked cerebral affection during the first stage; pulse small, weak, often irregular; skin harsh and dry, covered with a scanty dark-bluish rash, more profuse on forehead and face; violent vomiting, dizziness, photophobia, stupor and insensibility; pupils dilated; great thirst, with dry, parched tongue; throat inside swollen, dark-colored, even ulcerated, with infiltration of the cellular tissue about the neck; excoriating nasal discharge; great exhaustion and stoical indifference to whatever happens; petechiae, torpor, eruption is slow to make its appearance, remains livid even on forehead and face; skin dry, but never hot; irregular, patchy, livid eruption, disappearing on pressure and returning very slowly, interspersed with small vesicles, < forehead, neck and chest.

Ailanthus - lividity, stupor and **malignancy**.

Ailanthus - symptoms remarkably alike to **malignant** scarlatina.

Amm-carb. (Scarlatina) - miliary scarlatina of a **malignant** type from deficient oxygenation; throat swollen internally and externally, with enlargement of glands and bluish, dark-red swelling of tonsils; infiltration of cellular tissue around engorged cervical lymphatics; gangrenous, putrid ulceration of tonsils, covered with rapidly decomposing, sticky, offensive, muco-pus; burning pains in the throat, sticky salivation; nose obstructed, particularly at night, causing the child to start from its sleep as if smothering, has to lie with its mouth wide open in order to breathe; mental confusion, gloom, inclined to shed tears; chill and heat often alternate till towards midnight; continuous day or night-sweat; upper half of the body covered by eruption with violent itching, or faintly developed eruption; stertorous breathing; involuntary defaecation and urination; threatening paralysis of brain with excessive vomiting; hard swelling of right parotid and lymphatic glands of the neck.

Amm-carb. - **malignant** scarlatina, with somnolence, swollen glands, dark red sore throat, faintly developed eruption.

Ant-tart. (Ulcers) - deeply penetrating, **malignant** ulcers; broad and deep sloughing ulcers; gangrenous ulcers with hectic fever; ulcers surrounded with black pustules, which break down into deep ulcers; no pus. Merely oozing of foetid humor.

Anthracinum - this nosode has proven a great remedy in epidemic spleen diseases of domestic animals, and in septic inflammation, carbuncles and **malignant** ulcers. in boils and boil-like eruptions, acne.

Arnica (Tumors) - tumor following a contusion or a similar injury, but not becoming **malignant**; dull tingling pain in indurated part; red, blue or yellow spots, like ecchymosis; pus thin and bloody.

Arnica - maintains the system under the stress of **malignancy** regardless of location.

Arnica montana - **malignant** symptoms. **malignant** pustules.

Ars-alb. (Duodenitis and duodenal catarrh) - great restlessness and anxiety; ulceration of duodenum, involving pancreas, following burns or **malignant** diseases; neuralgia of coeliac plexus.

Ars-alb. (Glaucoma) - glossitis, with constant thirst, drinking but a little at a time; gangrene of tongue, spots on tongue, burning like fire; gangrenous ulcers of mouth and fauces; **malignant** aphthae of children.

Ars-alb. (Pancreas, diseases of) - organic degenerations with great restlessness and despair; ulceration of duodenum, which, by extension, involves the pancreatic duct, perhaps the result of burns, of **malignant** disease, etc.; neuralgia of the coeliac plexus; stools undigested, containing fat.

Ars-alb. (Sore throat) - restlessness, anxiety, prostration; gangrene in throat, burning like hot coals in throat; tonsils swollen, dark-red; vesicles in throat; tongue, throat, oesophagus inflamed; paralysis of pharynx; drinks come out of nose; **malignancy** (Ars.-iod.).

Ars-alb. (Stomatitis, inflammation and ulceration of buccal cavity.) **malignant** ulceration in mouth; edges of tongue ulcerated; aphthae with violent burning pains; ulcers and blisters turn livid and black; swollen and readily-**bleeding** gums; looseness of teeth; ptyalism; restlessness and great exhaustion.

Ars-alb. (Syphilis and sycosis) - phagedenic chancres, livid hue, with intense burning, even sloughing; chancres (after mercury), with too florid granulations; margins of ulcers hard and **bleeding** at least touch, with a thin, offensive discharge; bubo when assuring a gangrenous aspect; inguinal glands painful, swollen, indurated; constitutional syphilis, with indescribable feeling of weakness, or with dropsy and **malignant** ulcerations; coffee-colored eruptions on skin, burning pimples or pustular eruption. (Ars. brings out dormant syphilis.) Ars-iod, secondary syphilis, mucous plaques; tertiary syphilis, cutaneous ulcers discharging a greenish pus, corroding every spot over which it passes.

Arum-t. (Uraemia) - uraemia in **malignant** cases of scarlatina, diphtheria, etc.; child tosses about the bed unconsciously, picking at one spot, boring finger in nose; profuse urination is the sign that the remedy acted well.

Aur-mur.-nat. (Ophthalmia) - chronic ophthalmia, **malignant**, cancerous, at the same time nose scurfy, ulcerated; violent pains in whole left side of head, mostly over eyes; glaucoma; retinal congestion; syphilitic iritis, with sore, bruised sensation around the eyes; scrofulous ophthalmia; amaurosis.

Aur-mur.-nat. (Scrofulosis) - scrofulous **malignant** ophthalmia, even cancerous; at the same time nose scurfy; destruction of nasal bones, ozaena with ichorous, bloody, foetid discharge; epithelioma; cynanche cellularis; uterine and ovarian enlargements; indurations and chronic suppuration of glands and bones (Aur, Ars.).

Aurum met. (Tumors) - **malignant** ulceration of palate and nasal bones (syphilis, lupus); mental despondency, with suicidal disposition; pus greenish, ichorous, putrid; worse at night and morning; on getting cold, while reposing; better from warmth, moving, while walking.

Baryta carbonica - gastric weakness in the aged with possible **malignancy** present.

Bromium (Diphtheria) - **malignant** forms of diphtheria, invading larynx down respiratory organs, leaving great weakness and lassitude; no fever, cool skin, sweating and spasm; husky tone of voice, rattling of mucus in larynx when coughing, cough has a croupy sound, with strangling rattling mucus in breathing; face ashy-gray, cheeks sunken, stiffness of neck, prostration. suits children with fair hair and skin, blue eyes, etc., and teste affirms that milk neutralizes the action of brom. and iod. (Kali-bi., no spasm).

Bromium (Favus, tinea maligna) - **malignant** scaldhead, oozing profusely; where the skin is dry, extreme tenderness of the scalp; unbearable foetor of the discharge.

Bromium (Tinea capitis. Scald head) - **malignant** scald head, oozing profusely; in places, where eruption is dry, skin throws off flakes; extreme tenderness of scalp; unbearable offensive smell of eruption; especially in children with light hair and blue eyes.

Bufo (Carbuncle. see boils) - carbuncle at the commencement already pestilential, with blueness far around, and red and purplish streaks in neck, back and other parts (ant. crud. and lach., redness and swelling along course of lymphatics); **malignant** pustule (Malandrinum).

Carbo-an. (Ozaena) - scrofulous ozaena; swelling of nose, with pimples inside and outside, forming crusts which last a long time; vesicle at right nostril with **malignant** ulceration; little boils inside of nose, with tense and burning sensation, < during menses; saddle across nose with copper-colored eruption. cancer nasi.

Carbo-an. (Uterus complaints) - induration of neck of uterus; menorrhagia from chronic induration of uterus; scirrhus of uterus, with pressive pains in loins, groins and thighs; distention of abdomen; flatulence, frequent eructations and desire to vomit; leucorrhoea leaving yellow stains on linen; numbness of limbs; ulcers, scrofulous or **malignant**, with foul discharge; tearing transversely across pubes and then through pudendum as far as anus; stitches in the groins; burning pains down the thighs; alternate cheerfulness and despondency.

China-ars. (Scarlatina) - **malignant** scarlatina; pallor of skin with rapid exhaustion; anxiety; nightly delirium; diphtheritic angina, threatening to invade larynx.

Cistus canadensis - **malignant** disease of the glands of the neck.

Crotalus hor. (Cancer) - **cancer of the tongue with great haemorrhagic tendency;** putrid sore mouth with bloody salivation; cancer of stomach, **much haemorrhage** or much vomiting of mucus, slimy or bloody, with distressing sensation of sinking, and craving for stimulants; cancer uteri, fungoid, **malignant sarcoma,** cauliflower excrescence, **with much tendency to haemorrhage;** weak, debilitated constitutions.

Crotalus hor. (Hepatic derangements) - **malignant** jaundice, dark **haemorrhages** from nose, mouth, etc.; dark, scanty urine.

Crotalus hor. (Jaundice) -**malignant, black jaundice;** stitches in hepatic region on drawing a long breath, < on pressure; complete loss of taste, constipation; urine jellylike and red like blood; skin very dark-brown; **dark haemorrhages from nose, mouth, bowels, uterus,** etc.; confused speech, rapid pulse, coldness of skin.

Crotalus hor. (Scarlatina) - **malignant scarlatina with haemorrhagic tendency, oozing of blood from every** orifice and even from the pores; vomiting of bile and blood; scanty; great infiltration of connective tissue, especially at throat. indicated when at the beginning of the invasion there is overwhelming toxication with convulsions or without them, but steady collapse, and also for late stage or sequelae, especially dropsy, when urine is dark, smoky, bloody, albinous.

Crotalus hor. (Sore throat) -**malignant sore throat,** which is greatly swollen, with tendency to gangrene; neck swollen; puffy face; violent pain in constricted throat; tongue trembles; prostration; **haemorrhages** from dissolution of blood; nervous sore throat, pain out of all proportion to visible trouble; fauces dry; great sensitiveness to dry or cold air.

Crotalus hor. (Uterus complaints) - cancer; fungoid, **malignant sarcoma;** cauliflower excrescence, **with haemorrhagic tendency; very degraded state in patient.**

Crotalus horridus - **blood decomposition, haemorrhages,** tendency to carbuncles, **malignant scarlatina,** yellow fever, the plague, cholera, give opportunity to use this remedy.

Crotalus horridus - **malignant fevers of a haemorrhagic** or putrescent character.

Curare (Cancer) - **malignant** ulcers in different parts of the body; cancer of the cheeks, healing over very slowly and passing easily into gangrene; funnel-shaped ulcer of os uteri, with corroding, ichorous, foetid discharge, smarting in vulva and thighs, shooting and digging pains in womb.

Curare (Uterus complaints) - lips thick and full of scirrhous tubercles; sores healing very slowly and passing easily into gangrene; **malignant** ulcers in different parts of body; corroding, cancerous ulcers; smarting in vulva and thighs; shooting and digging pains in womb; swelling of rectum and anus; very sensitive haemorrhoidal fissures; anxious and despairing expression.

Diphtherinum - **malignancy** from the start.

Dulcamara - tendency to **malignancy** in acute and subacute disorders.

Eucalyptus - **malignant** disease of stomach with vomiting of blood and sour fluid.

Fluoric acid - it seems to have the peculiar property of eating into **malignant** tumors, leaving the surrounding healthy tissue uncharred and unchanged.

Hippozaeninum - **malignant** erysipelas, particularly if attended with large formation of pus, destruction of parts.

Hippozaeninum - putrescence, destructive, quasi **malignant** ulcerative tendency to decomposition of generals, rare-strange-peculiars: g.1

Kali-bich. - man, aged 82, lived for thirsty years in india, had fever, dysentery, bronchitis; bowels generally loose, habitual snuff taker; **malignant** ulceration of nose.

Kali-phos. (Scarlatina) - desquamation; discharges of foul, offensive, ichorous pus from ears; ulceration of drumhead and middle ear suppuration; foetid discharge from mucous membrane of nose; breath offensive; face livid and sunken; **malignant** gangrenous conditions with excessive nervous prostration, feeling of goneness and faintness.

Kali-ars. - skin cancer, where suddenly an alarming **malignancy** without any external signs sets in.

Kali-ars. - the Kali-ars. patient tends towards **malignancy**, and inveterate skin diseases.

Kali-phos. - remember it in the treatment of suspected **malignant** tumors.

Kreosotum (Cancer) - shooting stitches in the vagina; burning and swelling of the external and internal labia; profuse discharge of dark coagulated blood, or of a pungent bloody ichor, preceded by pain in the back; aggravation of the pains at night; fainting on rising from the bed; she always feels chilly at the menstrual period; complexion livid; disposition sad, irritable; cauliflower excrescences; wretched complexion, great debility, sleeplessness. Tightness of the pit of the stomach, cannot bear the weight of her clothing; painful hard place on the left side of her stomach; constipation in uterine cancer; soreness and smarting between labia and vulva, with excessive pruritus and ulcerative pain in neck of uterus; epithelial cancer on nose; **malignant** induration of stomach.

Kreosotum (Diphtheria) - putrid odor from mouth; **malignant** diphtheria, when confined to fauces, especially in scrofulous and lymphatic patients; black softening and decomposition of mucous membrane with atony and extension of softening to oesophagus; fever, vomiting, loss of appetite, restless sleep; swelling of glands.

Lachesis - girl, infant, aged 6 months; **malignant** erysipelas.

Lachesis - **malignant** local inflammations, with secondary blood infection and nervous prostration; **malignant** pustule.

Lanciolatus - **malignant** erysipelas.

Ledum (Sore throat) - sore throat with fine stinging pains, < when not swallowing; sensation as from a lump in throat, when swallowing, a stinging pain; great heat in throat, when moving in the open air; **malignant** sore throat; oedema.

Manganum acet. - **malignant** ulcers with blue border, following slight injury.

Merc-cyanatus (Heart, diseases of) - ulcerated endocarditis (Lach.); rapid heart failure due to **malignant** cardiac disease. Threatening paralysis of heart in diphtheria or zymotic diseases. Need more provings.

Mercurius cyanatus - **malignant** types, with prostration.

Mercurius solubilis - this **malignant** medicinal force is converted into useful life saving and life preserving service if employed homoeopathically, guided by its clear cut symptoms.

Mezereum (Leucorrhoea) - leucorrhoea resembling alben, **malignant**, chronic; discharge of mucus from the vagina; menses too early and protracted; prolapsus ani; constipation.

Nitric acid. (Coryza) - coryza, especially when associated with some **malignant** disease, as scarlatina or diphtheria; discharge watery, offensive, excoriating every part it touches; foetor in throat, with sensation of a splinter there; intermittent pulse (arum).

Phosphorus (Hepatic derangements) - hyperaemia, at first enlargement, fatty degeneration and finally atrophy of the liver with jaundice and dropsy; waxy liver dependent upon long-lasting bone disease; fatty liver in consequence of cardiac troubles; acute yellow atrophy of liver; suppurating hepatitis with hectic fever, night-sweats, enlargement in right hypochondrium and marked soreness of liver; **malignant** jaundice from venous obstruction, often from alcoholism; gall-bladder full of pale-yellow, slimy fluid; loss of appetite, unquenchable thirst, < after eating and drinking; abdomen flaccid, with chronic loose bowels; haemorrhoidal **bleeding** and **haemorrhages** from different parts of body; profuse sweat immediately after falling asleep; worse during atmospheric changes, thunderstorms, windy weather, after midnight.

Phosphorus (Jaundice) - acute, yellow atrophy of liver, fatty liver from heart affection; **malignant** jaundice from organic affections; in complication with pneumonia or deep-seated brain diseases, during pregnancy, from nervous excitement; painful feeling of weakness across abdomen; stools profuse, watery, light-colored; dry cough and involuntary discharge of urine; constant chilliness, even in a warm room.

Phytolacca (Anthrax) - tendency to boils, carbuncles or **malignant** pustule, very painful, and appearing especially on the back and behind the ears.

Secale - **malignant** pustule.

Sempervivum tectorum - **malignant** ulcers of mouth.

Silicea - boils, carbuncles, felons, and **malignant** pustule, during suppurative stage.

Silicea - **malignant** and gangrenous inflammations.

Silicea (Nails, diseases of) - affection of periosteum; moderate redness or heat, deep-seated inflammation, violent shooting pain deep in the finger, worse in the warm bed, sleepless at night, pain being unbearable, with great restlessness, irritability, even unto convulsive jerks; opening with a surrounding wall of proud flesh, pus **malignant**, discolored; it promotes expulsion of necrotic bones; ingrowing toe-nail; tearing pains as if the bones would be actually torn out, preventing all sleep; frequent crops of boils; chronic foetid foot-sweats; slightest draught unbearable.

Silicea (Tumors) - semi-**malignant** and cancerous tumors; scirrhus induration of the upper lip and face; sebaceous and synovial cysts, fibroid tumors; epulis; encephaloma oculi; blood-boils and warts; gliomatosis.

Silicea (Scrofulosis) - **malignant** pustule;

Stramonium - boy, aged 6; **malignant** scarlatina.

Tarentula cubensis - various forms of **malignant** suppuration.

Thuja (Aphthae, thrush; gangrene of mouth in children) - **malignant** aphthae on a sycotic basis.

Thuja (Ophthalmia) - **malignant** ophthalmo-blennorrhoea; frequently repeating scrofulous ophthalmia.

Vaccininum; variolin; malandrinum; thuja are powerful adjuvants in treatment of **malignant** disease.

Zincum met. - after an abscess in left mammae, the right became hard and tender, the left being opened instead of cured by inward medicine; the right became swollen and red, pitted on pressure, the horrible cut with the knife brought no matter; three days later the lancet was plunged in again, pus and blood came, but not freely; towards night breast got painful, middle of night tremendously swollen. Finally the cut closed, but left an angry bright redness of surrounding skin, which changed to a **malignant** purple hue, the woman became greatly exhausted and shivered. Arnica lotion relieved at once and very soon there followed a healthy discharge from the abscess.

Zincum met. - after having taken homoeopathic medicine for **malignant** ulcers, suddenly the greatest malaise, and a black blister formed below knee with swelling all around, and feverish shaking chill through whole body.

Zincum met. - chronic ophthalmia; **malignant**, cancerous; at same time, nose scurfy.

Zincum met. - constitutional syphilis, with indescribable feeling of weakness, or with dropsy and **malignant** ulcerations.

Zincum met. - hands and lower half of forearm dark and livid, as in **malignant** cholera.

Zincum met. - **malignant** forms of diphtheria.

Zincum met. - **malignant** scald head.

Zincum met. - **malignant** scarlatina with somnolence, starting from sleep; dark red or putrid sore throat; sticky salivation; parotitis; external throat swollen; stertorous breathing; involuntary stools with excessive vomiting; body red, with miliary rash, or faintly developed eruption; threatened paralysis of brain.

Zincum met. - **malignant** scarlet fever. **malignant** sore throat. Scarlatina.

Zincum met. - **malignant** swelling of parotid glands in scarlet fever, when remissions occur in which patient is better, but soon spell of great prostration returns.

Zincum met. - most **malignant** gangrenous ulcers. **malignant** ulceration of mammae, mouth.

Zincum met. - parotitis in scarlatina; discharge ichorus, **malignant**.

Zincum met. - scarlatina, eruption delays, or suddenly pales, becomes livid, or intermixed with petechiae; **malignant** sore throat; dropsy; or eruption well out, but with disproportionate weakness, mild delirium, vomiting, etc.

Zincum met. - sulphur; in **malignant** pustule, Antim. crud., Lach.; in bullae, panaritia, etc., Hepar, Lach., Phosph-ac., Silicea.

Zincum met. - **malignant** fevers. **malignant** pustule. **malignant** puerperal fever.

Zincum met. - Dr. C. Hering applied, in his first cases of **malignant** scarlatina, in a damp cellar, in cherry street, the alcoholic tincture made from the dried bulb, and Dr. Lippe, who has given us all the characteristics used only potencies in alcohol, mostly the higher.

Pathological condition associated with malignancy

(Abscesses) For chronic abscesses, whether cold or occasioned by congestions, to: Asa., Aur., Calc., Carb-v., Con., Hep., Iod., Laur., Lyc., Mang., Merc., Merc-cor., Nitr-ac., Phos., Sep., Sil., Sulph. - further, if there arises on any internal or external part a painful, red, inflamed swelling, which may point and form a suppurating swelling, Bell., or if this does not succeed in twenty-four or forty-eight hours, Hep. will often disperse the whole swelling and keep suppuration off;

but when once matter has formed, merc. will bring on the discharge of the pus and frequently finish up the case, its chief indication being that suppuration must have already taken place should the open wound not heal under the continuation of Merc. give Hep. or Sil., which are the real specifics against all benign or **malignant** suppurations. if the abscess looks erysipelatous, Apis, Bell.; if bluish, Lach.

(Anthrax) - The **malignant** pustule generally yields to: 1, Ars. Bell. Sil., Rhus, or, perhaps, Chin., Hyosc., Mur-ac., Sec., Sep.; 2, Anthrac., Apis, Carb-v., Kreos., Hydr., Tarent-cubana.

(Anthrax) Phytolacca - tendency to boils, carbuncles or **malignant** pustule, very painful, and appearing specially on the back and behind the ears.

(Aphthae, thrush; gangrene of mouth in children) Thuja - **malignant** aphthae on a sycotic basis.

(Cancer) Crotalus hor. - cancer of the tongue with great **haemorrhagic** tendency; putrid sore mouth with bloody salivation; cancer of stomach, much **haemorrhage** or much vomiting of mucus, slimy or bloody, with distressing sensation of sinking, and craving for stimulants; cancer uteri, fungoid, **malignant** sarcoma, cauliflower excrescence, with much tendency to **haemorrhage**; weak, debilitated constitutions.

(Cancer) Curare - **malignant** ulcers in different parts of the body; cancer of the cheeks, healing over very slowly and passing easily into gangrene; funnel-shaped ulcer of os uteri, with corroding, ichorous, foetid discharge, smarting in vulva and thighs, shooting and digging pains in womb.

(Cancer) Kreosotum - shooting stitches in the vagina; burning and swelling of the external and internal labia; profuse discharge of dark coagulated blood, or of a pungent bloody ichor, preceded by pain in the back; aggravation of the pains at night; fainting on rising from the bed; she always feels chilly at the menstrual period; complexion livid; disposition sad, irritable; cauliflower excrescences; wretched complexion, great debility, sleeplessness. Tightness of the pit of the stomach, cannot bear the weight of her clothing; painful hard place on the left side of her stomach; constipation in uterine cancer; soreness and smarting between labia and in vulva, with excessive pruritus and ulcerative pain in neck of uterus; epithelial cancer on nose; **malignant** induration of stomach.

(Carbuncle—see also boils) Bufo sahytiensis - carbuncle at the commencement already pestilential, with blueness far around, and red and purplish streaks in neck, back and other parts (Ant-crud. and Lach., redness and swelling along course of lymphatics); **malignant** pustule (Malandrinum).

(Coryza) Nitric acid. - coryza, especially when associated with some **malignant** disease, as scarlatina or diphtheria; discharge watery, offensive, excoriating every part it touches; foetor in throat, with sensation of a splinter there; intermittent pulse (arum).

(Diphtheria) Bromium - **malignant** forms of diphtheria, invading larynx down respiratory organs, leaving great weakness and lassitude; no fever, cool skin, sweating and spasm; husky tone of voice, rattling of mucus in larynx when coughing, cough has a croupy sound, with strangling rattling mucus in breathing; face ashy-gray, cheeks sunken, stiffness of neck, prostration. suits children with fair hair and skin, blue eyes, etc., and teste affirms that milk neutralizes the action of Brom. and Iod. (Kali-bi., no spasm).

(Diphtheria) Kreosotum - putrid odor from mouth; **malignant** diphtheria, when confined to fauces, especially in scrofulous and lymphatic patients; black softening and decomposition of mucous membrane with atony and extension of softening to oesophagus; fever, vomiting, loss of appetite, restless sleep; swelling of glands.

(Duodenitis and duodenal catarrh) Ars-alb. - great restlessness and anxiety; ulceration of duodenum, involving pancreas, following burns or **malignant** diseases; neuralgia of coeliac plexus.

(Favus, tinea maligna) Bromium - **malignant** scaldhead, oozing profusely; where the skin is dry, extreme tenderness of the scalp; unbearable foetor of the discharge.

(Glaucoma) Ars-alb. - glossitis, with constant thirst, drinking but a little at a time; gangrene of tongue, spots on tongue, burning like fire; gangrenous ulcers of mouth and fauces; **malignant** aphthae of children.

(Haemorrhoids) Acetic acid. - **malignant** diseases of rectum; profuse haemorrhoidal **bleeding**; **haemorrhage** from bowels after checked metrorrhagia; obstinate constipation.

(Heart, diseases of) Merc-cyanatus - ulcerated endocarditis (Lach.); rapid heart failure due to **malignant** cardiac disease. threatening paralysis of heart in diphtheria or other zymotic diseases. needs more provings.

(Hepatic derangements) Crotalus hor. - shooting and stitches in hepatic region when taking a long breath, also on top of right shoulder; pressive hepatic congestion, especially when from heart disease or from imperfect performance of uterine functions, or if a sequel of malarial fever. acute yellow atrophy; **malignant** jaundice, dark **haemorrhages** from nose, mouth, etc.; dark, scanty urine.

(Hepatic derangements) Phosphorus - hyperaemia, at first enlargement, fatty degeneration and finally atrophy of the liver with jaundice and dropsy; waxy liver dependent upon long-lasting bone disease; fatty liver in consequence of cardiac troubles; acute yellow atrophy of liver; suppurating hepatitis with hectic fever, night-sweats, enlargement in right hypochondrium and marked soreness of liver; **malignant** jaundice from venous obstruction, often from alcoholism; gall-bladder full of pale-yellow, slimy fluid; loss of appetite, unquenchable thirst, < after eating and drinking; abdomen flaccid, with chronic loose bowels; haemorrhoidal **bleeding** and **haemorrhages** from different parts of body; profuse sweat immediately after falling asleep; worse during atmospheric changes, thunderstorms, windy weather, after midnight.

(Jaundice) Aconite - severe and constant pain in epigastrium, pressing outward; pain going to the navel or changing from stomach to liver; yellowish-white thick fur in mouth. jaundice from a cold with catarrh of the small intestines, after fright, during pregnancy, in newborn children. from atrophy of liver **malignant** jaundice (tincture according to jousset); constipation or diarrhoea.

(Jaundice) Crotalus hor. - **malignant**, black jaundice; stitches in hepatic region on drawing a long breath, < on pressure; complete loss of taste, constipation; urine jelly-like and red like blood; skin very dark-brown; dark **haemorrhages** from nose, mouth, bowels, uterus, etc.; confused speech, rapid pulse, coldness of skin.

(Jaundice) Phosphorus - acute, yellow atrophy of liver, fatty liver from heart affection; **malignant** jaundice from organic affections; in complication with pneumonia or deep-seated brain diseases, during pregnancy, from nervous excitement; painful feeling of weakness across abdomen; stools profuse, watery, light-colored; dry cough and involuntary discharge of urine; constant chilliness, even in a warm room.

(Leucorrhoea) Mezereum - leucorrhoea resembling alben, **malignant**, chronic; discharge of mucus from the vagina; menses too early and protracted; prolapsus ani; constipation.

(Nails, diseases of) Silicea - affection of periosteum; moderate redness or heat, deep-seated inflammation, violent shooting pain deep in the finger, worse in the warm bed, sleepless at night, pain being unbearable, with great restlessness, irritability, even unto convulsive jerks; opening with a surrounding wall of proud flesh, pus **malignant**, discolored; it promotes expulsion of necrotic bones; ingrowing toe-nail; tearing pains as if the bones would be actually torn out, preventing all sleep; frequent crops of boils; chronic foetid foot-sweats; slightest draught unbearable.

(Ophthalmia) Aur-mur.-nat. - chronic ophthalmia, **malignant**, cancerous, at the same time nose scurfy, ulcerated; violent pains in whole left side of head, mostly over eyes; glaucoma; retinal congestion; syphilitic iritis, with sore, bruised sensation around the eyes; scrofulous ophthalmia; amaurosis.

(Ophthalmia) Thuja - **malignant** ophthalmo-blennorrhoea; frequently repeating scrofulous ophthalmia; potbelliedness of children; bulimy alternating with inappetency; excessive flatulence; obstinate constipation, or obstinate diarrhea; iritis, with condylomata on iris, much heat above and around the eye; amblyopia, blurred sight, better from rubbing; aching back into the head; conjunctivitis trachomatosa, granulations like warts or blisters, with burning; photophobia and suffusion of eyes in tears; tinea ciliaris, eyelashes irregular and imperfectly grown, fine scales covering the skin, eyes weak and watery; tarsal tumors and styes; better by warmly covering eyes.

(Ozaena) Carbo-an. - scrofulous ozaena; swelling of nose, with pimples inside and outside, forming crusts which last a long time; vesicle at right nostril with **malignant** ulceration; little boils inside of nose, with tense and burning sensation, < during menses; saddle across nose with copper-colored eruption. cancer nasi.

(Pancreas, diseases of) - **malignant** or epidemic form: Calc-ars., Rhus-t.

(Pancreas, diseases of) Ars-alb. - organic degenerations with great restlessness and despair; ulceration of duodenum, which, by extension, involves the pancreatic duct, perhaps the result of burns, of **malignant** disease, etc.; neuralgia of the coeliac plexus; stools undigested, containing fat.

(Parotitis) Mumps: for **malignant** parotitis, passing over into ichoration.

(Puerperal fever) Ailanthus - **malignant** puerperal fever; ichorous and foetid lochia; deliria; diarrhoea; eruption all over body; constant thirst, longing for brandy; soreness, irritability, pricking and tingling everywhere.

(Scarlatina) Ailanthus - adynamic **malignant** scarlatina from the start; general prostration and marked cerebral affection during the first stage; pulse small, weak, often irregular; skin harsh and dry, covered with a scanty dark-bluish rash, more profuse on forehead and face; violent vomiting, dizziness, photophobia, stupor and insensibility; pupils dilated; great thirst, with dry, parched tongue; throat inside swollen, dark-colored, even ulcerated, with infiltration of the cellular tissue about the neck; excoriating nasal discharge; great exhaustion and stoical indifference to whatever happens; petechiae, torpor, eruption is slow to make its appearance, remains livid even on forehead and face; skin dry, but never hot; irregular, patchy, livid eruption, disappearing on pressure and returning very slowly, interspersed with small vesicles, < forehead, neck and chest.

(Scarlatina) Amm-carb. - miliary scarlatina of a **malignant** type from deficient oxygenation; throat swollen internally and externally, with enlargement of glands and bluish, dark-red swelling of tonsils; infiltration of cellular tissue around engorged cervical lymphatics; gangrenous, putrid ulceration of tonsils, covered with rapidly decomposing, sticky, offensive, muco-pus; burning pains in the throat, sticky salivation; nose obstructed, particularly at night, causing the child to start from its sleep as if smothering, has to lie with its mouth wide open in order to breathe; mental confusion, gloom, inclined to shed tears; chill and heat often alternate till towards midnight; continuous day or night-sweat; upper half of the body covered by eruption with violent itching, or faintly developed eruption; stertorous breathing; involuntary defaecation and urination; threatening paralysis of brain with excessive vomiting; hard swelling of right parotid and lymphatic glands of the neck.

(Scarlatina) China ars. - **malignant** scarlatina; pallor of skin with rapid exhaustion; anxiety; nightly delirium; diphtheritic angina, threatening to invade larynx.

(Scarlatina) Crotalus hor. - **malignant** scarlatina with **haemorrhagic** tendency, oozing of blood from every orifice and even from the pores; vomiting of bile and blood; dry skin; dark-brown, dry tongue; insatiable thirst; low muttering delirium, drowsiness; urine dark, scanty; great infiltration of connective tissue, especially at throat. Indicated when at the beginning of the invasion there is overwhelming toxication with convulsions or without them, but steady collapse, and also for late stage or sequelae, especially dropsy, when urine is dark, smoky, bloody, albinous.

(Scarlatina) Kali-phos. - desquamation; discharges of foul, offensive, ichorous pus from ears; ulceration of drumhead and middle ear suppuration; foetid discharge from mucous membrane of nose; breath offensive; face livid and sunken; **malignant** gangrenous conditions with excessive nervous prostration, feeling of goneness and faintness.

(Scrofulosis) Aethiops antimonialis - scrofulous glandular and skin diseases; blepharitis, conjunctivitis and keratitis scrofulosa, even with a **malignant** tendency; boils and furuncles.

(Scrofulosis) Aur-mur.-nat. - scrofulous **malignant** ophthalmia, even cancerous; at the same time nose scurfy; destruction of nasal bones, ozaena with ichorous, bloody, foetid discharge; epithelioma; cynanche cellularis; uterine and ovarian enlargements; indurations and chronic suppuration of glands and bones (Aur.-ars.).

(Scrofulosis) - decided want of vital heat even when taking exercise; imperfect nutrition, not from want of food, but from imperfect assimilation; canine hunger, in nervous, irritable people; desires only cold things; swelling and induration of parotid and cervical glands; difficult dentition; offensive-smelling sweat of feet and head; headache, > by wrapping head up warmly (Magn.-mur.); rachitis; ozaena; swelling and soreness in old cicatricial tissues about neck and throat; curvature of bones; caries of vertebral column with lateral curvature; disposition of skin to ulcerate; tendency to boils, which leave indurations; carbuncles; **malignant** pustule; eczema, impetigo, herpes; blepharitis; otorrhoea; face pale and bloated; abdomen large and hard; diarrhoea with thin, offensive stools, containing partially digested food. (Calc.-fluor. follows well after Sil.)

(Sore throat) Ars-alb. - restlessness, anxiety, prostration; gangrene in throat, burning like hot coals in throat; tonsils swollen, dark-red; vesicles in throat; tongue, throat, oesophagus inflamed; paralysis of pharynx; drinks come out of nose; **malignancy** (Ars.-iod.).

(Sore throat) Crotalus hor. - **malignant** sore throat, which is greatly swollen, with tendency to gangrene; neck swollen; puffy face; violent pain in constricted throat; tongue trembles; prostration; **haemorrhages** from dissolution of blood; nervous sore throat, pain out of all proportion to visible trouble; fauces dry; great sensitiveness to dry or cold air.

(Sore throat) Ledum - sore throat with fine stinging pains, < when not swallowing; sensation as from a lump in throat, when swallowing, a stinging pain; great heat in throat, when moving in the open air; **malignant** sore throat; oedema.

(Stomatitis, inflammation and ulceration of buccal cavity.) Ars-alb. **malignant** ulceration in mouth; edges of tongue ulcerated; aphthae with violent burning pains; ulcers and blisters turn livid and black; swollen and readily-**bleeding** gums; looseness of teeth; ptyalism; restlessness and great exhaustion.

(Suppuration) - **malignant**: 1, Asa., Chin., Hep., Merc., Phos., Pyrogen., Sil.; 2, Ars., Calc., Carb-v., Caust., Kreos., Nitr.-ac., Rhus, Sulph., Sulph-ac.

(Syphilis and sycosis) Ars-alb. - phagedenic chancres, livid hue, with intense burning, even sloughing; chancres (after mercury), with too florid granulations; margins of ulcers hard and **bleeding** at least touch, with a thin, offensive discharge; bubo when assuring a gangrenous aspect; inguinal glands painful, swollen, indurated; constitutional syphilis, with indescribable feeling of weakness, or with dropsy and **malignant** ulcerations; coffee-colored eruptions on skin, burning pimples or pustular eruption. (Ars. brings out dormant syphilis.) Ars-iod, secondary syphilis, mucous plaques; tertiary syphilis, cutaneous ulcers discharging a greenish pus, corroding every spot over which it passes.

(Tinea capitis. Scald head) Bromium - **malignant** scald head, oozing profusely; in places, where eruption is dry, skin throws off flakes; extreme tenderness of scalp; unbearable offensive smell of eruption; especially in children with light hair and blue eyes.

(Tumors) Semi - **malignant** Fibroid: Bry., Con., Led., Sil.

(Tumors) Arnica - tumor following a contusion or a similar injury, but not becoming **malignant**; dull tingling pain in indurated part; red, blue or yellow spots, like ecchymosis; pus thin and bloody.

(Tumors) Aurum met. - **malignant** ulceration of palate and nasal bones (syphilis, lupus); mental despondency, with suicidal disposition; pus greenish, ichorous, putrid; worse at night and morning; on getting cold, while reposing; better from warmth, moving, while walking.

(Tumors) Silicea - semi-**malignant** and cancerous tumors; scirrhus induration of the upper lip and face; sebaceous and synovial cysts, fibroid tumors; epulis; encephaloma oculi; blood-boils and warts; gliomatosis.

(Ulcers) Ant-tart. - deeply penetrating, **malignant** ulcers; broad and deep sloughing ulcers; gangrenous ulcers with hectic fever; ulcers surrounded with black pustules, which break down into deep ulcers; no pus. merely oozing of foetid humor.

(Uraemia) Arum-t. - uraemia in **malignant** cases of scarlatina, diphtheria, etc.; child tosses about the bed unconsciously, picking at one spot, boring finger in nose; profuse urination is the sign that the remedy acted well.

(Uterus complaints) Carbo-an. - induration of neck of uterus; menorrhagia from chronic induration of uterus; scirrhus of uterus, with pressive pains in loins, groins and thighs; distention of abdomen; flatulence, frequent eructations and desire to vomit; leucorrhoea leaving yellow stains on linen; numbness of limbs; ulcers, scrofulous or **malignant**, with foul discharge; tearing transversely across pubes and then through pudendum as far as anus; stitches in the groins; burning pains down the thighs; alternate cheerfulness and despondency.

(Uterus complaints) Crotalus-hor. - cancer; fungoid, **malignant** sarcoma; cauliflower excrescence, with **haemorrhagic** tendency; very degraded state in patient.

(Uterus complaints) Curare - lips thick and full of scirrhous tubercles; sores healing very slowly and passing easily into gangrene; **malignant** ulcers in different parts of body; corroding, cancerous ulcers; smarting in vulva and thighs; shooting and digging pains in womb; swelling of rectum and anus; very sensitive haemorrhoidal fissures; anxious and despairing expression.

Cancer, Cancerous diathesis, Cancerous constitution, Cancerous cachexia

(Note: If, in a patient, cancer appears repeatedly or it lasts for several years or more than one member in the family has or had cancer, the following list may be of help.)

Bromium (Gangrene) - hospital gangrene; death of the edges of the wound; cancerous ulcer in face; stony-hard swelling of glands, especially on lower jaw and throat; decayed teeth and gums; foul breath; much prostration and emaciation; psoric constitution (mcfarlan recommends its internal use and applies the fuming destructive liquid externally to remove the sloughs).

Calc-phos. - cancer in scrofulous constitutions.

Calc-phos. (Glands, diseases of, adenitis) - incipient mesenteric tabes, with foetid diarrhoea and emaciation; tuberculosis; cancer in scrofulous, psoric constitutions.

Carbo-an. (Cancer) - cachexia fully developed. Scirrhous cancer on the forehead; sudden and short aching from colloid cancer in the pit of the stomach, on taking a deep inspiration, clawing and griping in stomach; violent pressing in loins, small of back and thighs during menses, with chilliness and yawning; weak, empty feeling in the pit of the stomach;

it checks the putrid taste, the waterbrash, and contracting, spasmodic burning; scirrhus mammae with dirty bluish, loose skin or red spots on skin, burning and drawing towards axilla; axillary glands indurated.

Carbo-an. (Haemorrhage from uterus) - menses too early, not too profuse, but last too long; great weakness of the thighs. after the appearance of the menses she feels so tired she is scarcely able to speak; menorrhagia from chronic induration of uterus, also in cachectic women with glandular affections, cancer, etc.; blood black, clotted, putrid.

Carcinosinum - indigestion accumulation of gas in stomach and bowels; rheumatism - cancerous cachexia.

Conium - cancerous diathesis.

Corydalis - cancer cachexia pronounced.

Crotalus hor. (Cancer) - cancer of the tongue with great haemorrhagic tendency; putrid sore mouth with bloody salivation; cancer of stomach, much haemorrhage or much vomiting of mucus, slimy or bloody, with distressing sensation of sinking, and craving for stimulants; cancer uteri, fungoid, malignant sarcoma, cauliflower excrescence, with much tendency to haemorrhage; weak, debilitated constitutions.

Cundurango (Cancer) - most efficacious in open cancer or cancerous ulcers, where it effectually moderates the severity of the pain; epithelial cancer on lower eyelid, on left side of nose; cancer of lip, an unclean and sinuous ulcer, with surrounding hardness and swelling, burning pains, lip inverted; painful cracks at the angle of the mouth; ulcer on chin, perforating the gums; lumps on chin; cancer of tongue; cancer of stomach, severe pains, vomiting of coffee-ground masses; hard, knobby, large swelling in pylorus, complete loss of appetite, emaciation, cachectic look, constipation;

scirrhus mammae, whole breast, skin and axillary glands; tumor hard, immovable, with severe lancinating pains, nipple retracted; skin purple in spots and wrinkled: ulceration with foetid sanious discharge and much sloughing.

Hydrastis - emaciation; scrofula; cancer cachexia.

Hydrastis (Dyspepsia, weakness of stomach) - atonic dyspepsia; cancerous diathesis. Great lassitude, debility, exhaustion; obstinate constipation, and its attendant dull headache in the forehead; urging to urinate, and sensation as if bowels would move, but only wind passes; large, flabby, slimy-looking tongue; sour eructations; cannot digest bread and vegetables; empty, aching, gone feeling in stomach, aggravated by eating; weakness of digestion, with heavy, dull, hard, thumping fulness of chest and dyspnoea, palpitation of heart; even light pressure of hand reveals strong pulsations in pit of stomach; faintings from exhaustion; eructations of a bitter fluid; pyrosis; burning pains in umbilical region, with stitches in epigastrium, extending to testicles, appearing after stool and accompanied by great weakness; constipation, faeces hard, knotty, stool followed by pain and weakness; haemorrhoids; sympathetic sore throat; chronic mucous discharges; like Nux-v. after abuse of drugs.

Hydrastis (Scrofulosis) - chronic catarrhs of mucous membranes wherever situated; constipation from weakened and congestive state of the lower bowel; cancerous cachexia; cancers hard, adherent; skin mottled, puckered, with lancinating cutting pains; atony of muscles.

Kali-mur. (Cancer) - epithelioma of lip; ulceration of mouth has perforated cheeks and threatens to become cancer of the face; discharge ichorous and foetid; scurvy in cachectic people.

Trifolium pratense - cancerous diathesis.

Remedies for cancer with bleeding

(Note: Haemorrhage or bleeding in cancer patient invariably ends fatal. Therefore, the practitioner should keep the following in finger tips. For example, we have completely and permanently cured several cases of cancer of prostate or bladder with haematuria with one single dose of Crotalus horridus-10M. Similarly in uterus cancer with bleeding we should not forget Thlaspi bursa pastoris. In leucaemia where bleeding occurs, again Crotalus horridus).

Carcinosinum - carcinoma of the mammary glands with great pain and induration of glands; of uterus, the offensive discharge, haemorrhage and pain are greatly relieved.

Cistus - bleeding cancer on lower lip; lupus exedens about face, nose and mouth; cancer of mammae with amenorrhoea; chronic catarrhs with strumous diseases of glands.

Cistus - lupus, caries; open, bleeding cancer.

Conium - bleeding of ulcers with a secretion of foetid ichor; cancerous swelling and induration of glands; induration of lymphatics of lip after contusion; cancer of lip from pressure of pipe; cancer of face and lips, spreading ulcers; cancer of stomach with contractive, spasmodic pains extending from pit of stomach into back and shoulders; swelling in pyloric region; hardness of abdomen from swelling of mesenteric glands; induration and enlargement of ovaries or womb, with lancinating pains; or burning, stinging, darting pains in neck of uterus; with indurations and scirrhosities and profuse excoriating leucorrhoea; scirrhous cancer of mammae, hard as cartilage and uneven, sharp, shooting pains and occasional twinges and sense of great heaviness in breast, axillary glands swollen; concealed cancer of bones; effects of contusions and bruises; it acts best in the first stage of scirrhus.

- Conium - bleeding of ulcers, with secretion of fetid ichor; a portion becomes gangrenous; concealed cancer of bones; cancerous swelling and induration of glands; cancer of lips; spreading cancerous ulcers in face; cancer and cancerous ulcers after contusions, burning stitches; stinging in affected parts.
- Crotalus horridus - cancer of the tongue with great haemorrhagic tendency; putrid sore mouth with bloody salivation; cancer of stomach, much haemorrhage or much vomiting of mucus, slimy or bloody, with distressing sensation of sinking, and craving for stimulants; cancer uteri, fungoid, malignant sarcoma, cauliflower excrescence, with much tendency to haemorrhage; weak, debilitated constitutions.
- Crotalus horridus (Haematuria, haemorrhage from urinary organs) haematuria with cancer of bladder or prostate; haemorrhage from urethra; blood degeneration (Lach.), as in adynamic diseases.
- Crotalus horridus (Uterus complaints) - cancer; fungoid, malignant sarcoma; cauliflower excrescence, with haemorrhagic tendency; very degraded state in patient.
- Curare (Uterus complaints) - lips thick and full of scirrhous tubercles; sores healing very slowly and passing easily into gangrene; malignant ulcers in different parts of body; corroding, cancerous ulcers; smarting in vulva and thighs; shooting and digging pains in womb; swelling of rectum and anus; very sensitive haemorrhoidal fissures; anxious and despairing expression.
- Fuligo ligni - chronic irritations of mucous membranes of mouth; pruritus-vulvae; uterine haemorrhage; cancer, especially of scrotum-chimney sweeper's cancer; epithelial cancers; cancer of womb with metrorrhagia; sadness, thoughts of suicide.

Graphites (Uterus complaints) - cancer of womb, with warmth and painfulness of vagina, engorgement of lymphatic vessels and mucous follicles, hardness of neck of womb, which is swollen and covered with fungous excrescences; heaviness of abdomen, with exacerbation of pains and fainting while standing; stitches through thighs and hypogastrium, like electric shocks; retarded and painful menses, with discharge of black, coagulated and foetid blood, constipation, earthy complexion, sadness and restlessness. Tumor, size of an orange, in right and left iliac fossa, hard, round, slightly movable, not painful to pressure, only producing inconvenience from weight; os uteri standing backward, can only be reached with difficulty; pain in uterus when reaching high with arms; bearing-down pains in uterus to back, with weakness and sickness; vagina cold; cicatrical tissue easily cracks and bleeds.

Hepar-sulph. - corrosive pain in a cancerous ulcer, bleeding at the slightest touch; yellow skin and complexion; eruptions around the mouth, lips and chin, which are converted into cancerous ulcers, rapidly spreading; pressure and dull aching pain in the stomach after moderate eating; cancerous ulcer of the mamma, with stinging burning in the edges; pus, copious or scanty, smells like old cheese.

Iodum - uterine haemorrhage at every stool, with cutting in the abdomen and pains in the loins and small of the back; great weakness during the menses, particularly in going up stairs; long-lasting uterine haemorrhage; dwindling and falling away of the mammae; aggravation from external warmth; complete prostration of strength and general emaciation; violent vomiting, renewed by eating; pulsations in pit of the stomach; cancer uteri; leucorrhoea yellow and corrosive.

Iodum (Uterus complaints) - induration and swelling of uterus and ovaries; dropsical affection of ovaries, with pressing down towards genitals; cancerous degeneration of neck of uterus; acrid leucorrhoea, corroding the limbs, < at time of menses; uterine haemorrhage, renewed at every stool; numb feeling in thighs and legs; emaciation, hectic fever, canine hunger or no appetite; constipation or looseness of bowels; emaciation.

Kali-iod. - ulcers: vegetations bleed easily and are unhealthy; canceroid; deep; involving bone structure.

Kreosotum - haemorrhages, ulcerations, cancerous affections.

Lachesis - melanotic, colloid and encephalotic cancer; ulcers sensitive to touch, with ichorous, offensive discharge; blood dark, non-coagulable; violent burning, gangrenous spots; cancer of lower lip, dry, cracked, bleeding; cancer of stomach, the pit very sensitive to touch, with a gnawing pressure, > by eating, but coming on again in a few hours, and the more violent the emptier the stomach; cancer of the breast with lancinating pains and a constant painful feeling of weakness and lameness in left shoulder and arm; open cancer has a dark, bluish-red appearance, with blackish streaks of decomposed blood; uterine cancer developing itself at climaxis; pains increase rapidly until relieved by a profuse discharge of blood; violent pains as if a knife were thrust through abdomen, which has to be relieved from all pressure; coughing or sneezing causes stitches in affected parts.

Merc-sol. - ulcerations: very superficial and widespread; with whitish grey bases, bleeding easily and exuding thin matter; spreading, spongy, readily bleeding and extremely painful; unequal elevations and depressions in floor of ulcer; cancerous, with severe shooting, lancinating pain, not > by either hot or cold applications; fungous, chancrous, phagedenic, carious and syphilitic.

Phosphorus - epigastric region sensitive to touch; constant nausea and fullness in the stomach; after eating, or drinking even a swallow of water, vomiting of a sour, foul-smelling fluid, looking like a mixture of water, ink and coffee-grounds; cutting pains through abdomen, < by pressure and motion; a circumscribed hard swelling in the sunken abdomen; belching up of large quantities of wind after dinner; fine gurgling noise in abdomen; haematemesis; pale, earthy complexion, emaciation. cancer of womb with frequent and profuse flooding, pouring out freely and then ceasing for a short time; heat in back; chlorotic appearance; cancer of breast, when ulcer bleeds easily very vascular encephaloma.

Phosphorus (Tumors) - open cancers, bleeding profusely; polypi bleeding readily on slight provocation; lipoma; encephaloma; colloid cancer; condylomata of large size, rough and dry, filling the vagina; painfulness of stomach to touch, and when walking; worse after eating anything warm; pus thin, ichorous; hectic, desires to be magnetized; lymphoma on neck with hectic fever.

Sepia - suspicious tubercle on lip of a cartilaginous appearance, sometimes bleeding and having a scirrhous appearance, with a broad base; epithelial cancer of lower lip, with a burning pain and a pricking as from a splinter of wood; complexion yellow and earthy; cancer of rectum; indurations, ulcerations and congestion of the os and cervix uteri; cutting pains in abdomen and a pressure on uterus downward as if everything would fall out; sinking sensation at pit of stomach.

Strychnos gaultheriana - removes fetor and haemorrhage in cancer, revives the healing process.

Thlaspi bursa pastoris (Haemorrhage from uterus) - haemorrhage with severe uterine colic, with clots of blood, following miscarriage.

Sterility, Infertility

(The causes of sterility are varied. If cause is known removal of that cause would cure the patient. For example, we do not find the remedy Thuja in this list. It does not mean this remedy is not useful for sterility. We have cured several cases of sterility caused by ovarian cyst with Thuja).

Sterility: Agn., Amm., Bor., Calc., Cann., Croc., Caust., Cic., Con., Dulc., Fer., Graph., Hyosc., Merc., Natr-carb. and M., Phos., Plat., Ruta, Sulph., Sulph-ac.

Agnus castus - sterility.

Agnus castus (Hysteria) - despairing sadness, peevish, inclined to be angry, sometimes on account of her sterility.

Aletris (Chlorosis) - sterility from uterine atony.

Aletris (Hysteria) - sterility, amenorrhoea or delayed menses from uterine atony, abdomen distended, bearing down.

Aletris (Uterus complaints) - sterility from uterine atony.

Aurum met. - great depression of spirits, accompanied by sterility.

Aurum met. (Sexual complaints) - sterility from lowered vitality of the parts with great mental depression.

Aurum met. - sterility; vaginismus.

Baryta-mur. (Ovaries, diseases of) - sterility.

Borax (Leucorrhoea) - sterility.

Sterility, Infertility

Borax (Menses complaints) - after: gastralgia, stitches in uterus dysmenorrhoea with sterility.

Borax - sterility.

Calcarea carb - sterility with copious menses.

Calc-carb. (Hysteria) - sterility.

Cannabis indica - sterility.

Cannabis sat (Nymphomania) - increased sexual desire with sterility.

Cantharis (Ovaries, diseases of) - sterility.

Conium (Ovaries, diseases of) - atrophy of ovaries with sterility

Conium (Uterus complaints) - ovarian depression, with scanty menstruation and sterility.

Eupatorium purp. - impotency and sterility.

Ferr-met. (Amenorrhoea) - sterility, nervousness and debility.

Ferr-met. (Haemorrhage from uterus) - sterility.

Helonias (Amenorrhoea) - loss of sexual desire, with or without sterility.

Helonias (Chlorosis) loss of sexual desire and power, with or without sterility.

Helonias (Menses complaints) - loss of sexual desire with or without sterility.

Helonias (Ovaries, diseases of) - atony of sexual organs and loss of all sexual desire with or without sterility.

Helonias (Sexual complaints) - impotence. in women, loss of sexual desire and power, with sterility.

Iodum (Ovaries, diseases of) - atrophy with sterility (Con.).

Iodum (Sexual complaints) - atrophy of ovaries and mammae, with sterility.

Medorrhinum - sterility.

Millefolium (Haemorrhage from uterus) - sterility with too profuse menstruation.

Millefolium (Menses complaints) - sterility from profuse menstruation.

Natrum phos. - sterility, with acid secretions from vagina.

Natrum carb. (Menses complaints) - sterility from discharge of mucus from vagina after an embrace.

Natrum carb. (Sexual complaints) - discharge of mucus from vagina after an embrace, causing sterility.

Natrum carb. (Vaginismus) - discharge of mucus from vagina after an embrace, causing sterility.

Natrum mur. (Sexual complaints) - sterility, with too early and too profuse menstruation, or too late and scanty.

Natrum mur. (Uterus complaints) - sterility, with too early and too profuse menstruation.

Natrum phos. (Menses complaints) - sterility, with acid secretions from vagina.

Nux moschata (Sexual complaints) - sterility.

Phosphorus (Menses complaints) - aversion to sexual intercourse, or excessive voluptuousness with sterility.

Phosphorus (Uterus complaints) - sterility from excessive voluptuousness, or with profuse and too late menses.

Platina - woman, aged 32, married twelve years, under old school treatment was cured of hypertrophy and ulceration of cervix; suspected ovarian disease and sterility.

Platina - ovaritis with sterility.

Plumbum met. (Ovaries, diseases of) - atrophy and sterility.

Sepia - woman, aged 38, tall, slim, dark hair and eyes, bilionervous temperament, married fourteen years, has never conceived; sterility.

Sulphur (Sexual complaints) - sterility, with too early and too profuse catamenia.

Sulphur (Uterus complaints) - sterility with too early and profuse menses

Viburnum op. (Miscarriage, abortion) - frequent and very early miscarriages, so that the ovum is expelled at every menstrual period, thus causing sterility.

Viburnum ops - frequent and very early miscarriage causing seeming sterility.

X-ray - sterility.

Diseases accompanied by 'Sterility':

(Amenorrhoea) Ferr-met. - sterility, nervousness and debility

(Amenorrhoea) Helonias - loss of sexual desire, with or without sterility.

(Chlorosis) Aletris - sterility from uterine atony.

(Chlorosis) Helonias - loss of sexual desire and power, with or without sterility.

(Haemorrhage from uterus) Ferr-met. - sterility.

(Haemorrhage from uterus) Millefolium - sterility with too profuse menstruation.

(Hysteria) Agnus castus - despairing sadness, peevish, inclined to be angry, sometimes on account of her sterility.

(Hysteria) Aletris - sterility, amenorrhoea or delayed menses from uterine atony, abdomen distended, bearing down.

(Hysteria) Calc-carb. - sterility.

(Leucorrhoea) Borax - sterility.

(Menses complaints) Borax - after: gastralgia, stitches in uterus. dysmenorrhoea with sterility.

(Menses complaints) Helonias - loss of sexual desire with or without sterility.

(Menses complaints) Millefolium - sterility from profuse menstruation.

(Menses complaints) Natrum carb. - sterility from discharge of mucus from vagina after an embrace.

(Menses complaints) Natrum phos. - sterility, with acid secretions from vagina.

(Menses complaints) Phosphorus - aversion to sexual intercourse, or excessive voluptuousness with sterility.

(Miscarriage, abortion) Viburnum op. - frequent and very early miscarriages, so that the ovum is expelled at every menstrual period, thus causing sterility.

(Nymphomania) Cannabis sat. - increased sexual desire with sterility.

(Ovaries, diseases of) Baryta-mur. - sterility.

(Ovaries, diseases of) Cantharis - sterility.

(Ovaries, diseases of) Conium - atrophy of ovaries with sterility.

(Ovaries, diseases of) Helonias - atony of sexual organs and loss of all sexual desire with or without sterility.

(Ovaries, diseases of) Iodum - atrophy with sterility (Con.).

(Ovaries, diseases of) Phosphorus - sterility from excessive voluptuousness.

(Ovaries, diseases of) Plumbum-met. - atrophy and sterility.

(Sexual complaints) Aurum-met. - sterility from lowered vitality of the parts with great mental depression.

(Sexual complaints) Helonias - impotence. in women, loss of sexual desire and power, with sterility.

Sterility, Infertility

(Sexual complaints) Iodum - atrophy of ovaries and mammae, with sterility.

(Sexual complaints) Natrum carb. - discharge of mucus from vagina after an embrace, causing sterility.

(Sexual complaints) Natrum mur. - sterility, with too early and too profuse menstruation, or too late and scanty.

(Sexual complaints) Nux moschata - sterility.

(Sexual complaints) Phosphorus - sterility.

(Sexual complaints) Sulphur - sterility, with too early and too profuse catamenia.

(Uterus complaints) Aletris - sterility from uterine atony.

(Uterus complaints) Conium - ovarian depression, with scanty menstruation and sterility.

(Uterus complaints) Natrum mur. - sterility, with too early and too profuse menstruation.

(Uterus complaints) Phosphorus - sterility from excessive voluptuousness, or with profuse and too late menses.

(Uterus complaints) Sulphur - sterility with too early and profuse menses.

(Vaginismus) Natrum carb. - discharge of mucus from vagina after an embrace, causing sterility.

Gout—Retrocedent, Metastatic, Constitutional

In the treatment of chronic diseases, we must keep in mind the following:

When a patient has any one or more of the following: diabetes, heart complaints, lesions, insanity, still birth/abortion, allergy migraine, suicidal disposition, running away from home, never to return, etc. we may consider the remedies under 'syphilis' in the chapter GENERALITIES in Kent's Repertory.

When a patient has any one or more of the following: chronic affections of glands (tonsillitis, thyroid, tuberculosis (phthisis pulmonum) or bone affections, such as spondylitis we must consider 'scrofula'.

(Note: boring pains in bones at night is again syphilis.)

Note: If thyroid complaints are in more than one member in the family, it is both scrofula and syphilis. (Scrofulosis from hereditary syphilis) The remedy for this is Nit-ac. etc.

Now, let us learn about 'gout'. In Boericke's Repertory (page 875) we find the terms 'gout of eyes' 'gout of stomach' 'metastatic gout to heart' etc. etc.

(Metastasis = a change in the seat of a disease. The transfer of a disease from one part of the body to another, through the blood vessels, via lymph channels or across the body cavities. E.g., Septic infection may arise in other organs from some original focus. E.g. arthritis caused by decayed teeth.)

With a family history of tuberculosis (of lungs or bones) in the following generation it causes chronic affections of glands or bones and the term for this is 'scrofula'. So also, with a family history of gout, in the following generations it may affect mainly stomach, eye, chest, heart, nerve throat or uterus.

In very difficult cases of chronic affections of stomach, heart, chest, nerve, throat or uterus you may ask whether in the family* (*'family' means patients brothers/sisters, their children, the patient's parents and their brothers/sisters and their children, then grand parents and their brothers/sisters and their children and so on.) whether there was any one of the following complaints:

1. Gout;
2. Chronic colic or abdominal complaints;
3. Loss of vision that defied treatment of best doctors.

If the reply of the patient is in the affirmative you may make use of this chapter. Let us repeat, despite your best efforts to find the remedy if you are not able to cure any complaint in chest, heart, eye, abdomen, nerve, throat or uterus you may suspect gout and so make use of this chapter.

Debility after attack—Bellis., Cyprip.

Gout of chest—Colch.

Gout of eyes—Nux-v.

Gout of hands, feet, little swelling, subacute—Led.

Gout of heart—Aur., Mur., Cact., Conv., Cupr-m., Kal.

Gout of nerves (neuralgia)—Colch., Col., Sul.,

Gout of stomach—Hydroc-ac., Nux-m., Nux-v., Puls.

Gout of throat—Colch., Merc-s., Melastases to heart—Colch., Kal. Metastases to stomach—Ant-c.,

Nux-v. Nervous restlesness—Ign. Retrocedent or suppressed—Cajup., Nat-m., Ox-ac., Rhus-t. Sub-acute—Gualac., Led., Puls. Uterine disorders—Sab. Suppressed gout: Colch., Lith., Natr.-phos.,— if to the heart; Ant-crud., Lyc., if to the stomach.

Gout affecting the head or eyes: 1, Bry., Coloc., Ipec., Kali-iod., Nux-v.; 2, Colch., Lyc., Rhus, Sep., Staph., Sulph.

Gout affecting the head and ears: Fer.-pic.

Gout affecting the heart: Abrot., Ars., Benz-ac., Colch., Kalm., Lith., Phos.

Gout affecting the kidneys: 1, Benz-ac., Berb., Kali-iod (contracted kidney), Lyc., Sarsap., Sulph.; 2, Ars., Colch., Plumb., Phos., Tereb., Zinc.

Epilepsy: in gouty patients: Bry., Colch., Kali-iod., Lyc., Natr-salicyl. Back pain–spinal irritation - pains in back from rheumatism and gout: Acon., Ant-tart., Calc-phos., Colch., Gels., Guaiac., Hep., Hydr., Kali-bi., Kali-carb., Kalm., Merc., Puls., Rhus.

Gout affecting the stomach and abdomen: Ant-crud., Bry., Ars., Coloc,. Lyc., Nux-m., Nux-v., Sulph. Migraine (headache) Sick-headache: - gouty hemicrania: Colch., Coloc., Guaic., Kali-bi., Lyc., Magn-mur., Natr-m.

Gout — amblyopia, from metastasis: Puls. — alternates with asthma: Sulph. — old atomic: Form., Ter. — with irritable bladder: Nux-v. — with morbus Brightii: Kali-i. — arthritic deposits: Aur. — calcareous deposits, with painful spasmodic jerking of legs: Meny. — with chronic catarrh: Kali-c. — disposition to formation of chalkstones: Coff-t. — chronic: Aur-m-n., Form. — during chronic form acute paroxysms set in: Colch. — chronic, without fever: Ant-c. — chronic, rheumatic: Lyc.

— during climacteric period: Sal-ac. — concretions: Benz-ac. — with contractions: Bry., Calc., Caust., Coloc., Guaj., Rhus-t., Sil., Sulph., Thuj. — disposition to: Sep.

— from eating rich food: Ant-c., Calc., Iod., Nux-v., Puls., Sulph. — with fibrous exudation in great toe joint: Rhod. — with slight fever and great debility: Indg.

— suppressed, causes gastralgia: Abrot.

— with gleet: Mez.

— disturbing general health: Amm-c.

— incipient, in drunkards: Nux-v.

— with inflammation and swelling: Bell.

— after acute inflammatory conditions: Carbn-s.

— lame-like pain, now in shoulder and elbow joint, now in hip and knee, worse in warm room, better in open air, generallly in one side of body, worse on right: Sabin.

— lies upon back with bent knees: Kali-i.

— attacking many joints: Colch.

— metastasis: Acon., Bell., Nux-v., Sars., Sulph.

— metastasis, in gastric catarrh: Ant-c.

— metastasis, to intestines or stomach: Cinnm.

— worse from motion, heat of bed and evenings: Led.

— affections of nerve branches: Chel.

— thin fluid, profuse discharge from nose: Rhod.

— gouty pains: Anag., Caust.

— severe paroxysms: Hydrc.

— rheumatic: Rhus-t.

— rheumatic, in corpulent men, advanced in life: Staph.

— worse after sleep: Ant-s-aur.

— deposits cause stiffness: Caust.

— with stiffness and swelling of hands and feet: Colch.

— retrocession to stomach: Nux-m.

— with sweats: Merc.

— with swelling: Puls.

— with or without swelling: Sulph.

— shining red swelling: Merc.

— swelling not of long standing: Carbn-s.

— tearing and stitching with contractions of parts: Guaj.

— with tension, worse from contact and motion: Bry.

— fluid in great toe joint, or with lithates: Am-be.

— wandering: Arn., Cinnb., Mang-c., Nux-m., Nux-v., Puls.

Remedies for gout

Abrotanum - after suppressed gout —gastralgia.

Abrotanum - compare : scrophularia; bryonia; stellaria; benzoic acid, in gout.

Abrotanum - ill effects of suppressed conditions especially in gouty subjects.

Abrotanum (Arthritis, gout) - chronic arthritis. gouty deposits about finger-joints, < during cold, stormy weather, painful, sore and hot at that time; metastasis to heart; piercing pain in heart; high fever; emaciation, though appetite is good.

Abrotanum (Arthritis, gout) - painful and inflamed wrist and ankle-joints, stiff, with pricking sensation; ailments after suppressed gout. (See also *Urtica Urens*.)

Abrotanum (Gastralgia) - gnawing hunger; craves bread boiled in milk; appetite sometimes ravenous while emaciating; burning in stomach as from acidity; sensation as if the stomach were hanging or swimming in water, with a peculiar feeling of coldness and a dullness to all irritants; pains cutting, gnawing, burning, sometimes contracting and stinging, mostly < at night; never entirely free from pain, even in the intervals of the spasms; constipation; haemorrhoids; gastralgia after suppressed gout.

Abrotanum (Heart diseases) - metastasis of gout or rheumatism to heart; endocarditis with piercing pains across chest, < in cardiac region; dyspnoea, profuse sweat; sinking as if dying, feeble pulse.

Aesculus hip (Bronchitis chronica) - bronchitis complicated with gouty diathesis and a tendency to piles with constipation; rapid, labored breathing with pain in right lung.

Agnus-c. - gouty nodosities.

Alumina (Paralysis) - locomotor ataxia; inability to walk except when the eyes are open and in daylight; loss of sensibility of feet; numbness of heel when stepping; tearing in thighs and legs when sitting or lying, < at night; pain in sole of foot on stepping, as if it were too soft and swollen; drawing pains in extremities; rheumatic and traumatic paralysis in gouty patients; palsy from spinal disease; arms feel heavy and go to sleep; lower limbs heavy, can scarcely drag them; feeling of weakness in bladder and genitals; bowels inactive; mistakes in speaking; consciousness of his identity confused; strength all exhausted after walking in fresh air, with yawning, stretching, drowsiness and inclination to lie down, which only increases the lassitude.

Ammoniacum - gout not developing in usual form of attacks, but disturbing general health.

Ammoniacum (Bronchitis chronica) - bronchorrhoea respiration short, quick, with anguish, especially at night; oppression and obstruction in the chest from the accumulation of mucus; stitches in the left side of the chest when taking a deep inspiration; tickling in throat without cough; frontal headache, dimness of sight; in rheumatic or gouty subjects.

Ammonium benz. - gout, with deposits in joints; - One of the remedies for albuminuria, especially in the gouty.

Ammonium phos. - a remedy for chronic gouty patients uric acid diathesis, indicated in bronchitis and nodosities of the joints of the fingers and backs of the hands.

Amm-phos. (Bronchitis chronica) - bronchitis chronica arthritica when patients suffering from gout or rheumarthritis are attacked with bronchial catarrhs or bronchitis.

Anantherum (Sciatica) - sciatic, gouty and rheumatic pains in legs and feet, especially in heels; stiffness, lancinating and crampy pains in sacrum and iliac bones; offensive foot-sweat.

Anthrokokali - chronic rheumatism, gout, caries, scrofulosis.

Ant-crud. - acute gout having left deposits, with gastric symptoms; inveterate (chronic) gout without fever; - metastasis of gout and rheumatism causing gastric catarrh; - rheumatism and gout if parts are inflamed or swollen.

Ant-crud. (Dyspepsia, weakness of stomach) - overloading the stomach and gastric derangement in children, women and old people; thickly coated white tongue, with anorexia, slow digestion and foetid eructations, often followed by diarrhoea, particularly after acid wines or new beer; habitual sensation in stomach as if overloaded, excessive crossness, even hypochondriasis with suicidal tendencies; dryness of mouth with great thirst, < at night; constipation alternating with diarrhoea; helminthiasis; caused by overeating, hot weather, bathing, during measles; metastasis of gout and rheumatism.

Ant-crud. (Rheumatism) - acute and chronic rheumatism or gout; pains drawing, shooting, tensive; shortening of the muscles and tendons with bending of limbs and great tenderness and soreness of soles of feet, < by warm air and heat of sun; gastric symptoms, nausea, vomiting, white tongue, great thirst at night.

Ant-crud. - gout with gastric symptoms.

Ant-crud. - gouty metastasis to stomach and bowels.

Ant-tart. - gastric affections of drunkards and gouty subjects.

Apis - gout; gouty nodes.

Apis - rheumatism and gout.

Apoc-andr. (Rheumatism) - rheumatism and gout; pain especially in right shoulder and knee; pains in the joint of the big toe; bilious vomiting, with or without diarrhoea; pain and stiffness in back of head and neck; dull heavy pain in chest, while breathing; rheumatic headaches; worse after sleep or continued quiet; joints feel stiff, especially on moving in the morning.

Arbutus andrachne - a remedy for eczema associated with gouty and rheumatic symptoms.

Arnica - fears being struck by those coming towards him; fears even the possibility of being touched —gout.

Arnica - gout and rheumatism.

Asimina - gout of drinking people.

Asparagus off. (Dropsy) - old people with heart disease; weak action of heart; when urinating the last drops, constricting pain in cardiac region, turns blue in face, urine has an unpleasant odor; must sit up in bed to relieve dyspnoea. hydrothorax in senility on a gouty diathesis.

Asparagus off. (Heart diseases) - cardiac affections of the aged, with weak pulse and pain about left acromion, heart's stroke twofold, irregular, quickened; disinclination to any work and languor. hydrothorax with heart disease or gouty diathesis of old people.

Aurum mur natronatum - old cases of rheumatism and gouty pains.

Baptisia - he thinks his gouty legs are holding a conversation with each other; a man, aged 60 —gout.

Baptisia - he thinks his toe is holding a confab with his gouty thumb.

Belladonna - rheumatic and gouty complaints, with inflammation and swelling.

Belladonna (Headache) - congestion of blood to head, with danger of apoplexy; gouty and hysterical headaches; throbbing pains, especially on right side, with intolerance of light and noise; hot head and cold feet, not relieved by lying down, but by sitting propped up, > by holding head in the opposite direction to the part of head affected; sensation as if the brain were pressed to the forehead, disappearing quickly on bending the head backward; in walking feels as if with every step brain rose and fell in forehead; soreness in forehead, stiffness in occiput, eyeballs feel as if starting from their sockets; stabbing as with a knife, from one temple to the other; violent pressing in whole head, from within outward, as if it would burst; pains come suddenly, last indefinitely, but cease suddenly; intense headache makes him first blind, then unconscious; sun-headache; headaches < when leaning forward, from warmth, > during menses, from pressure, tight bandaging and wrapping up; headache from abuse of coffee, from overheating and from cold.

Bellis perennis - after gout, debility of limbs.

Benzoic-acid. - gout with arthritic nodosities.

Benzoic-acid. - gouty diathesis; arthritis vaga.

Benzoic-acid. (Arthritis, gout) - tearing in joints with nearly clear urine; old nodes become painful, and as the pains abate palpitation sets in, ceasing only when pains increase; gout going from left to right or commencing in right great toe; urine of offensive odor, depositing a reddish cloudy sediment. chronic rheumarthritis, wandering pains (Puls.).

Benzoic-acid. (Bone diseases, osteitis, periostitis, exostosis, caries, necrosis, etc.) - swelling and cracking of knee-joint; gouty deposits between metacarpal bones; tearing pain in anterior surface of thigh; ulcerative pain in whole leg.

Benzoic-acid. (Heart diseases) - gout or rheumatism affecting the heart and nodular swellings in the joints; pains change place incessantly, but are more constant about heart; awakens after midnight with violent palpitation of heart and temporal arteries; at times tearing rheumatic pains in extremities relieve the heart; palpitation and trembling while sitting, < after drinking, at night; undulating or intermitting beats of heart; dysuria senilis; urine dark and of an offensive odor.

Benzoic-acid. (Kidney/bladder stone) - nephritic colic; morbid condition of urine in persons with calculous or gouty diathesis; urine containing urates of ammonia and having a strong ammoniacal smell. dysuria senilis from irritability of the bladder and mucopurulent discharge.

Benzoic-acid. (Rheumatism) - arthritis deformans; painful nodes in joints, especially in syphilitic or gonorrhoeal patients, with rheumatic diathesis; pains go from right to left side and from below upward; < from heat and joints cracking on motion; gout or rheumatism affecting heart or alternating one with the other; wandering pains, but most constant about heart; irritable bladder, freshly voided urine of strong ammoniacal smell and highly colored.

Benzoic-acid. (Urinary difficulties) - vesicular catarrh; irritability of the bladder; nocturnal enuresis in children; too frequent desire to evacuate the bladder, urine being normal; decrease of the quantity of urine, which is thick and bloody; urine has strong odor like that of horses and contains excess of hippuric acid (Nitr-ac.); urine brownish, cloudy, alkaline or dark-reddish, high specific gravity and acid reaction, sometimes of a putrid, cadaverous smell; morbid condition of urine, as in persons with calculous or gouty diathesis; dysuria senilis, when gravel is trifling and the irritable state of bladder and pains are induced by other causes, with too frequent desire to urinate, though urine appears normal.

Benzoic-acid. - gouty and asthmatic.

Benzoic-acid. - gouty deposits.

Benzoic-acid. - it produces and cures symptoms of a uric acid diathesis, with urine highly colored and very offensive, and gouty symptoms.

Benzoic-acid. - rheumatic gout; nodes very painful.

Benzoic-acid. - useful after colchic. fails in gout; after copavia in gonorrhoea.

Berberis vul. - rheumatic and gouty complaints, with diseases of urinary organs.

Berberis vul. (Albuminuria) - gouty or rheumatic diathesis; burning in back; urine of dark, bloody appearance and largely supplied with Alben; tough mucus in mouth and throat; constant nausea and loss of sleep; frequent palpitation, slow, weak pulse; painful pressure and tension in the lumbar and renal regions, with sensation of numbness, puffiness, warmth, stiffness and lameness, extending at times into the lower limbs, especially indicated in persons addicted to the use of alcoholic beverages.

Berberis vul. - old gouty constitutions.

Berberis vul. - tearing pain in auricle, and gouty concretions.

Bryonia - gouty, red, shining swelling of single parts, with stinging when moving them.

Bryonia (Paralysis) - paralysis, generally of both sides, in rheumatic and gouty patients; < from motion and contact; legs so weak they will scarcely hold him, knees totter and knock together when walking.

Cajuputum - retrocedent gout.

Calcarea fluor. - diarrhoea in gouty subjects.

Calcarea fluor. - gouty enlargements of the joints of the fingers.

Calc-carb. - a widow, aged 40, large figure, round form, brown hair, blue eyes, white and delicate skin, constantly red cheeks, irritable —gout.

Calc-carb. - gouty people.

Calc-carb. (Rheumatism) - is the chronic rhus, and often comes in where the latter fails. rheumatism from working in water or by a long continuance in it; chronic cases with swelling of joints, < with every change of weather; crackling or crepitation of joints, as if they were dry; weakness and weariness of all the limbs; sensation of coldness on top of head; profuse sweat and cold, damp feet; omodynia in right shoulder or from left shoulder down left arm towards the heart; lumbago; cold feeling in various points, as gluteal region; pains confined to small spots; gouty nodosities about fingers; arthritis nodosa deformans.

Calc-phos. - a constituent of teeth, bones, connective tissue and blood corpuscles, and to be given in corresponding disturbances,; in true chlorosis from anemia; chronic swelling of glands; chronic articular rheumatism; gout; exostoses, osteophytes and similar new growths on bone;

scrofulosis; suppuration of bones and joints; dropsy from loss of blood or of other fluids, or depending on diseases of heart, liver and kidneys.

Calc-phos. - gouty constitutions: catarrh; pains; skin diseases.

Capsicum - gout, stiffness, painfulness and cracking of joints.

Carbon-sul. - gout, but not gouty dyscrasia.

Carbon-sul. - gouty swellings when not of too long standing.

Carbon-sul. - rheumatism and gout; after the relief of acute and inflammatory conditions.

Carlsbad - famous for its action on the liver and in the treatment of obesity, diabetes, and gout.

Causticum (Headache) - torpid gout (Colch., gout in vigorous constitutions); constant succession of shocks and jerks through the head.

Causticum (Syphilis and sycosis) - vesicles under prepuce changing into suppurating ulcers; phagedenic chancre; watery, greenish, corroding discharge with jerking pains; chancre with fungous excrescences; buboes secreting an acrid, corrosive ichor, with systemic complications, such as scurvy or gout.

Chamomilla - incipient gout; gouty ophthalmia.

Chelidonium - in rheumatic and gouty affections of single joints or nerve branches, with frequent headache, attacks of vertigo, dimness of vision.

China (Rheumatism) - later stages of inflammatory rheumatism, when the fever has become intermittent in its character, joints still swollen; jerking and pressing pains, excited by merely moving the affected part and gradually rising to a most fearful state, < at night and accompanied by a sensation of weakness in affected parts, < by contact more than by motion; rheumatic pains in metatarsal bones and phalanges; rheumatic gout.

China - chronic gout.

Chininum sulph. - polyarticular gout.

Chloralum - rheumatism and gout.

Cinnabaris - wandering gout.

Clematis - rheumatic and gouty affections of joints; catarrhal and rheumatic affections of bladder; rheumatic affections of eyes and ears.

Cocculus - gouty pains or cracking in joints.

Cochlearia - gout; also in suppression, followed by colic and retention of urine (used in footh bath).

Colchicum - cachectic appearance —dysentery —gout.

Colchicum - gout attacking many joints; muscular pains like torticollis; lumbago; tearing pains in joints; pains in all bones.

Colchicum - gout in persons of vigorous constitution.

Colchicum - it hastens relapses of gout if abused.

Colchicum - mind depressed —dropsy —gout.

Colchicum - vesical irritability depending upon gouty diathesis.

Colchicum - when during chronic form of gout acute paroxysms set in, also in metastasis to heart.

Colchicum - woman, aged 22, of dissipated habits, and mother of three illegitimate children; gout.

Colchicum (Albuminuria) - first stage; flatulent distention of stomach; stools watery, jellylike, mucous or bloody, and mingled with a stringy substance; gouty pains in joints; urine dark and scanty, discharged in drops and depositing a whitish sediment; urine as black as ink, containing blood, and loaded with alben and tube-casts, smoky in appearance; pericarditis rheumatica with violent cutting, stinging pain in chest, with great oppression and dyspnoea; sensation as if the chest or heart were squeezed by a tight bandage; relapses from taking cold in damp weather or from suppressed perspiration; patient cannot stand up straight or lie down with stretched-out legs without causing pain in renal region and vomiting, especially in albuminuria of pregnancy.

Colchicum (Arthritis, gout) - gout attacking many joints; shifting from one to another, with burning and tearing pains, < from any external impression, noise, odor, touch or bright light. the joint becomes inflamed, dark red, hot and intensely painful, patient nearly beside himself with agony; oedema and coldness of legs and feet, with weariness, heaviness and inability to move; urine acid, dark and scanty; even the smell of food nauseates; frequent, ineffectual inclination to sneeze on waking in the morning; uric acid diathesis; gout in persons of vigorous constitution.

Colchicum (Asthma) - oppression of chest, dyspnoea, tensive feeling in chest, high up or low down; with anxiety, > by bending forward; extreme anxiety of face; cheeks, lips and eyelids purple; anxious feeling in praecordia; flatulency and meteorism; rheumatic gout.

Colchicum (Cystitis, inflammation of bladder) - vesical irritability depending upon a gouty diathesis; strangury with haemorrhage from bladder; micturition accompanied and followed by tenesmus of bladder and burning pain in urethra; as if urine were hot.

Colchicum (Diaphragm, diseases of) - similar to Bry.; gouty diathesis; albuminosis; uneasiness at epigastrium, extremely sensitive to touch and pressure; pain in epigastrium as if pierced with a knife; violent vomiting accompanied by intense straining and loud, hollow belching, > by bending himself up and lying quiet; limbs cold, hands and feet cold.

Colchicum (Dropsy) - dropsy after scarlatina, with suppression of urine, or urine black, containing alben and destroyed blood-corpuscles; acute dropsy with renal affections, constant urging to urinate, but only a little is voided and that with great pain, as from spasm in the bladder. dropsy of cavities and internal organs, especially hydropericardium, hydrothorax, hydrometra, ascites. lower limbs oedematous and cold; skin dry and pale; emaciated sensitive persons, disposed to rheumatism and catarrh, always < when it is damp, in spring and fall; gout with nervous weakness and oversensitiveness.

Colchicum (Dyspepsia, weakness of stomach) - appetite for different things, but as soon as he sees them or still more smells them, he shudders from nausea and is unable to eat anything (Cocc., extreme aversion to food, even the smell of food nauseates, although feeling hungry); the smell of fish, eggs or fat meat makes him faint; frequent copious eructations of tasteless gas; on assuming an upright position qualmishness in stomach and inclination to vomit; violent retching, followed by copious and forcible vomiting of food and then of bile, renewed by every motion; burning sensation in stomach more frequently than an icy coldness, accompanied by great pains and debility. (retrocession of gout.)

Colchicum (Headache) - gout in vigorous constitutions (caust., torpid gout); grinding, boring, arthritic headache, usually parietal or occipital; tearing, drawing, pressing headache, often semilateral; severe pressing pain deep in the substance of the cerebellum from the slightest intellectual exertion, especially in overtaxed brains; as soon as he loses any rest, as by night-watching, he becomes mentally tired and suffers with headache, nausea, bitter taste, becomes irritable and intolerant even to slight pain; painful drawing, tearing, beginning in one eyeball and extending to occiput, < by motion or jar, > by physical rest, from warmth, after supper; frequent ineffectual inclination to sneeze on waking in the morning.

Colchicum (Insanity) - gouty diathesis; alternately excited or depressed; loss of memory; great desire for mental and bodily rest; intense melancholia, peevish and dissatisfied.

Colchicum (Iris, affections of) - gouty or rheumatic iritis, with great soreness of eyeballs; violent, short, sharp, tearing pain in and around eyeball; excoriating lachrymation, < in open air.

Colchicum (Nephritis) - nephritis with bloody, ink-like, albuminous urine, pain in renal region; urine turbid; leaves an orange-colored ring on vessel; after scarlatina or from gouty troubles.

Colchicum (Pericarditis) - violent palpitations with anxiety, and sensation as if chest were squeezed by a tight bandage; vertigo on assuming upright position; palpitation and stitches about heart, loss of consciousness. effusion into pericardium, with heart's action muffled, indistinct, very weak; pulse threadlike, imperceptible-following gout or acute rheumatism; sharp, rending pains along sternum and into left shoulder; distressing restlessness and sleeplessness; hot, dry skin, vomiting and purging, with coated tongue and thirst.

Colchicum (Tympanitis) - great distention of abdomen with gas, as if he had eaten too much, contracts spasmodically when touched, > from bending double; metastasis of gout.

Colchicum (Urinary difficulties) - constant burning in urinary organs, with diminished secretion; passing of urine attended and followed by tenesmus of bladder and burning pain in urethra as if urine were very warm; frequent micturition with diminished discharge; urethra hurts while urine passes, as if raw; constriction in neck of bladder; feeling of soreness in kidneys, < by straightening out legs, > by doubling them upon himself, has to keep quiet to prevent vomiting; feeling of icy coldness in stomach with nausea; brown-black urine; whitish deposit in urine; gouty diathesis.

Colchicum - gouty gastralgia.

Colchicum - has specific power of relieving the gouty paroxysms.

Colchicum - inflammation of great toe, gout in heel, cannot bear to have it touched or moved.

Colocynth - neuralgia of the small branches of the infraorbital nerves, in plethoric, choleric, irritable men, from 40 to 50 years of age, and disposed to hemorrhoidal and gouty affections and to congestions towards head; most frequent cause was vexation, but sometimes too close application to business; but once produced, this neuralgia was apt to recur many days successively at same hour, in forenoon.

Colocynth - rheumatic or gouty rheumatic diathesis.

Colocynth - woman, aged 56, suffering from gastralgia and gout, followed by inflammation of eyes; choleric temperament, venous, hemorrhoidal constitution; choroiditis.

Colocynth (Headache) - bilious headaches; gouty or nervous headaches, of excruciating severity; violent tearing pain, digging through the whole brain, increased particularly when moving the upper eyelid; frontal and coeliac neuralgia alternating; intermittent headaches; severe boring burning pain in one or both temples; compressive sensation in forehead; worse when stooping or lying on back; aggravation afternoon and evening, with great restlessness and anguish, especially when the sweat smells urinous; little urine is passed, or very foul-smelling during the interval, and copiously and clear during the pain, > by firm pressure and lying on affected side; great restlessness and anxiety.

Colocynth (Headache) - intermittent, paroxysmal, bilious or gouty headaches of great severity, > by firm pressure and by lying on affected side; sweat smells vinous and urine foul during interval, clear during paroxysm and copious.

Colocynth [Migraine (headache)] - hemicrania from anger with indignation, after suppression of menses, pains extending towards forehead and left side of head, with nausea, vomiting or diarrhoea, especially towards evening; violent periodical or intermittent headache; bilious, gouty or nervous migraine (headache) of great severity.

Colocynthis - gouty affections of eyes.

Crotalus hor. - rheumatic, gouty, albuminuric, or amenorrheic subjects.

Cypripedium - debility after gout.

Daphne indica - rheumatic and gouty affections in muscles and bones.

Daphne indica - wandering gout, < from cold air.

Digitalis - gouty nodosities.

Digitalis - woman, aged 48, unmarried, gouty diathesis, had two attacks of gout, in consequence of which abnormalities in tricuspid areas developed.

Dulcamara - man, aged 72, gouty, with tendency to emaciation after catching cold; myelitis.

Elaterium - gouty pain in great toes.

Euonymus - chronic rheumatism and gout.

Eupatorium per. - rheumatism and gouty affection.

Eupatorium per. - gouty soreness and inflamed nodosities of joints, associated with headache.

Euphrasia - old woman, gouty; obscuration of cornea.

Ferr-picr. (Hearing, defective) - deafness or hard hearing with eczema in meatus; gouty dyspepsia, dry tongue, constipation; oppression of chest; gout in legs.

Ferrum picric - chronic deafness and tinnitus due to gout.

Formica rufa - the best field for the formic acid treatment are cases of atypical gout.

Formica rufa - acute outbursts of gouty poisons, especially when assuming the neuralgic forms.

Formica rufa - chronic gout and stiffness in joints.

Formica rufa - gout and articular rheumatism; pains worse, motion; better, pressure.

Formica rufa - the most satisfactory cases are chronic arthritis in connection with gouty diathesis.

Fragaria vesca - prevents formation of calculi, removes tartar from teeth and prevents attacks of gout.

Geranium - subacute gouty state.

Glycerinum - gouty concretions.

Glycerinum - gouty pains in big toes.

Gnaphalium (Arthritis, gout) - gouty pains in big toes; sciatica.

Granatum - gouty nodosities.

Gratiola - diarrhoea; green, frothy water, followed by anal burning, forcibly without pain. constipation, with gouty acidity.

Guaiacum - promotes the spontaneous breaking of gouty abscesses, greatly relieving sufferings of patient.

Guaicum (Arthritis, gout) - arthritic lancinations and contraction of limbs; < by slightest motion and accompanied by heat on affected parts. gouty inflammation and abscess of the knee; immovable stiffness of the contracted parts; pinching in abdomen from incarcerated flatulence; pyrosis; constipation.

Guaicum (Back pain–spinal irritation) - rheumatic stiffness of whole left side of back, with intolerable pain on slightest motion or turning the part, not noticed on touch or during rest, drawing limbs out of shape; gouty nodes on joints.

Guaicum (Headache) - attacks of gout in head; sensation as if the brain were detached and loose; drawing and lacerating in occiput and forehead; violent sharp stitches in brain; pulsative throbbing in outer parts of head, with stitches in temples; > by external pressure and walking, < by sitting and standing; gouty tearing and stitching in limbs, with contracting of affected parts; gets up with a headache.

Guaicum (Headache) - gout in head, gets up with headache and sharp stitches in brain.

Guaicum (Rheumatism) - follows well after caust. when there are contractions of tendons, drawing the limbs out of shape, < by any attempt at motion, in daytime, > by warmth, particularly where there are well-developed gouty nodosities on the joints; pains in all joints, even in chest; tearing, drawing lancinations; followed by exhaustion; syphilitic and mercurial dyscrasia.

Guaicum - gouty and rheumatic pain in head and face, extending to neck.

Guaicum - gouty tearing, with contractions.

Hepar-sul. - gout with arthritis, without tophus.

Heracleum sphondylium - recommended as a spinal stimulant; in epilepsy with flatulency, gouty and skin symptoms.

Hydrocotyle - gout with very severe paroxysms.

Ichthyolum - externally, it is used as an ointment, with lanoline 20 to 50 per cent.; for chronic eczema and psoriasis, also acne rosacea and gouty joints.

Ignatia - girl, aged 10, after catching cold, pain in limbs, followed by gouty swellings of joints; chorea.

Indigo - rheumatic and gouty affections of nerves and joints, accompanied by slight fever and great debility.

Insulin. - in the gouty, transitory glycosuria when skin manifestations are persistent give three times daily after eating.

Iridium met. - rheumatism and gout.

Kali-ars. - gouty nodosities.

Kali-ars. - rheumatic, gouty and syphilitic pains.

Kali-ars. - gouty nodosities; worse, change of weather.

Kali-bich. (Arthritis, gout) - gouty pains, especially of fingers, alternate with gastric ailments; periodical wandering pains, shooting, pricking; stiff all over, < mornings; audible cracking in joints on slight motion in the wrists or ankles; lumbago, ischias, periostitis.

Kali-bich. - man, aged 40, in bad health for two years, has had rheumatic gout and rheumatic iritis; inflammation of eyes.

Kali-brom. - nodular form of chronic gout.

Kali-carb. - use cautiously in old gouty cases, advanced bright's and tuberculosis.

Kali-carb. - chronic catarrh, ozaena, with rheumatism or gout.

Kali-carb. - rheumatism, often attacking heart, generally going from upper to lower parts; painful swelling; gout.

Kali-iod. (Nephritis) - scanty dark urine; painful micturition; sediment dirty, yellowish, great thirst, heat in the head, deliria; granulated kidney from gout or mercurio-syphilis.

Kali-iod. - gout and rheumatism; synovitis.

Kali-mur. - rheumatic, gouty pains.

Kali-mur. - woman, aged 44, gouty; faceache.

Kalmia (Heart diseases) - especially useful when gout or rheumatism, after external applications, shifts from joints to heart sharp, severe pains about heart, taking away the breath and shooting down into stomach and abdomen, with slow pulse (Dig.) and numb feeling in left arm. Pericarditis rheumatica, first stage, with tumultuous, rapid and visible beating of the heart, paroxysms of anguish with great dyspnoea, febrile excitement, pains in limbs, stitch in lower part of chest, right-sided face-ache; pressure as of a stone from epigastrium towards the heart, with a strong, quick heart-beat, > by sitting erect, < when bent over or lying on left side. Hypertrophy and valvular insufficiency, or thickening after rheumatism; arms feel numb and weak, limbs cold; weariness in all muscles, shuns all exertion; pulse slow and weak; albinuria; ascites.

Kalmia - gouty and rheumatic metastasis of heart.

Lac-can. - neuralgia and acute pains; rheumatism; gout; syphilitic sciatica; sexual debility.

Ledum - rheumatic, gouty diathesis; constitutions abuse by alcohol

Ledum (Arthritis, gout) - low, asthenic cases (maltreated by large doses of Colch.); lancinating, tearing pains; < by motion than by touch and at midnight, when joints feel so hot that he throws off all covering; oedematous swelling of joint, which may feel cold to the touch; affects chiefly left shoulder and right hip-joint; habitual gout in the articulations of hands and feet; ball of great toe swollen and painful; soles very sensitive; tendons stiff; gouty nodosities in joints; fine tearing pains in toes; face bloated; pimples on forehead; after abuse of alcoholic drinks.

Ledum (Cough) - chronic cases, characterized by cold and deficiency of animal heat; spasmodic cough, preceding for a few days the eruption of eczema or an attack of gout;

hollow, racking, spasmodic cough from tickling in larynx; before cough he loses his breath; after cough dizziness and staggering; double sobbing inspiration; expectoration of bright-red, foaming blood, or foetid purulent matter.

Ledum (Dropsy) - gout, constant chilliness, only at midnight sense of suffocation, patient throwing off all covering and becoming restless and cross; dry skin, want of perspiration. Ailments, as dropsy, from abuse of alcoholic drinks.

Ledum (Haemorrhage from lungs, hacmoptysis) - copious discharge of bright-red and foamy blood, accompanied by violent cough in paroxysms, caused by tickling in larynx and trachea; congestion to chest and head; hardness of hearing; pulse strong and hard; burning pain in some point of chest, from which the blood seems to come; stagnation in liver and portal system; hot hands and hot feet; heat of whole body; coxalgia alternating with haemopto; suits rheumatic or gouty persons who are weak from abuse of Colch.; also drunkards.

Ledum (Headache) - raging, pulsating headache, as if something were gnawing in her temples, occiput and ears; beating, tearing pain in head, with red, bloated-looking face and eyes; cannot bear to have head covered; head affected after getting wet; syphilitic and mercurial headaches; chronic rheumatic gout.

Ledum (Rheumatism) - arthritic nodosities, with violent pains; growing < in evening, or at night when getting warm in bed and last till midnight; gout and rheumatism affecting the smaller joints where cellular tissue is wanting; < by motion; pains travel upward; oedema of feet; blisters on heels, acute tearing pains in joints, with great weakness of limbs, and numbness and coldness of surface; rheumatic or gouty inflammation of the great toe, with scanty effusion, which tends to harden into nodosities; < at night, from warmth of bed and covering up, > by cold; boring pains in bones; stiffness affecting the muscles of back, neck and loins; pains change location quickly, accompanied by little or no swelling; rheumatic pains in joints of arms; emaciation; coldness of affected parts; erythema nodosum, < in cold damp weather.

Ledum - cataract with gout.

Ledum - gouty nodosities.

Ledum - gouty pains shoot all through the foot and limb, and in joints, but especially small joints.

Lithium carb. - arthritis; gouty diathesis.

Lithium carb. - gout and tophi.

Lithium carb. - obesity with gout; dyspnoea.

Lithium carb. - woman, aged 52; gouty diathesis, puffing, swelling and itching of body and limbs.

Lithium carb. (Arthritis, gout) - gout in knees, sides of feet and soles; ankle-joints pain on walking; profuse urine, with uric acid deposit; painful urination; pain in heart before and at time of urinating; valvular deficiencies; < from mental agitation, which causes a fluttering and trembling of heart, general puffiness of body and limbs; **increase of bulk and weight;** clumsiness in walking at night and weariness in standing; swelling, tenderness, sometimes redness of last joints of fingers; intense itching of feet and hands at night from no apparent cause; uric acid deposits in urine.

Lithium carb. (Heart diseases) - hypertrophy from valvular deficiencies, especially of the aortic valves, in persons of a gouty diathesis; rheumatic soreness about heart; mental agitation causes fluttering of heart, < by bending forward; shocks and jerks about heart, > by urinating; finger-joints tender and painful; paralytic stiffness in all limbs and whole body.

Lycopodium - gouty lithemia.

Lycopodium - man, aged 81; gout.

Lycopodium - woman, aged 58, large, corpulent, gouty diathesis; flatulent dyspepsia.

Lycopodium (Diabetes) - peevish and depressed in mind; thirst and hunger constant, but worse at night; flatulence; faeces small in quantity; want of natural warmth; sexual desire and power gone; lithic acid gravel; pulmonary phthisis, pituitosa and purulenta, with hectic; great emaciation; mental, nervous and bodily exhaustion; gouty lithaemia.

Lycopodium - chronic gout, with chalky deposits in joints.

Manganum aceticum - gout.

Medorrhinum - a maiden lady, no suspicion of sycotic poisoning, a long line of ancestors had rheumatism and gout; chronic rheumatism.

Medorrhinum - gouty concretions.

Menyanthes (Arthritis, gout) - painful spasmodic jerking of lower extremities in gouty persons; with calcareous deposits in joints.

Menyanthes (Rheumatism) - painful spasmodic jerking of lower extremities, from hip down; stitching pains in gouty persons, with calcareous deposits in joints.

Merc-sol. - gouty and rheumatic pains, with sweats without relief,

Merc-sol. - gouty, shining red swellings,

Merc-sol. - strong man, aged 50, subject to gouty pains in joints; iritis,

Merc-sol. - woman, aged 24, unmarried, gouty tendency; gout,

Natrum mur. - there seems also to be a retention in the tissues of effected materials giving rise to symptoms loosely described as gouty or rheumatic gout.

Natrum sulph. - chronic gout.

Natrum sulph. - gout.

Nitric acid. (Eczema) - after abuse of mercurial ointments; eczema ani with long-lasting pain in rectum after stool and itching at night; humid, stinging eruption on vertex and temples, bleeding easily when scratched and feeling very sore when lain on, also in auditory meatus, on genitals, about the anus and on hand (left); chronic swelling of tonsils; < nights, in open air, from change of weather and during sweat; > in cold air. gouty inheritance; child likes sweets.

Nux moschata - retrocession of gout to stomach.

Nux moschata (Dyspepsia, weakness of stomach) - dyspepsia of hysterical women, given to sleepiness, fainting or laughing hysteria, with feeling as though the food formed itself into small hard lumps, with hard surfaces and angles, which produce soreness of stomach; dyspeptic symptoms come on at once, while patient is still at the table; she eats with appetite, but a few mouthfuls satisfy her; turning in stomach with some nausea; mouth and throat dry, no thirst, saliva like cotton; chalky taste; vomiting of digested food, with tough mucus of somewhat bitter or sour taste (Nux-v.); immediately after eating or while person is still at table there is enormous abdominal distention with sensation as if food in the stomach had formed into hard lumps; heartburn; distended condition of stomach and abdomen, with sensation of warmth not only after a meal, but also from least contradiction, showing its nervous character; retrocession of gout to stomach, < from cool moisture, > by external warmth; syncope from nervous weakness.

Nux vomica [Migraine (headache)] - gouty and haemorrhoidal patients. Attack sets in the morning when awaking, getting worse during the day; nausea and vomiting during attack; becoming often most severe in occiput; drawing, aching feeling as of a nail driven into the head, or as if the brain were dashed to pieces; face pale, or sallow on a red ground; < from mental exercise, by motion and by rest, from stimulants; patient irritable with his abdominal plethora.

Nux vom. - gout in incipient stage in habitual drinkers; oversensitiveness to pain, constipation; during hard stool, violent pain in affected part; scanty, dark urine; heat mixed with chilliness, especially when moving; perspiration relieves; torticollis.

Nux vom. - man, aged 22, father gouty, leads an active life, uses coffee and tobacco to excess, suffers with hemorrhoids; angina pectoris.

Nux vom. - man, aged 25, beer drinker, father subject to gout, suffering six months; disordered stomach, enlarged liver, tuberculosis.

Nux vom. - woman, aged 40, gouty, suffering several months; headache.

Nux vom. - woman, suffering many years with gout and profuse leucorrhoea; epilepsy.

Oleum jec. - chronic gout and rheumatism of elderly persons, with rigidity of muscles and tendons, joint nearly inflexible.

Pareira brava - rheumatic or gouty subjects suffering from renal colics.

Phosphorus (Diabetes) - diabetes, with phthisis; urine profuse, pale, watery; or turbid, whitish, like curdled milk, with brickdust sediment and variegated cuticle on surface; gouty diathesis; cerebral disease; cheesy degeneration of lungs.

Phosphorus - man, aged 62, formerly had gout, apparently in articulo mortis; cerebral oedema.

Phytolacca - arthritis vaga, or wandering gout; passing from one joint and place to another, with swelling and redness.

Phytolacca (Headache) - headache of gouty aged people and of syphilitic patients; migraine (headache) with backache and bearing down once a week, dull pressive pain with vertigo and impairment of vision; sensation of soreness deep in the brain; sensation as if the brain were bruised when stepping from a high step down to the ground; pain from frontal region to vertex, shooting from left eye to vertex (cimicif., shooting from vertex to eyes); mental depression, painful pressure deep in head, temple and vertex; foul tongue, disinclination to food; disgust of life, for everybody and everything, < in wet weather; constipation.

Phytolacca (Headache) - headache of gouty old people or of syphilitic patients; sensation as if brain were bruised when stepping from a high step to the ground; < wet weather.

Pinus silvestris - stiffness; gouty pain in all joints, especially finger-joints.

Platina - suits hysterical and hemorrhoidal patients and, perhaps, such as suffer from gout or worms, especially those of mournful mind, or alternately sad and gay, who cry easily, are pale, easily fatigued, suffer from wandering pains, are inclined to spasms.

Plumb-met. - gout is more frequent in persons suffering from lead-poisoning.

Podophyllum - man, aged 45, bilious temperament; gout.

Podophyllum - useful in gout after acute symptoms have subsided, or in cases where attack is preceded by premonitory symptoms it is indicated at once; it will ward off an impending attack of gout.

Primula veris - cerebral congestion, with neuralgia; migraine; rheumatic and gouty pains.

Pulsatilla - man, plethoric habit, subject to attacks of rheumatic gout; rheumatism in hand.

Pulsatilla - rheumatic and gouty affections; also with swelling.

Pulsatilla - woman, aged 70, belonging to upper class of society, small, choleric temperament, suffering for years with hemorrhoids and gout; glossitis.

Pulsatilla (Ophthalmia) - blepharo-adenitis, with tendency to formation of styes and abscesses on the margin of lids, accompanied by acne on face; granular lids, dry, or with excessive bland secretion; pustular conjunctivitis, discharge thick, yellow, bland, profuse, > in open air, but not in wind; gonorrhoeal ophthalmia, when the gonorrhoea became suddenly suppressed; ophthalmia neonatorum, with profuse yellow, purulent discharge, gluing the lids; amblyopia from suppression of any bloody discharge, from gastric derangement, from metastasis of gout or rheumatism; fistula lachrymalis, discharging pus when pressed; frequent rubbing of eyes for relief.

Pulsatilla (Synovitis) - joint swollen, with sharp, erratic pains, accompanied by a feeling of soreness or of subcutaneous ulceration; tearing, stinging, erratic pains force the patient to move the affected joint, > by pressure and slowly moving about, jerking pains down the limbs, < evening and from warmth, > by cold; gonorrhoeal or traumatic synovitis or gouty, especially in affections of the knee, ankle and tarsal joints.

Pulsatilla (Vision complaints) - amblyopia from suppression of any bloody discharge; from metastasis of gout or rheumatism; from gastric derangement; with heart disease; with coexisting diminished hearing; diminished sight especially on getting warm from exercise; blindness at twilight and sensation as if the eyes were bandaged; shining or flashing rings before eyes; mistiness of sight or sensation as if the dimness could be removed by wiping; frequent and copious lachrymation.

Quercus gland spirit. - useful in gout, old malarial cases with flatulence.

Radium brom. - found effective in the treatment of rheumatism and gout, in skin affections generally, acne rosacea, naevi, moles, ulcers and cancers.

Ranunculus sceleratus - gout in fingers and toes.

Rhododendron (Hearing, defective) - hard hearing; every pulsation felt in the ear, surring and noises in the ear; gouty dyspepsia; pain and numbness in extremities.

Rhododendron - gouty inflammation of great toe-joint.

Rhododendron - rheumatic and gouty symptoms well marked.

Sabina - gout; arthritic complaints; tearing, stinging in joints after they become swollen; < in heated room; > in cool air or cool room; arthritic nodes.

Sabina - gout; worse, in heated room.

Sabina - gouty diathesis.

Sabina - gouty nodosities.

Sabina - has a special action on the uterus; also upon serous and fibrous membranes; hence its use in gout.

Salicylic-acid - acute gout.

Secale - woman, aged 70, gouty; diarrhoea.

Sepia - disposition to gout and hemorrhoids.

Sepia (Apoplexy) - in men addicted to drinking and sexual excesses, with a disposition to gout and haemorrhoids; or in women, from affections of the reproductive system. venous apoplexy. headache coming on in terrific shocks; dizziness in walking; with staggering; forgetfulness; cold feet; intermitting pulse, uses wrong words in writing.

Sepia (Arthritis, gout) - anomalous or regular gout; urates in blood and deposited in or near the joints; pains in hepatic region, >

by lying on affected side (Magn-mur. <); bleeding, painful piles; after stool weakness and emptiness in abdomen.

Silicea - chronic gouty nodosities.

Silicea - hard lumps on neck, not of glands, extending to left side, in a gouty subject.

Silicea (Rheumatism) - chronic hereditary rheumatism and gouty nodosities, causing such tenderness of soles that patient cannot walk (Ant-crud.); shoulder pains, < at night and by uncovering (Led., opposite); rheumatism of lower cervical vertebrae; violent tearing between shoulder-blades; pressure and tension in small of back; stiff back after sitting; coccyx hurts after riding; drawing in limbs with tearing and sticking pains in joints, < after motion.

Spigelia (Headache) - neuralgic and rheumatic headaches, eyeballs involved, < by stooping; headache rises and declines with the sun; when moving facial muscles sensation as if head would split. Gouty pains and stiffness of joints.

Staphisagria (Arthritis, gout) - arthritic nodes from deposition of urates of soda; pain from the eyes to the teeth; eyes burn and feel dry despite profuse lachrymation; patient weak and exhausted from dissipation; face sallow. chronic gout of men advanced in life, corpulent with feeble pulse, palpitation, dyspnoea on exertion; pains in smaller joints of hands and feet, with much swelling and hardness; skin affections alternating with pains in joints; weakness of knees; soles of feet tender.

Staphisagria (Constipation) - retarded stool on account of lack of peristaltic action; hard, scanty stool, with cutting and burning in anus; hard stool and flatus alternately; difficult stool with great distress, as if the rectum or anus were constricted, first with hard, then with soft faeces, or with only soft stool. Gouty persons of a strumous diathesis, who lived too well for their own benefit. colic with incarcerated flatus and gnawing, darting pains, > by passing flatus.

Stellaria - enlarged and inflamed gouty finger joints.

Sulphur - aged 62; gouty ophthalmia.

Sulphur - miss h, aged 50, suffering sixteen years; rheumatic gout

Sulphur - rheumatic gout, with itching.

Sulphur (Arthritis, gout) - habitual gout, especially of drunkards and those who indulge in rich food and take but little exercise, red blotches in face, nose habitually red; disgust for animal food; dyspnoea with desire to take a deep inspiration; uric acid urine; dull, aching, pressive pain in joints; as soon as he falls asleep the affected limbs jerk and arouse him; pain serratic and leave a sensation of numbness; alternate constipation or diarrhoea, with excessively foetid stools and foetid flatulence; haemorrhoids.

Sulphur (Headache) - abdominal plethora (Sep.); gouty and rheumatic headaches; periodical headaches.

Sulphur (Headache) - heat on top of head, flushes in face, feet cold, vertigo when going up stairs; headache from abdominal plethora, from suppressed skin diseases, or chronic gouty and rheumatic headaches, increased by mental exertion, motion, coughing, sneezing; periodical headaches, every seventh day; dull headache, commencing in the morning, increasing until noon or a little later and then gradually decreasing; throbbing headache at night; sick-headache, very weakening, once a week or every two weeks, pains generally lacerating, stupefying, benumbing; headache every day, as if the head would burst; nightly headache, < from slightest motion in bed; < in wet cold weather and when at rest, > from motion; hypochondriasis.

Taxus baccata - also in gout and chronic rheumatism.

Terebinth. - atonic gout; rheumatism and gout; asthenic inflammation; passive hemorrhages; purpura haemorrhagica; burns; hospital gangrene; cold gangrene; hydrophobia, gangrenous wound from bite of a dog; wounds of skin, tendons and nerves; dissection wounds; old ulcers.

Terebinth. - chronic rheumatic and gouty complaints.

Uran-nit. - diabetes mellitus and insipidus; brights disease, and kindred renal maladies; contracted, gouty kidneys, with gastric disturbances; irritable condition of renal plexus, of sympathetic.

Urea pura. - gouty eczema.

Urtica urens - fever of gout.

Urtica urens - gout and uric acid diathesis.

Urtica urens - pain in acute gout deltoid; pain in ankles, wrists.

Verat-alb. - woman, aged 56, medium height, weak, gouty; colic.

Viola tricolor - rheumatism or gout.

Viscum alb. (Hearing, defective) - gouty and rheumatic deafness, tearing pains in ears, < by sharp cold winds in winter.

Viscum alb. - asthma if connected with gout or rheumatism.

Viscum alb. - the symptoms point especially to rheumatic and gouty complaints; neuralgia, especially sciatica.

Diseases associated with 'Gout'

(Albuminuria) Berberis-vul. - gouty or rheumatic diathesis; burning in back; urine of dark, bloody appearance and largely supplied with Alben; tough mucus in mouth and throat; constant nausea and loss of sleep; frequent palpitation, slow, weak pulse; painful pressure and tension in the lumbar and renal regions, with sensation of numbness, puffiness, warmth, stiffness and lameness, extending at times into the lower limbs, especially indicated in persons addicted to the use of alcoholic beverages.

(Albuminuria) Colchicum - first stage; flatulent distention of stomach; stools watery, jelly-like, mucous or bloody, and mingled with a stringy substance; gouty pains in joints; urine dark and scanty, discharged in drops and depositing a whitish sediment; urine as black as ink, containing blood, and loaded with alben and tube-casts, smoky in appearance; pericarditis rheumatica with violent cutting, stinging pain in chest, with great oppression and dyspnoea; sensation as if the chest or heart were squeezed by a tight bandage; relapses from taking cold in damp weather or from suppressed perspiration; patient cannot stand up straight or lie down with stretched-out legs without causing pain in renal region and vomiting, especially in albuminuria of pregnancy.

(Apoplexy) Sepia - in men addicted to drinking and sexual excesses, with a disposition to gout and haemorrhoids; or in women, from affections of the reproductive system. Venous apoplexy. Headache coming on in terrific shocks; dizziness in walking; with staggering; forgetfulness; cold feet; intermitting pulse, uses wrong words in writing.

(Arthritis, gout) Abrotanum - chronic arthritis. Gouty deposits about finger-joints, < during cold, stormy weather, painful, sore and hot at that time; metastasis to heart; piercing pain in heart; high fever; emaciation, though appetite is good.

(Arthritis, gout) Artemisia abrotan. - painful and inflamed wrist and ankle-joints, stiff, with pricking sensation; ailments after suppressed gout.

(Arthritis, gout) Benzoic-acid. - tearing in joints with nearly clear urine; old nodes become painful, and as the pains abate palpitation sets in, ceasing only when pains increase; gout going from left to right or commencing in right great toe; urine of offensive odor, depositing a reddish cloudy sediment. Chronic rheumarthritis, wandering pains (Puls.).

(Arthritis, gout) Colchicum - gout attacking many joints; shifting from one to another, with burning and tearing pains, < from any external impression, noise, odor, touch or bright light. the joint becomes inflamed, dark red, hot and intensely painful, patient nearly beside himself with agony; oedema and coldness of legs and feet, with weariness, heaviness and inability to move; urine acid, dark and scanty; even the smell of food nauseates; frequent, ineffectual inclination to sneeze on waking in the morning; uric acid diathesis; gout in persons of vigorous constitution.

(Arthritis, gout) Gnaphalium - gouty pains in big toes; sciatica.

(Arthritis, gout) Guaicum - arthritic lancinations and contraction of limbs; < by slightest motion and accompanied by heat on affected parts. Gouty inflammation and abscess of the knee; immovable stiffness of the contracted parts; pinching in abdomen from incarcerated flatulence; pyrosis; constipation.

(Arthritis, gout) Kali-bich. - gouty pains, especially of fingers, alternate with gastric ailments; periodical wandering pains, shooting, pricking; stiff all over, < mornings; audible cracking in joints on slight motion in the wrists or ankles; lumbago, ischias, periostitis.

(Arthritis, gout) Ledum - low, asthenic cases (maltreated by large doses of colch.); lancinating, tearing pains; < by motion than by touch and at midnight, when joints feel so hot that he throws off all covering; oedematous swelling of joint, which may feel cold to the touch; affects chiefly left shoulder and right hip-joint; habitual gout in the articulations of hands and feet; ball of great toe swollen and painful; soles very sensitive; tendons stiff; gouty nodosities in joints; fine tearing pains in toes; face bloated; pimples on forehead; after abuse of alcoholic drinks.

(Arthritis, gout) Lithium carb. - gout in knees, sides of feet and soles; ankle-joints pain on walking; profuse urine, with uric acid deposit; painful urination; pain in heart before and at time of urinating; valvular deficiencies; < from mental agitation, which causes a fluttering and trembling of heart, general puffiness of body and limbs; increase of bulk and weight; clumsiness in walking at night and weariness in standing; swelling, tenderness, sometimes redness of last joints of fingers; intense itching of feet and hands at night from no apparent cause; uric acid deposits in urine.

(Arthritis, gout) Menyanthes - painful spasmodic jerking of lower extremities in gouty persons; with calcareous deposits in joints.

(Arthritis, gout) Sepia - anomalous or regular gout; urates in blood and deposited in or near the joints; pains in hepatic region, > by lying on affected side (magn. mur. <); bleeding, painful piles; after stool weakness and emptiness in abdomen.

(Arthritis, gout) Staphisagria - arthritic nodes from deposition of urates of soda; pain from the eyes to the teeth; eyes burn and feel dry despite profuse lachrymation; patient weak and exhausted from dissipation; face sallow. Chronic gout of men advanced in life, corpulent with feeble pulse, palpitation, dyspnoea on exertion; pains in smaller joints of hands and feet, with much swelling and hardness; skin affections alternating with pains in joints; weakness of knees; soles of feet tender.

(Arthritis, gout) Sulphur - habitual gout, especially of drunkards and those who indulge in rich food and take but little exercise, red blotches in face, nose habitually red; disgust for animal food; dyspnoea with desire to take a deep inspiration; uric acid urine; dull, aching, pressive pain in joints; as soon as he falls asleep the affected limbs jerk and arouse him; pain serratic and leave a sensation of numbness; alternate

Gout—Retrocedent, Metastatic, Constitutional

constipation or diarrhoea, with excessively foetid stools and foetid flatulence; haemorrhoids.

(Asthma) Colchicum - oppression of chest, dyspnoea, tensive feeling in chest, high up or low down; with anxiety, > by bending forward; extreme anxiety of face; cheeks, lips and eyelids purple; anxious feeling in praecordia; flatulency and meteorism; rheumatic gout.

(Back pain–spinal irritation) Guaicum - rheumatic stiffness of whole left side of back, with intolerable pain on slightest motion or turning the part, not noticed on touch or during rest, drawing limbs out of shape; gouty nodes on joints.

(Back pain–spinal irritation) pains in back from rheuma and gout: Acon., Ant-tart., Calc-phos., Colch., Gels., Guaiac., Hep., Hydr., Kali-bi., Kali-carb., Kalm., Merc., Puls., Rhus.

(Bone diseases, osteitis, periostitis, exostosis, caries, necrosis, etc.) Benzoic-acid. - swelling and cracking of knee-joint; gouty deposits between metacarpal bones; tearing pain in anterior surface of thigh; ulcerative pain in whole leg.

(Bronchitis chronica) Aesculus hip. - bronchitis complicated with gouty diathesis and a tendency to piles with constipation; rapid, labored breathing with pain in right lung.

(Bronchitis chronica) Ammoniacum - bronchorrhoea respiration short, quick, with anguish, especially at night; oppression and obstruction in the chest from the accumulation of mucus; stitches in the left side of the chest when taking a deep inspiration; tickling in throat without cough; frontal headache, dimness of sight; in rheumatic or gouty subjects.

(Bronchitis chronica) Amm-phos. - bronchitis chronica arthritica when patients suffering from gout or rheumarthritis are attacked with bronchial catarrhs or bronchitis.

(Constipation) Staphisagria - retarded stool on account of lack of peristaltic action; hard, scanty stool, with cutting and burning in anus; hard stool and flatus alternately; difficult stool with great distress, as if the rectum or anus were constricted, first with hard, then with soft faeces, or with only soft stool. gouty persons of a strumous diathesis, who lived too well for their own benefit. colic with incarcerated flatus and gnawing, darting pains, > by passing flatus.

(Cough) Ledum - chronic cases, characterized by cold and deficiency of animal heat; spasmodic cough, preceding for a few days the eruption of eczema or an attack of gout; hollow, racking, spasmodic cough from tickling in larynx; before cough he loses his breath; after cough dizziness and staggering; double sobbing inspiration; expectoration of bright-red, foaming blood, or foetid purulent matter.

(Cystitis, inflammation of bladder) Colchicum - vesical irritability depending upon a gouty diathesis; strangury with haemorrhage from bladder; micturition accompanied and followed by tenesmus of bladder and burning pain in urethra; as if urine were hot.

(Debility) Bar-c. - suits first childhood and senility (old age) with mental or physical debility; old people, especially when fat or when they suffered from gout; constantly weak and weary, wishes to lean on something, to sit or lie down, and still feels weak and weary; deficient memory, absent-mindedness.

(Diabetes) Lycopodium - peevish and depressed in mind; thirst and hunger constant, but worse at night; flatulence; faeces small in quantity; want of natural warmth; sexual desire and power gone; lithic acid gravel; pulmonary phthisis, pituitosa and purulenta, with hectic; great emaciation; mental, nervous and bodily exhaustion; gouty lithaemia.

(Diabetes) Phos. - diabetes, with phthisis; urine profuse, pale, watery; or turbid, whitish, like curdled milk, with brickdust sediment and variegated cuticle on surface; gouty diathesis; cerebral disease; cheesy degeneration of lungs.

(Diaphragm, diseases of) Colchicum - similar to Bry.; gouty diathesis; albuminosis; uneasiness at epigastrium, extremely sensitive to touch and pressure; pain in epigastrium as if pierced with a knife; violent vomiting accompanied by intense straining and loud, hollow belching, > by bending himself up and lying quiet; limbs cold, hands and feet cold.

(Dropsy) Asparagus off. - old people with heart disease; weak action of heart; when urinating the last drops, constricting pain in cardiac region, turns blue in face, urine has an unpleasant odor; must sit up in bed to relieve dyspnoea. hydrothorax in senility on a gouty diathesis.

(Dropsy) Colchicum - dropsy after scarlatina, with suppression of urine, or urine black, containing alben and destroyed blood-corpuscles; acute dropsy with renal affections, constant urging to urinate, but only a little is voided and that with great pain, as from spasm in the bladder. dropsy of cavities and internal organs, especially hydropericardium, hydrothorax, hydrometra, ascites. lower limbs oedematous and cold; skin dry and pale; emaciated sensitive persons, disposed to rheumatism and catarrh, always < when it is damp, in spring and fall; gout with nervous weakness and oversensitiveness.

(Dropsy) Ledum - gout, constant chilliness, only at midnight sense of suffocation, patient throwing off all covering and becoming restless and cross; dry skin, want of perspiration. Ailments, as dropsy, from abuse of alcoholic drinks.

(Dyspepsia, weakness of stomach) Ant-crud. - overloading the stomach and gastric derangement in children, women and old people; thickly coated white tongue, with anorexia, slow digestion and foetid eructations, often followed by diarrhoea, particularly after acid wines or new beer; habitual sensation in stomach as if overloaded, excessive crossness, even hypochondriasis with suicidal tendencies; dryness of mouth with great thirst, < at night; constipation alternating with diarrhoea; helminthiasis; caused by overeating, hot weather, bathing, during measles; metastasis of gout and rheumatism.

(Dyspepsia, weakness of stomach) Colchicum - appetite for different things, but as soon as he sees them or still more smells them, he shudders from nausea and is unable to eat anything (cocc., extreme aversion to food, even the smell of food nauseates, although feeling hungry); the smell of fish, eggs or fat meat makes him faint; frequent copious eructations of tasteless gas; on assuming an upright position qualmishness in stomach and inclination to vomit; violent retching, followed by copious and forcible vomiting of food and then of bile, renewed by every motion; burning sensation in stomach more frequently than an icy coldness, accompanied by great pains and debility. (retrocession of gout.)

(Dyspepsia, weakness of stomach) Nux moschata - dyspepsia of hysterical women, given to sleepiness, fainting or laughing hysteria, with feeling as though the food formed itself into small hard lumps, with hard surfaces and angles, which produce soreness of stomach; dyspeptic symptoms come on at once, while patient is still at the table; she eats with appetite, but a few mouthfuls satisfy her; turning in stomach with some nausea; mouth and throat dry, no thirst, saliva like cotton; chalky taste; vomiting of digested food, with tough mucus of somewhat bitter or sour taste (Nux-v.); immediately after eating or while person is still at table there is enormous abdominal distention with sensation as if food in the stomach had formed into hard lumps;

heartburn; distended condition of stomach and abdomen, with sensation of warmth not only after a meal, but also from least contradiction, showing its nervous character; retrocession of gout to stomach, < from cool moisture, > by external warmth; syncope from nervous weakness.

(Eczema) Nitric acid. - after abuse of mercurial ointments; eczema ani with long-lasting pain in rectum after stool and itching at night; humid, stinging eruption on vertex and temples, bleeding easily when scratched and feeling very sore when lain on, also in auditory meatus, on genitals, about the anus and on hand (left); chronic swelling of tonsils; < nights, in open air, from change of weather and during sweat; > in cold air. Gouty inheritance; child likes sweets.

(Epilepsy) - Gouty: Colch., Nux-v.

(Epilepsy): in gouty patients: Bry., Colch., Kali-iod., Lyc., Natr.-salicyl.

(Gastralgia) Abrotanum - gnawing hunger; craves bread boiled in milk; appetite sometimes ravenous while emaciating; burning in stomach as from acidity; sensation as if the stomach were hanging or swimming in water, with a peculiar feeling of coldness and a dullness to all irritants; pains cutting, gnawing, burning, sometimes contracting and stinging, mostly < at night; never entirely free from pain, even in the intervals of the spasms; constipation; haemorrhoids; gastralgia after suppressed gout.

(Haemorrhage from the lungs, haemoptysis) Ledum - copious discharge of bright-red and foamy blood, accompanied by violent cough in paroxysms, caused by tickling in larynx and trachea; congestion to chest and head; hardness of hearing; pulse strong and hard; burning pain in some point of chest, from which the blood seems to come; stagnation in liver and portal system; hot hands and hot feet; heat of whole body; coxalgia alternating with haemopto?; suits rheumatic or gouty persons who are weak from abuse of colch.; also drunkards.

[Migraine (headache)] Sick-headache - gouty hemicrania: Colch., Coloc., Guaic., Kali-bi., Lyc., Magn. Mur., Natr-m.

(Headache) Belladonna - congestion of blood to head, with danger of apoplexy; gouty and hysterical headaches; throbbing pains, especially on right side, with intolerance of light and noise; hot head and cold feet, not relieved by lying down, but by sitting propped up, > by holding head in the opposite direction to the part of head affected; sensation as if the brain were pressed to the forehead, disappearing quickly on bending the head backward; in walking feels as if with every step brain rose and fell in forehead; soreness in forehead, stiffness in occiput, eyeballs feel as if starting from their sockets; stabbing as with a knife, from one temple to the other; violent pressing in whole head, from within outward, as if it would burst; pains come suddenly, last indefinitely, but cease suddenly; intense headache makes him first blind, then unconscious; sun-headache; headaches < when leaning forward, from warmth, > during menses, from pressure, tight bandaging and wrapping up; headache from abuse of coffee, from overheating and from cold.

(Headache) Causticum - torpid gout (Colch., gout in vigorous constitutions); constant succession of shocks and jerks through the head.

(Headache) Colchicum - gout in vigorous constitutions (Caust., torpid gout); grinding, boring, arthritic headache, usually parietal or occipital; tearing, drawing, pressing headache, often semilateral; severe pressing pain deep in the substance of the cerebellum from the slightest intellectual exertion, especially in overtaxed brains; as soon as he loses any rest, as by night-watching, he becomes mentally tired and suffers with headache, nausea, bitter taste, becomes irritable and intolerant even to slight pain; painful drawing, tearing, beginning in one eyeball and extending to occiput, < by motion or jar, > by physical rest, from warmth, after supper; frequent ineffectual inclination to sneeze on waking in the morning.

(Headache) Colocynth - bilious headaches; gouty or nervous headaches, of excruciating severity; violent tearing pain, digging through the whole brain, increased particularly when moving the upper eyelid; frontal and coeliac neuralgia alternating; intermittent headaches; severe boring burning pain in one or both temples; compressive sensation in forehead; worse when stooping or lying on back; aggravation afternoon and evening, with great restlessness and anguish, especially when the sweat smells urinous; little urine is passed, or very foul-smelling during the interval, and copiously and clear during the pain, > by firm pressure and lying on affected side; great restlessness and anxiety.

(Headache) Colocynth - intermittent, paroxysmal, bilious or gouty headaches of great severity, > by firm pressure and by lying on affected side; sweat smells vinous and urine foul during interval, clear during paroxysm and copious.

(Headache) Guaicum - attacks of gout in head; sensation as if the brain were detached and loose; drawing and lacerating in occiput and forehead; violent sharp stitches in brain; pulsative throbbing in outer parts of head, with stitches in temples; > by external pressure and walking, < by sitting and standing; gouty tearing and stitching in limbs, with contracting of affected parts; gets up with a headache.

(Headache) Guaicum - gout in head, gets up with headache and sharp stitches in brain.

(Headache) Ledum - raging, pulsating headache, as if something were gnawing in her temples, occiput and ears; beating, tearing pain in head, with red, bloated-looking face and eyes; cannot bear to have head covered; head affected after getting wet; syphilitic and mercurial headaches; chronic rheumatic gout.

(Headache) Phytolacca - headache of gouty aged people and of syphilitic patients; migraine (headache) with backache and bearing down once a week, dull pressive pain with vertigo and impairment of vision; sensation of soreness deep in the brain; sensation as if the brain were bruised when stepping from a high step down to the ground; pain from frontal region to vertex, shooting from left eye to vertex (Cimic-if., shooting from vertex to eyes); mental depression, painful pressure deep in head, temple and vertex; foul tongue, disinclination to food; disgust of life, for everybody and everything, < in wet weather; constipation.

(Headache) Phytolacca - headache of gouty old people or of syphilitic patients; sensation as if brain were bruised when stepping from a high step to the ground; < wet weather.

(Headache) Spigelia - neuralgic and rheumatic headaches, eyeballs involved, < by stooping; headache rises and declines with the sun; when moving facial muscles sensation as if head would split. Gouty pains and stiffness of joints.

(Headache) Sulphur - abdominal plethora (Sep.); gouty and rheumatic headaches; periodical headaches.

(Headache) Sulphur - heat on top of head, flushes in face, feet cold, vertigo when going up stairs; headache from abdominal plethora, from suppressed skin diseases, or chronic gouty and rheumatic headaches, increased by mental exertion, motion, coughing, sneezing; periodical headaches, every seventh day; dull headache, commencing in the morning, increasing until noon or a little later and then gradually decreasing; throbbing headache at night; sick-headache, very weakening, once a week or every two weeks, pains generally lacerating, stupefying, benumbing; headache every day, as if the head would burst; nightly headache, < from slightest motion in bed; < in wet cold weather and when at rest, > from motion; hypochondriasis.

(Hearing, defective) Ferr-picr. - deafness or hard hearing with eczema in meatus; gouty dyspepsia, dry tongue, constipation; oppression of chest; gout in legs.

(Hearing, defective) Rhododendron - hard hearing; every pulsation felt in the ear, surring and noises in the ear; gouty dyspepsia; pain and numbness in extremities.

(Hearing, defective) Viscum alb. - gouty and rheumatic deafness, tearing pains in ears, < by sharp cold winds in winter.

(Heart diseases) Abrotanum - metastasis of gout or rheumatism to heart; endocarditis with piercing pains across chest, < in cardiac region; dyspnoea, profuse sweat; sinking as if dying, feeble pulse.

(Heart diseases) Asparagus off. - cardiac affections of the aged, with weak pulse and pain about left acromion, heart's stroke twofold, irregular, quickened; disinclination to any work and languor. Hydrothorax with heart disease or gouty diathesis of old people.

(Heart diseases) Benzoic-acid. - gout or rheumatism affecting the heart and nodular swellings in the joints; pains change place incessantly, but are more constant about heart; awakens after midnight with violent palpitation of heart and temporal arteries; at times tearing rheumatic pains in extremities relieve the heart; palpitation and trembling while sitting, < after drinking, at night; undulating or intermitting beats of heart; dysuria senilis; urine dark and of an offensive odor.

(Heart diseases) Kalmia - especially useful when gout or rheumatism, after external applications, shifts from joints to heart sharp, severe pains about heart, taking away the breath and shooting down into stomach and abdomen, with slow pulse (Dig.) and numb feeling in left arm. Pericarditis rheumatica, first stage, with tumultuous, rapid and visible beating of the heart, paroxysms of anguish with great dyspnoea, febrile excitement, pains in limbs, stitch in lower part of chest, right-sided face-ache; pressure as of a stone from epigastrium towards the heart, with a strong, quick heart-beat, > by sitting erect, < when bent over or lying on left side. Hypertrophy and valvular insufficiency, or thickening after rheumatism; arms feel numb and weak, limbs cold; weariness in all muscles, shuns all exertion; pulse slow and weak; albinuria; ascites.

(Heart diseases) Lithium carb. - hypertrophy from valvular deficiencies, especially of the aortic valves, in persons of a gouty diathesis; rheumatic soreness about heart; mental agitation causes fluttering of heart, < by bending forward; shocks and jerks about heart, > by urinating; finger-joints tender and painful; paralytic stiffness in all limbs and whole body.

(Insanity) Colchicum - gouty diathesis; alternately excited or depressed; loss of memory; great desire for mental and bodily rest; intense melancholia, peevish and dissatisfied.

(Iris, affections of) Colchicum - gouty or rheumatic iritis, with great soreness of eyeballs; violent, short, sharp, tearing pain in and around eyeball; excoriating lachrymation, < in open air.

(Kidney/bladder stone) Benzoic-acid. - nephritic colic; morbid condition of urine in persons with calculous or gouty diathesis; urine containing urates of ammonia and having a strong ammoniacal smell. Dysuria senilis from irritability of the bladder and mucopurulent discharge.

(Migraine) Sick-headache - gouty hemicrania: Colch., Coloc., Guaic., Kali-bi., Lyc., Magn.-mur., natr-m.

(Migraine) Colocynth - hemicrania from anger with indignation, after suppression of menses, pains extending towards forehead and left side of head, with nausea, vomiting or diarrhoea, especially towards evening; violent periodical or intermittent headache; bilious, gouty or nervous migraine (headache) of great severity.

(Migraine) Nux vomica - gouty and haemorrhoidal patients. attack sets in the morning when awaking, getting worse during the day; nausea and vomiting during attack; becoming often most severe in occiput; drawing, aching feeling as of a nail driven into the head, or as if the brain were dashed to pieces; face pale, or sallow on a red ground; < from mental exercise, by motion and by rest, from stimulants; patient irritable with his abdominal plethora.

(Nephritis) Colchicum - nephritis with bloody, ink-like, albinous urine, pain in renal region; urine turbid; leaves an orange-colored ring on vessel; after scarlatina or from gouty troubles.

(Nephritis) Kali-iod. - scanty dark urine; painful micturition; sediment dirty, yellowish, great thirst, heat in the head, deliria; granulated kidney from gout or mercurio-syphilis.

(Ophthalmia) Pulsatilla - blepharo-adenitis, with tendency to formation of styes and abscesses on the margin of lids, accompanied by acne on face; granular lids, dry, or with excessive bland secretion; pustular conjunctivitis, discharge thick, yellow, bland, profuse, > in open air, but not in wind; gonorrhoeal ophthalmia, when the gonorrhoea became suddenly suppressed; ophthalmia neonatorum, with profuse yellow, purulent discharge, gluing the lids; amblyopia from suppression of any bloody discharge, from gastric derangement, from metastasis of gout or rheumatism; fistula lachrymalis, discharging pus when pressed; frequent rubbing of eyes for relief.

(Paralysis) Alumina - locomotor ataxia; inability to walk except when the eyes are open and in daylight; loss of sensibility of feet; numbness of heel when stepping; tearing in thighs and legs when sitting or lying, < at night; pain in sole of foot on stepping, as if it were too soft and swollen; drawing pains in extremities; rheumatic and traumatic paralysis in gouty patients; palsy from spinal disease; arms feel heavy and go to sleep; lower limbs heavy, can scarcely drag them; feeling of weakness in bladder and genitals; bowels inactive; mistakes in speaking; consciousness of his identity confused; strength all exhausted after walking in fresh air, with yawning, stretching, drowsiness and inclination to lie down, which only increases the lassitude.

(Paralysis) Bryonia - paralysis, generally of both sides, in rheumatic and gouty patients; < from motion and contact; legs so weak they will scarcely hold him, knees totter and knock together when walking.

(Pericarditis) Colchicum - violent palpitations with anxiety, and sensation as if chest were squeezed by a tight bandage; vertigo on assuming upright position; palpitation and stitches about heart, loss of consciousness. effusion into pericardium, with heart's action muffled, indistinct, very weak; pulse threadlike, imperceptible-following gout or acute rheumatism; sharp, rending pains along sternum and into left shoulder; distressing restlessness and sleeplessness; hot, dry skin, vomiting and purging, with coated tongue and thirst.

(Rheumatism) Ant-crud. - acute and chronic rheumatism or gout; pains drawing, shooting, tensive; shortening of the muscles and tendons with bending of limbs and great tenderness and soreness of soles of feet, < by warm air and heat of sun; gastric symptoms, nausea, vomiting, white tongue, great thirst at night.

(Rheumatism) Apoc-andr. - rheumatism and gout; pain especially in right shoulder and knee; pains in the joint of the big toe; bilious vomiting, with or without diarrhoea; pain and stiffness in back of head and neck; dull heavy pain in chest, while breathing; rheumatic headaches; worse after sleep or continued quiet; joints feel stiff, especially on moving in the morning.

(Rheumatism) Benzoic-acid. - arthritis deformans; painful nodes in joints, especially in syphilitic or gonorrhoeal patients, with rheumatic diathesis; pains go from right to left side and from below upward; < from heat and joints cracking on motion; gout or rheumatism affecting heart or alternating one with the other; wandering pains, but most constant about heart; irritable bladder, freshly voided urine of strong ammoniacal smell and highly colored.

(Rheumatism) Calc-carb. - is the chronic rhus, and often comes in where the latter fails. rheumatism from working in water or by a long continuance in it; chronic cases with swelling of joints, < with every change of weather; crackling or crepitation of joints, as if they were dry; weakness and weariness of all the limbs; sensation of coldness on top of head; profuse sweat and cold, damp feet; omodynia in right shoulder or from left shoulder down left arm towards the heart; lumbago; cold feeling in various points, as gluteal region; pains confined to small spots; gouty nodosities about fingers; arthritis nodosa deformans.

(Rheumatism) China - later stages of inflammatory rheumatism, when the fever has become intermittent in its character, joints still swollen; jerking and pressing pains, excited by merely moving the affected part and gradually rising to a most fearful state, < at night and accompanied by a sensation of weakness in affected parts, < by contact more than by motion; rheumatic pains in metatarsal bones and phalanges; rheumatic gout.

(Rheumatism) Guaicum - follows well after caust. when there are contractions of tendons, drawing the limbs out of shape, < by any attempt at motion, in daytime, > by warmth, particularly where there are well-developed gouty nodosities on the joints; pains in all joints, even in chest; tearing, drawing lancinations; followed by exhaustion; syphilitic and mercurial dyscrasia.

(Rheumatism) Ledum - arthritic nodosities, with violent pains; growing < in evening, or at night when getting warm in bed and last till midnight; gout and rheumatism affecting the smaller joints where cellular tissue is wanting; < by motion; pains travel upward; oedema of feet; blisters on heels, acute tearing pains in joints, with great weakness of limbs, and numbness and coldness of surface; rheumatic or gouty inflammation of the great toe, with scanty effusion, which tends to harden into nodosities; < at night, from warmth of bed and covering up, > by cold; boring pains in bones; stiffness affecting the muscles of back, neck and loins; pains change location quickly, accompanied by little or no swelling; rheumatic pains in joints of arms; emaciation; coldness of affected parts; erythema nodosum, < in cold damp weather.

(Rheumatism) Menyanthes - painful spasmodic jerking of lower extremities, from hip down; stitching pains in gouty persons, with calcareous deposits in joints.

(Rheumatism) Silicea - chronic hereditary rheumatism and gouty nodosities, causing such tenderness of soles that patient cannot walk (Ant-crud.); shoulder pains, < at night and by uncovering (Led., opposite); rheumatism of lower cervical vertebrae; violent tearing between shoulder-blades; pressure and tension in small of back; stiff back after sitting; coccyx hurts after riding; drawing in limbs with tearing and sticking pains in joints, < after motion.

(Sciatica) Anantherum - sciatic, gouty and rheumatic pains in legs and feet, especially in heels; stiffness, lancinating and crampy pains in sacrum and iliac bones; offensive foot-sweat.

(Synovitis) Pulsatilla - joint swollen, with sharp, erratic pains, accompanied by a feeling of soreness or of subcutaneous ulceration; tearing, stinging, erratic pains force the patient to move the affected joint, > by pressure and slowly moving about, jerking pains down the limbs, < evening and from warmth, > by cold; gonorrhoeal or traumatic synovitis or gouty, especially in affections of the knee, ankle and tarsal joints.

(Syphilis and sycosis) Causticum - vesicles under prepuce changing into suppurating ulcers; phagedenic chancre; watery, greenish, corroding discharge with jerking pains; chancre with fungous excrescences; buboes secreting an acrid, corrosive ichor, with systemic complications, such as scurvy or gout.

(Tympanitis) Colchicum - great distention of abdomen with gas, as if he had eaten too much, contracts spasmodically when touched, > from bending double; metastasis of gout.

(Urinary difficulties) Benzoic-acid. - vesicular catarrh; irritability of the bladder; nocturnal enuresis in children; too frequent desire to evacuate the bladder, urine being normal; decrease of the quantity of urine, which is thick and bloody; urine has strong odor like that of horses and contains excess of hippuric acid (Nitr-ac.); urine brownish, cloudy, alkaline or dark-reddish, high specific gravity and acid reaction, sometimes of a putrid, cadaverous smell; morbid condition of urine, as in persons with calculous or gouty diathesis; dysuria senilis, when gravel is trifling and the irritable state of bladder and pains are induced by other causes, with too frequent desire to urinate, though urine appears normal.

(Urinary difficulties) Colchicum - constant burning in urinary organs, with diminished secretion; passing of urine attended and followed by tenesmus of bladder and burning pain in urethra as if urine were very warm; frequent micturition with diminished discharge; urethra hurts while urine passes, as if raw; constriction in neck of bladder; feeling of soreness in kidneys, < by straightening out legs, > by doubling them upon himself, has to keep quiet to prevent vomiting; feeling of icy coldness in stomach with nausea; brown-black urine; whitish deposit in urine; gouty diathesis.

(Vision complaints) Pulsatilla - amblyopia from suppression of any bloody discharge; from metastasis of gout or rheumatism; from gastric derangement; with heart disease; with coexisting diminished hearing; diminished sight especially on getting warm from exercise; blindness at twilight and sensation as if the eyes were bandaged; shining or flashing rings before eyes; mistiness of sight or sensation as if the dimness could be removed by wiping; frequent and copious lachrymation.

Treatment of chronic diseases—Miasms—Psora, Sycosis, Syphilis—Constitutional treatment—Generals—General symptoms

We make the prescription based on symptoms.

1. Felt and reported by the patient (subjective symptoms).
2. Observed by the practitioner and/or reported by the relatives/attendant, lab. findings (objective symptoms).
3. Constitutional symptoms: *i.e.* symptoms elicited by our questioning about the patient's past health history and that of his family.

If the routine or usual repertorisation as described in the preceding pages does not help, we must question the health history of the patient's family. This is more particularly in the case of chronic diseases, *e.g.,* diabetes that does not respond to insulin and other allopathic drugs etc.

How to treat the 'Constitution'?

You must ask the patient as under:

"In your family... ('family' means your brothers/sisters, their children; your parents, their brothers/sisters and their children; your grand parents, their brothers/sisters and their children) is (or was) there:

1. Diabetes, heart complaints, still birth, epilepsy, mind derangement (insanity, suicidal disposition etc.), migraine, sciatica, allergy, lesions, tonsillitis, thyroid? If any one or more of these complaints are in the family, you must write the word 'syphilis' on the case sheet.

   Apart from the above, if two or more family members are having one and the same complaint *e.g.,* cancer, baldness, migraine etc. it is also 'syphilis'.

2. Tonsillitis, thyroid, spondylitis and all bone complaints (except nightly boring pain in bones). If there are anyone or more of these complaints, you must write the word 'scrofula' on the case sheet. Suppose in a family if two or more members had thyroid complaint what is to be done? Because Thyroid = scrofula More than one family member having thyroid = syphilis In such a case we must keep both 'scrofula' and 'syphilis' in mind. For example (Lilienthal—page 943-949) under the remedy *Nitric-acid* we find the following:

   "scrofulosis from hereditary syphilis".

   i. For treating patients with diabetes/migraine/sciatica/ mental derangement/heart complaints/suicidal disposition/still birth/abortion/ epilepsy/lesions, boring pain in bones, vision complaints etc., you must take the 48 remedies given against SYPHILIS in Kent's Repertory—Generalities section.

   ii. For treating chronic tonsillitis/thyroid complaints, (other than boring pain in bones) first take the remedies given against "SCROFULOSIS—glandular affections" on page 943 of Lilienthal.

iii. For treating bone complaints (other than nightly boring pain in bone) first take the 15 remedies given against "SCROFULOSIS—affections of bones", (see page 943 of Lilienthal).

iv. In respect of children with birth defects or whose complaints are from birth or within nine months of birth—it is *syphilis* (in fact, all complaints from birth is *syphilis*) and also epilepsy since childhood where E.E.G. (electro encephalogram) report reads "epileptogenic regions seen" (is also *syphilis*.) For all these we must, first of all, take the twelve remedies given against "SYPHILIS—Infantile syphilis". (see page 1021 of Lilienthal)

In chronic diseases, after taking one of the respective above lists, compare it with other mind/general symptoms of the patient.

The symptoms on which we have to work out the case are: (i) Rare, strange, peculiar or uncommon (ii) Mind symptoms (iii) General symptoms. In respect of mind symptoms, it is difficult to classify a symptom as 'common' or 'uncommon'.

Also, there are 'grades' in the value of mind symptoms. In order of their importance are:

Will (Desires/aversions, arising independent of causation).

Intellect, Memory, All 'will' symptoms are uncommon, because the meaning of will is: "Faculty by which a person decides independent of causation" (Oxford). (Therefore 'will' symptoms are 'uncommon') Be that as it may.

In respect of (iii) above, *i.e.* 'general symptoms' ('generals' is different from 'general symptoms' and we shall elaborate on this later) we do not have any difficulty. Because here the question of 'common' or 'uncommon' does not arise.

"General symptoms" are those that do not belong to a particular part of body but pertain to the patient as a whole. Such general symptoms which are frequently useful in practice are: SLEEP, DREAMS. These do not belong to any part of the body. Sexual behaviour and sexual symptoms are generals because they affect the person as a whole though we call sexual parts. Ulcers, Unhealthy skin (slight wounds do not heal or ulcerate or suppurate etc.) Bathing, dread of Congestions (Let us now see when and where we would be using this rubric in Kent's Repertory under the last chapter *Generalities*. Whenever a patient gets a symptom in one organ while some other (in many cases, distant) part is exerted or diseased. E.g., cough with pain in chest. Excitement/emotion causes loose bowel movement or urging to urinate. In these cases YOU SHOULD NOT LOOK INTO THE REPERTORY FOR "Diarrhoea aggravated by emotion" but use the rubric CONGESTION under GENERALITIES in Kent's Repertory. Other examples are: Breast painful before menses. Mental tension causes eruption on skin, etc. Also, two or more complaints co-existing in one and the same part of body *e.g.,* vertigo and headache. For this you should not consider the rubric 'Vertigo' and 'Headache' but consider HEAD—CONGESTION.

Similarly pain, swelling, itching etc. all the three coexisting in leg. For this take the rubric CONGESTION in the chapter GENERALITIES.

Let us now list below other general symptoms more frequently useful. (Most of the rubrics under GENERALITIES in Kent's Repertory are general symptoms)

Mucous secretions (Profuse discharge from coryza or expectoration, frequent diarrhoea). For these, instead of looking under NOSE or DIARRHOEA you must take this rubric.

Aversion to or craving for a particular item of food.

Abscess.

Air, open, desire for.

Air, seashore agg.

Anaemia.

Analgesia (If injured or beaten up by others does not feel the pain— insensible to pain.).

Anxiety general physical.

Bathing, dread of.

Blackness of external parts.

Caries of bones.

Catalepsy.

Change of weather agg.

Chlorosis (complaints that are chronic and dating back to the onset of puberty.) Chlorosis is caused by tuberculosis in the family. When tuberculosis affects lungs we call it *phthisis pulmonum*. When it affects glands/bones it is called 'scrofula'. All chronic diseases dating back to puberty are due to tuberculosis and the term for this is "chlorosis".

Coition, after agg. Cold, tendency to take. Color and consistency of discharges. Constriction. Contradictory and alternating states. Convulsions. Convulsive movements. Cyanosis. Dropsy. Emissions agg. Faintness. Fasting, while: Food, milk agg. HEAT, flushes of. HEAT, sensation of. HEAVINESS HUNGER, from. INDURATIONS. INFLAMMATION. INJURIES, extravasations with. IRRITABILITY, excessive physical. IRRITABILITY, lack of. JAR, stepping agg. JERKING. LASSITUDE. LEAN people. LEUKAEMIA. LIFTING straining of muscles and tendons, from. LOSS of fluids. MENSES, after, before MENSES, at beginning of MENSES, during MENSES, amel. MENSES, after MERCURY, abuse of.

METASTASIS. MOONLIGHT agg. MOTION amel. MOTION at beginning of, agg. MOTION aversion to. MOTION continued, amel. MUCOUS secretions increased. NARCOTICS agg. NECROSIS bones. NON-UNION of bones. NUMBNESS externally. NURSING children. OBESITY OLD age, premature OLD people. ONANISM, from PAIN, bones PAIN, boring PAIN, burning externally PAIN, burning, internally. PAIN, constricting externally PAIN, constricting internally PAIN, drawing. PAIN, paralytic PAIN, paralytic internally.

PAINLESSNESS of complaints usually painful. PARALYSIS agitans. PARALYSIS internally. PARALYSIS organs, of. PARALYSIS, painless PERIODICITY. PERSPIRATION gives no relief. PERSPIRATION suppression of. PLETHORA. POLYPUS (Abnormal growth of soft tumour). PULSE QUININE, abuse of REACTION, lack of RELAXATION of muscles. SCURVY (Nutritional Disease), scorbutus SENSITIVENESS, externally. SENSITIVENESS, internally SENSITIVENESS, to pain. SEPTICAEMIA (Blood-Poisoning). SEXUAL excesses, after SHOCKS from injury.

SHOCKS electric-like. SIDE, symptoms on one side. SIDE, crosswise, left upper and right lower. SIDE, left lower and right upper. SLEEP, before, agg. SLEEP, at beginning of, agg. SLEEP, during, agg. SLEEP, after, agg. SLEEP, long agg. SLEEP, loss of, from. SLOW repair of broken bones. SYCOSIS. SYPHILIS. TREMBLING. ULCERS, cancerous. UNCOVERING agg. UNDRESSING, after, agg. VACCINATION, after. VARICOSE veins. WARM, room agg. WEAKNESS, enervation. WEAKNESS, paralytic. WINTER, in. WOUNDS, slow to heal, constitutional effects (chronic effects).

Some more general symptoms are: puberty, menopause, complaint in wisdom teeth, teething, pregnancy. The best time for constitutional treatment for a woman is during pregnancy. Altered color and consistency of discharges or secretions are also general symptoms.

Scrofulosis: Chronic bedwetting, Chronic tonsilittis, thyroid complaints, spondylitis are known as scrofulosis.

1, Sulph., Calc.; 2, Alnus-rub., Asa., Aur., Bad., Bar., Bell., Berb-aquif., Calc-ars., Calc-carb., Calc-phos., Calc-mur., Cist., Con., Graph., Hep., Hydrast, Iod., Lyc., Merc., Mez., Natr-m., Pinus, Phyt., Rhus, Rumex., Sep., Sil., Stilling., Therid., Thuj.

—**glandular affections:** Bar., Bell., Calc., Carb-an., Cist., Clem., Con., Dulc., Graph., Hep., Kali, Lapis, Lyc., Merc., Nitr-ac., Phos., Rhus, Sil., Staph., Sulph.

—**BONES, affections:** Asa., Aur., Bell., Calc., Cist., Hep., Merc., Mez., Nitr-ac., Phos., Rhus, Ruta, Sil., Staph., Sulph.

—**potbelliedness of children:** Ars., Bar., Bell., Calc., Cina, Lyc., Rhus, Sulph.

—at commencement of disease, when children have **great difficulty in learning to walk:** Bell., Calc., China, Cina, Fer., Lyc., Pinus, Puls., Sil., Sulph.

—**cutaneous affections (scrofulodermata):** Aur., Bar., Berb.-aquif., Calc., Cist., Clem., Con., Dulc., Hep., Lapis, Merc., Mez., Nitr-ac., Ol-jec., Petr., Ran., Rhus, Sil., Sulph.

Chronic Rheumatism, Rheumatic constitution/ Diathesis

Abies nigra - rheumatic pains and aching in bones; Abrotanum - painful, inflammatory rheumatism before swelling; Abrotanum - rheumatism from suddenly checked diarrhoea, cannot move her head, arms or limbs, and suffers much pain, no swelling; Actea spic - impatient and restless—rheumatism; Actea spic - rheumatic diathesis; Actea spic - rheumatism showing itself partly in small joints; pains in wrists or finger joints, very tender to touch, excruciating, < at night.

Agaricus - muscles feel bruised from touch; > from walking — chronic rheumatism.

Agnus castus - inflammatory, rheumatic swelling of joints.

Aletris - chronic rheumatism.

Alfalfa - the rheumatic diathesis seems especially amenable to its action.

Anagallis - rheumatic and gouty pains.

Angustura - rheumatic and paralytic complaints.

Ant-crud. - metastasis of gout and rheumatism causing gastric catarrh.

Ant-crud. - rheumatism and gout if parts are inflamed or swollen.

Anthrokokali - chronic rheumatism, gout, caries, scrofulosis.

Ant-tart. - acute articular rheumatism.

Ant-tart. - joints somewhat swollen, reddened, hot; very painful at every attempt to move them—rheumatism.

Ant-tart. - shifting rheumatism.

Apis - muscles stiff, tender on pressure, somewhat swollen; rigid; rheumatic inflammation.

Apocynum can. - rheumatic stiffness.

Arg-met. - articular rheumatism without swelling.

Arg-met. - man, aged 26, robust, active, intelligent; red hair, white skin, marked rheumatic diathesis.

Arnica - gout and rheumatism.

Arsenic alb. - tearing, burning pain in limbs, particularly in joints, with pale swelling of affected parts, preventing sleep — rheumatism.

Arsenic alb. - tearing, drawing pains in all joints of left side, with swelling; joints of fingers and left hand deformed, contracted, immovable - rheumatism.

Ars-sul-fl. - pain in joints - rheumatism.

Ars-sul-rub. - rheumatic symptoms first twenty-four hours after taking medicine in morning.

Asclepias syr. - acute rheumatism, confined to large joints, with much pain and swelling.

Asclepias syr. - chronic rheumatism.

Asclepias tub. - aching in bones and rheumatic pains in limbs, most in joints; almost always upper left and lower right or opposite.

Asclepias tub. - muscular and articulate rheumatism, with stitching pains, dark red urine and hot perspiring skin.

Asclepias tub - rheumatic pains in joints.

Atropinum sul. - rheumatic fever.

Aurum met. - rheumatism appears on back, sacrum, hands and feet, after the heat is relieved.

Aurum met. - rheumatism, erratic; attacking the heart.

Aurum met. - woman, aged 55, after third week of rheumatic fever - endocarditis.

Aurum mur. - a stout young man, subject to rheumatic attacks - endocarditis.

Aurum mur. - violent rheumatic fever, with painful swelling of joints; leaving joints and attacking heart.

Aurum mur. - woman, aged 40, after rheumatism and endocarditis, fatty degeneration - stenocardia.

Badiaga - chronic rheumatism.

Baptisia - stiffness of all joints, as though strained; rheumatic pains and soreness all over body.

Belladonna - rheumatic and gouty complaints, with inflammation and swelling.

Benzoic-acid. - rheumatic diathesis in syphilitic or gonorrhoeal patients.

Berberis vul. - hepatic, arthritic, and rheumatic affections, particularly with urinary, hemorrhoidal or menstrual complaints.

Berberis vul. - male, aged 34; for years indigestion from chronic gastritis, reduced in weight, pale, discouraged; after improvement by lycop; rheumatism of knee.

Berberis vul. - muscular rheumatism in chest, lumbar region, and upper and lower limbs.

Berberis vul. - rheumatic and gouty complaints, with diseases of urinary organs.

Bryonia - fixed, acute rheumatism, aggravated by motion; travels slowly from joint to joint.

Bryonia - rheumatism, muscular and articular.

Bryonia - rheumatism, with redness and swelling of joints; motion is intolerable.

Bryonia - soreness appears to be sheath of tendon, but principally in periosteum and ligaments; there do not appear to be that swelling of joints, stiffness and dread of motion that usually characterize rheumatism; but motion always increases pain.

Cactus - emaciation —low fever —rheumatic heart disease.

Cactus - feels she is dying and thinks she will not live till morning, but has no fear of death - cardiac rheumatism.

Cactus - man, aged 28, during service in our war, articular rheumatism in back and limbs; mustered out as incurable cactus 1 - cardiac rheumatism.

Cactus - miss, aged 60 cactus, (20) three doses —cardiac rheumatism.

Cactus - rheumatism of all joints of limbs, great deal of pain, stiffness and swelling; worse, in evening and again mornings on first rising —pain in heart.

Cactus - screaming with pains, or complete loss of consciousness - cardiac rheumatism.

Cactus - thinks she will not recover; weeps much; despondent - cardiac rheumatism.

Cactus - woman, aged 60, stout, robust, after exposure to water in cellar - rheumatism.

Cactus - woman, aged 28, tall, dark hair and eyes - rheumatic disease of heart cactus, (800) one dose followed by rapid improvement, without return of symptoms.

Calc-carb. - black hair, dark complexion, blue eyes - rheumatism

Calc-carb. - rheumatism - goitre.

Calc-carb. - with rheumatic pains hard welts are to be felt in muscles.

Calc-fluor. - a man, aged 50, blonde, lymphatic; for 10 years rheumatic arthritis; articular exostoses on fingers, feet and knees; after partial relief by Bryon and Calc-ostr, Calc-fluor (12), the supernumerary bones disappeared —osseous growths.

Calc-phos. - a constituent of teeth, bones, connective tissue and blood corpuscles, and to be given in corresponding disturbances,; in true chlorosis from anemia; chronic swelling of glands; chronic articular rheumatism; gout; exostoses, osteophytes and similar new growths on bone; scrofulosis; suppuration of bones and joints; dropsy from loss of blood or of other fluids, or depending on diseases of heart, liver and kidneys.

Calc-phos. - rheumatic pains in joints and various parts of body.

Calc-sul. - acute and chronic rheumatism.

Camphor - rheumatic fevers; pains changing place, persistently return.

Capsicum - chronic muscular rheumatism in patients of sedentary habits.

Carbo-veg. - cholera asiatica; yellow fever; typhus; epilepsy; rheumatism.

Carbon-sul. - chronic rheumatism, sensitive and cold.

Carbon-sul. - chronic rheumatic and arthritic affections, which, of themselves, are without fever.

Carbon-sul. - rheumatism and gout; after the relief of acute and inflammatory conditions.

Caulophyllum - rheumatism, particularly of small joints, which has a tendency to shift.

Causticum - manifests its action mainly in chronic rheumatic, arthritic and paralytic affections, indicated by the tearing, drawing pains in the muscular and fibrous tissues, with deformities about the joints; progressive loss of muscular strength, tendinous contractures.

Causticum - rheumatic and arthritic inflammations, with contraction of flexors and stiffness of joints.

Chamomilla - a girl, aged 20, robust build, short in stature, quiet, even temperament; rheumatism.

Chamomilla - adults, even aged persons with arthritic or rheumatic diathesis.

Chamomilla - muscular or articular rheumatism, with great nervous excitability.

Chamomilla - rheumatism; drawing, tearing pains, accompanied by sensation of lameness or numbness; pain more in tendons, ligaments and bones (not in muscles), without swelling of parts; pain < at night; they do not change location.

Chelidonium - a bleacher, aged 50, who had to watch bleaching ground, every other night, summer and winter, was attacked with rheumatism, finally amaurosis.

Chelidonium - a girl, aged 6; rheumatism.

Chelidonium - a widow, aged 44, ceased menstruating for seven years, has suffered from rheumatism in hands, the wrists particularly swollen and painful on change of weather a year ago, ten weeks ill of pneumonia for last nine weeks, prosopalgia.

Chelidonium - in rheumatic and gouty affections of single joints or nerve branches, with frequent headache, attacks of vertigo, dimness of vision.

Chelidonium - mr w, shopkeeper, aged 30; acute rheumatism.

Chelidonium - mrs e b, aged 23, blonde complexion, healthy and strong; acute rheumatism.

Chelidonium - muscular and articular rheumatism; the least touch on any part of body is exceedingly painful.

Chimaphila umb. - useful in scrofula and chronic, rheumatic, and nephritic affections.

China - a thin, weakly woman; rheumatic ophthalmia during confinement.

China - hannah p, aged about 35, complexion dark, medium height, had a child five weeks ago, and had for some months past pain in loins; never had rheumatism; heart normal; acute dropsy following parturition.

China - lymphatic, scrofulous woman; rheumatic ophthalmia during lactation.

China - man, aged 40, subject to hemorrhoids; rheumatism of thigh.

China - man, aged 70; nocturnal rheumatism in hip.

China - rheumatic, hard, red, inflammatory swellings; painful to touch, not to pressure.

China - woman, aged 52; rheumatism.

China-ars. - lady, aged 58; hydrogenoid constitution; rheumatic headache.

China-sulph. - a man, aged 34; acute rheumatism.

Chloralum - rheumatism and gout.

Cimicifuga - chorea from rheumatic irritation.

Cimicifuga - rheumatic persons.

Clematis - rheumatic and gouty affections of joints; catarrhal and rheumatic affections of bladder; rheumatic affections of eyes and ears.

Coca - rheumatism, coming on from slightest cold.

Cocculus - g, aged 43, strong, muscular, formerly suffered from rheumatic pains in limbs; rheumatic ophthalmia.

Cocculus - girl, aged 19; acute articular rheumatism.

Cocculus - man, aged 34, had scabies all over, later rheumatism of l. arm, also had pneumonia; heart disease.

Cochlearia - rheumatism, wandering, chronic.

Colchicum - boy, aged 10, subject to frequent attacks of rheumatism, has for last fourteen days been suffering from rheumatic fever; pericarditis.

Colchicum - emaciated, sensitive individuals, disposed to rheumatism and catarrh.

Colchicum - emaciation, oedema, anasarca, complicated with rheumatism.

Colchicum - gastric rheumatic genus epidemicus.

Colchicum - m, aged 30, male; rheumatism.

Colchicum - m, aged 65, coachman; rheumatism.

Colchicum - male, aged 46; acute articular rheumatism.

Colchicum - muscular rheumatism and loss of muscular power.

Colchicum - rheumatism: articular, acute or chronic; with or without fever; after getting thoroughly wet; complicated with gastric affections; occurring immediately after moist weather; in later stages.

Colchicum - woman, aged 55; rheumatism.

Colocynth - a young countryman, aged 18, had suffered for several weeks; rheumatic sciatica.

Colocynth - boy, aged 13, after catching cold; rheumatism.

Colocynth - man, aged 34, suffering for eight days from periodical recurrence of pain in right eye; rheumatic inflammation of eye.

Colocynth - potter, aged 40, had rheumatism and lead colic, suffering all winter and spring; lumbago.

Colocynth - rheumatic and arthritic conditions; coxalgia.

Colocynth - rheumatic or gouty rheumatic diathesis.

Colocynth - seldom indicated in rheumatism, is, however, useful in rheumatoid pains or pains along course of sciatic nerve, from reflex nervous action, during or after an attack of rheumatism.

Comocladia - rheumatic pains and swellings, < by rest, > by continued motion.

Copaiva - gonorrhoeal rheumatism.

Crotalus hor. - rheumatic, gouty, albuminuric, or amenorrheic subjects.

Croton tig. - farmer, aged 40, formerly healthy; rheumatism.

Daphne indica - rheumatic and arthritic pains, especially after suppressed gonorrhoea.

Daphne indica - rheumatic and gouty affections in muscles and bones.

Digitalis - woman, aged 50, unmarried, sentimental and very excitable, rheumatic tendency; palpitation of heart.

Dolichos - woman, unmarried, aged 36, suffered from chronic rheumatism; skin disease.

Dulcamara - anasarca after fever and ague, scarlatina, or rheumatic fever.

Dulcamara - chronic rheumatism, < from a little exposure to cold, or any change of temperature from warm to cold; rheumatic pains after acute cutaneous eruptions, or when chronic form alternates with attacks of intestinal catarrh.

Dulcamara - woman, aged 35; another, aged 63; muscular rheumatism.

Elaps - man, aged 61, rheumatic symptoms in legs; amaurosis.

Elaps - rheumatic constitutions.

Eugenia jambos - rheumatic pain wanders from place to place, with catarrh.

Euonymus - chronic rheumatism and gout.

Eupatorium perf. - rheumatism and gouty affection.

Eupatorium pur. - through the spinal nervous system it produces a state of muscular system similar to rheumatism; it probably affects the anterior portion of spinal cord the most.

Ferrum iod. - rheumatism without fever.

Ferrum met. - man, aged 45, dyer, thin, muscular, choleric, dark complexion; rheumatism.

Ferrum mur. - scrofula; rheumatism; rachitis and emaciation.

Ferrum phos. - boy, aged 5, very fair; pleurisy and rheumatism.

Ferrum phos. - rheumatic fevers; acute articular rheumatism.

Ferrum phos. - woman, aged 37; nervous temperament; acute rheumatism.

Formica - rheumatic affections; so-called rheumatic inflammation of eyes; aural affections and sequela.

Formica rufa - chronic arthritis following an attack of acute rheumatic fever shows also remarkable results although often pains of a neuralgic character persisting in certain spots are very stubborn.

Gambogia - feeling of soreness all over body; rheumatism.

Gelsemium - pains in back, shoulders, neck and occiput, preceding or following attacks of ague; also when these or similar pains are of a neuralgic nature, arising from some form of spinal irritation, or come on as the result of a cold, having something of a rheumatic character.

Geranium - of use in sub-acute and chronic rheumatism.

Glycerinum - chronic muscular rheumatism of back and neck.

Guaiacum - acts especially upon muscular tissues, producing rheumatic and arthritic pains.

Guaiacum - rheumatic affection, especially in syphilitic and mercurial patients.

Guaiacum officinale - chief action on fibrous tissue, and is especially adapted to the arthritic diathesis, rheumatism, and tonsillitis.

Hamamelis - rheumatism with great soreness of affected parts.

Helonias - rheumatism.

Hepar sul. - rheumatic swelling, with heat, redness and sensation as if sprained.

Hepar sul. - woman, aged 33, suffered severely from rheumatic pains, no history of syphilis; keratitis parenchymatosa.

Hydrastis - man, aged 46, during crimean campaign was attacked with rheumatic fever, consequent upon exposure; anasarca and constipation.

Hydrocotyle - rheumatic disorders.

Hyoscyamus - boy, aged 13; rheumatic endocarditis.

Ichthyolum - chronic rheumatism.

Ictodes - chronic rheumatism.

Indigo - rheumatic and gouty affections of nerves and joints, accompanied by slight fever and great debility.

Iodum - girl, aged 12, during attack of rheumatism; threatened inflammation of brain.

Jacaranda - gonorrhoeal rheumatism.

Kali ars. - rheumatic, gouty and syphilitic pains.

Kali-bich. - catarrh alternating with rheumatic pains.

Kali-bich. - man, aged 24, has gastric and rheumatic troubles; pain in back.

Kali-bich. - man, aged 40, in bad health for two years, has had rheumatic gout and rheumatic iritis; inflammation of eyes.

Kali-bich. - man, aged 50, rheumatic; general pains.

Kali-bich. - man, aged 62; chronic rheumatism.

Kali-bich. - rheumatism alternating with gastric symptoms, one appearing in the fall, the other in spring.

Kali-bich. - woman, aged 60, weak, rheumatic, for several weeks has been suffering from sudden and profuse discharges of clear, watery fluid from nose which suddenly ceased; affection of oesophagus.

Kali-carb. - chronic catarrh, ozaena, with rheumatism or gout.

Kali-carb. - farmer, aged 40; rheumatism.

Kali-carb. - rheumatism, often attacking heart, generally going from upper to lower parts; painful swelling; gout.

Kali-carb. - woman, aged 45, hard of hearing, rheumatic; gastric disorder.

Kali-iod. - chronic periosteal rheumatism of syphilitic or mercurial origin; intolerable nocturnal bone pains, driving patient to despair.

Kali-iod. - gout and rheumatism; synovitis.

Kali-mur. - inflammation of serous membranes in second stage of peritonitis, pleuritis and pericarditis; acute articular rheumatism and inflammation of lungs.

Kali-nit. - acute rheumatism, with endocarditis.

Kali-phos. - rheumatism, acute and chronic, with pains disappearing on moving about, severe in morning after rest, and on first rising from sitting position.

Kali-sulph. - man, aged 26, healthy, powerful; articular rheumatism.

Kali-sulph. - migratory rheumatism of joints.

Kalmia - acute rheumatism, going from joint to joint; violent fever; pains intense; ankles most painful and swollen; < from least movement.

Kalmia - boy, aged 12; rheumatism.

Kalmia - dropsy from cold with rheumatic complaints.

Kalmia - every joint and every muscle of body affected; high fever; every attempt to move attended with excruciating pains; afterwards paralysis of arms and legs - rheumatism.

Kalmia - man, aged 47, rheumatic; pressure in epigastrium.

Kalmia - pains shifting, pains suddenly changing position; tendency to metastasis to heart - rheumatism.

Kalmia - young german; chronic rheumatism.

Kreosotum - rheumatic pains in joints, also stitches, most of hip and knee; numbness of whole limb as if asleep.

Kreosotum - woman, aged 41; rheumatism.

Lac-can. - neuralgia and acute pains; rheumatism; gout; syphilitic sciatica; sexual debility.

Lac-can. - woman, after exposure to draft; acute rheumatism.

Lac-can. - woman, aged 50, suffers after each attack of quinsy; acute rheumatism.

Lachesis - affections of meagre, weak, melancholy persons, or of those who are chlorotic, with sickly complexion; women at climacteric period, with frequent metrorrhagia and hot flushes, burning vertex, headaches, pain in back, or hot flushes by day and cold flashes by night, insomnia, < in afternoon, evening and after sleep; throat diseases commence on left side rheumatism on right.

Lachesis - woman, aged 51, after sudden suppression of menses by a mental emotion; rheumatism of vagus.

Lactic acid. - articular rheumatism; dissolves many generals, rare-strange peculiars:

Lactic acid. - kidney affections; croup; diphtheria; morning sickness of pregnancy; emaciation; rheumatism.

Laurocerasus - boy, aged 13, had rheumatism; disease of heart.

Ledum - farmer, aged 50; rheumatism in hip.

Ledum - man, aged 49; rheumatic ophthalmia.

Ledum - needle-woman, aged 24, two years married, healthy and robust; rheumatism.

Ledum - rheumatic, gouty diathesis; constitutions abuse by alcohol.

Ledum - young man; haemoptysis alternating with rheumatism.

Ledum - affects especially the rheumatic diathesis, going through all the changes, from functional pain to altered secretions and deposits of solid, earthy matter in the tissues.

Lithium carb. - chronic rheumatism connected with heart lesions and asthenopia offer a field for this remedy.

Lycopodium - boy, aged 12; rheumatism.

Lycopodium - man, aged 37; rheumatism; another, aged 37, frequently tapped; ascites.

Lycopodium - man, aged 38, rheumatism ten years ago; chronic rheumatism.

Lycopodium - man, aged 40, psoric, after rheumatic catarrhal affection ran splinter into finger; affection of hand and arm.

Lycopodium - man, aged 60, brunette, large, strong; rheumatism.

Lycopodium - the pains are drawing in character and seem to be? Between the bones and skin? Pains < rainy or stormy weather and by cold; > by warmth and particularly by lying in bed; rheumatic tension and tearing in joints of upper and lower extremities, so that she cannot do anything, as if paralyzed; stiffness of limbs and coldness of feet - chronic rheumatism.

Lycopodium - woman, aged 30, sanguine temperament, lively disposition, suffering with rheumatism, headache and congestions; hemorrhage after abortion.

Lycopodium - woman, aged 40, sanguine temperament, in youth affected with glandular swelling after catching cold; rheumatism.

Lycopodium - woman, aged 50, not menstruated for two years, after catching cold three years ago; rheumatism.

Lycopodium - woman, aged 50; rheumatism.

Lycopodium - young woman, fair complexion, sanguine, lymphatic temperament; intermittent rheumatic pains.

Lycopus - rheumatoid pains; erratic, but returning to original location; > from warmth; < from cold air and movement.

Lyssin. - felt same rheumatic pain his brother complained of — lyssophobia.

Magnesia-carb. - rheumatic affection of groups of muscles and of joints.

Medorrhinum - a maiden lady, no suspicion of sycotic poisoning, a long line of ancestors had rheumatism and gout; chronic rheumatism.

Medorrhinum - man, aged 20, gonorrhoea nine months ago, used injections eight months; gonorrhoeal rheumatism.

Medorrhinum - man, aged 60, suffering six months; rheumatism.

Medorrhinum - man, aged 60; sequela of rheumatism.

Medorrhinum - sequela of acute articular rheumatism; walks leaning on a cane, bent over; muffled in wraps to ears, looking like a broken down man apparently soon to fall into his grave.

Merc-cor. - man, athletic build, five days after suppression of gonorrhoeal discharge by large doses of balsam Copaiva; rheumatism.

Merc-iod-rub. - a servant girl, after washing floor; rheumatic affection.

Merc-sol. - girl, aged 19, strong, blonde, blue eyes, delicate skin; rheumatic ophthalmia.

Merc-sol. - gouty and rheumatic pains, with sweats without relief.

Merc-sol. - man, aged 30, sanguine nervous temperament, delicate complexion and body, has lived for some time in brazil; syphilitic ophthalmia and rheumatism.

- Merc-sol. - man, aged 30, subject to rheumatism and gastric and intermittent fevers; typhoid fever.
- Merc-sol. - man, aged 35, robust, after catching cold; rheumatic fever.
- Merc-sol. - man, aged 40; rheumatism of shoulder.
- Merc-sol. - man, aged 41; muscular rheumatism.
- Merc-sol. - rheumatic-catarrhal inflammations, with disposition to sweat.
- Merc-sol. - rheumatism, especially in cases of syphilitic origin or complication, affecting joints, bones, or periosteum, swelling of joints, pale or slightly red, puffy or oedematous; pains tearing, drawing, shooting, pressing; in bones as if broken; in joints as if sprained; < evenings and at night, and insupportable in heat of bed; accompanied by profuse sweat (often sour or offensive smelling) without > pains.
- Merc-sol. - woman, aged 27, unmarried, subject every autumn to attacks of angina; rheumatic pains.
- Merc-sol. - woman, aged 36, unmarried, suffering three months from pain in stomach; rheumatism.
- Merc-sol. - woman, aged 50, married seven years, no children, nervous temperament, had rheumatism in her youth; toothache.
- Merc-sol. - woman, aged 50; rheumatism.
- Merc-sol. - woman, aged 53, sick last four years; rheumatism.
- Merc-sol. - woman, delicate, psoric; rheumatic ophthalmia.
- Mercurialis perennis - rheumatic affections, acute, subacute or chronic, particularly when pericardium or heart are sympathetically affected; rheumatic affection of muscular coats of stomach, of intestinal canal and bladder; rheumatic pains in head and limbs, accompanied by disturbance of vision or with a melancholic or hypochondriacal mood.

Mercurius-sul. - rheumatic pains.

Millefolium - rheumatic and arthritic complaints.

Natrum mur. - man, aged 29, suffering several years; rheumatic, catarrhal inflammation of eyes.

Natrum mur. - patient, aged 20, after an attack of inflammatory rheumatism during childhood; strabismus.

Natrum mur. - rheumatic affections, with shortening of tendons.

Natrum phos. - rheumatic arthritis.

Nux mos. - rheumatism after getting feet wet.

Nux mos. - rheumatism or rheumatic pain consequent upon taking cold, particularly from exposure to drafts of air while heated; pains are fugitive in character, now here now there; < in cold or wet weather, or by application of cold or wet cloths; > in warm, dry weather and from warm applications.

Nux vom. - girl, aged 13, four years ago caught severe cold by going about in bare feet and had an attack of rheumatism; lateral sclerosis.

Nux vom. - girl, aged 15, previously in good health, after attending church in winter seized with severe chill and pain in limbs; rheumatism.

Nux vom. - man, aged 59, drunkard, suffering six years with rheumatic pains, last four weeks confined to bed; rheumatism.

Nux vom. - rheumatism: especially of large joints and muscles; cannot bear least jar; of trunk or back; swelling in joints usually rather pale; symptoms almost always < towards morning; muscles palpitate and are cramped; parts feel torpid, paralytic.

Oleander - man, aged 44, merchant, five feet ten inches in height, sallow complexion, nervo-bilious temperament, ill a year and a half and considered himself incurable, father subject to rheumatism; lienteric stools; rheumatism.

Oleum cajeputi - chronic rheumatism.

Oleum jecoris aselli - chronic rheumatism, with rigid muscles and tendons.

Oleum jecoris aselli - chronic gout and rheumatism of elderly persons, with rigidity of muscles and tendons, joint nearly inflexible.

Oleum jecoris aselli - contraction of muscles; musculo-fibrous rheumatis jecoris aselli.

Oleum jecoris aselli - mrs m, aged 30, formerly of strong robust constitution; rheumatism.

Oleum jecoris aselli - rheumatism of long standing; patient confined to bed or room, and only in warm summer months experienced a slight alleviation of her sufferings; nearly whole body was attacked, but principally inferior extremities, sacrum, back and shoulders; walking was entirely prevented by the insupportable pains, stiffness and swelling of joints; a kind of hectic fever and constant nightly exacerbations destroyed all repose; patient was wasted, of a bleachy whiteness, of a cachetic appearance and habit, and had lost all hope of relief.

Oleum jecoris aselli - rheumatism, produced by protracted residence in damp and cold localities; affection confined to joints; gradual exhaustion of strength and impairment of nutrition.

Pareira brava - man, aged 50, suffers from rheumatic attacks when traveling; renal colic.

Pareira brava - rheumatic or gouty subjects suffering from renal colics.

Pareira brava - seafaring captain, suffering for years from rheumatism and later from endocarditis; renal colic.

Petroleum - brown spots on arms, neck, chest and lower limbs; falling off of hair; rheumatic stiffness of shoulders and ankles —secondary syphilis.

Petroleum - rheumatism; knees stiff, with sharp sticking pains; stiffness of neck and cracking sound when moving head.

Petroleum - sprains of joints, especially in old rheumatic patients.

Petroleum - strong healthy peasant, after a chill four months previously; rheumatic dysecoia.

Phosphorus - man, aged 30, for a long time has had pain in arm; rheumatism.

Phosphorus - man, aged 36, hunter, several months ago fell into a stream, since then suffering; rheumatism

Phosphorus - man, aged 44, accustomed to exposure, caught cold two years ago, since then suffering; rheumatism

Phosphorus - man, aged 50, hard worker mentally and physically, after unusual exposure; rheumatic neuralgia.

Phosphorus - master carpenter, aged 59, suffering one year; paralytic rheumatism.

Phosphorus - mr pellman, aged 46, master tiller, strongly built and of good constitution, subject to rheumatic and gastric disturbances; paralysis.

Phosphorus - rheumatic stiffness with morning aggravation.

Phosphorus - rheumatism: drawing, tearing, tight feeling in affected part; headache, vertigo; < from cold weather; affects chest with oppression, cough, dyspnoea, forcing patient to sit up (endocarditis).

Phosphorus - sailor, aged 44; rheumatism.

Phosphorus - soldier, had been exposed during the war to several drenching rains; paralytic rheumatism.

Phytolacca - gonorrhoeal rheumatism.

Phytolacca - man, aged 40, had similar attack fourteen years ago, from which he did not recover for over a year; rheumatism.

Phytolacca - man, subject to rheumatism; aching in heels.

Phytolacca - mr h, aged 40, blacksmith; chronic rheumatism.

Phytolacca - mrs b, aged 45, suffering several years; rheumatism.

Phytolacca - mrs s, aged 40, scrofulous diathesis, fifteen years ago had severe attack of inflammatory rheumatism which became chronic; rheumatism.

Phytolacca - mrs s, aged 43, suffering several weeks; rheumatism.

Phytolacca - pains shifting rapidly; swelling pale, puffy, anemic; no appetite; constipation; < from motion and at night — rheumatism.

Phytolacca - patient is of a rheumatic diathesis, and is frequently afflicted with rheumatism of the periosteal and fibrous tissues, or is suffering from secondary or tertiary syphilis.

Phytolacca - rev w, aged 50, suffering many months; rheumatism.

Phytolacca - rheumatic and neuralgic affections after diphtheria.

Phytolacca - rheumatic or syphilitic affections of fibrous tissues and periosteum, it not only affects the fibrous coverings of muscles but the fibrous envelopes or sheaths of the nerves.

Phytolacca - rheumatism affecting periosteum, sheaths of nerves and fasciae.

Phytolacca - rheumatism of back and hip joints; chronic form; obtuse; heavy, aching pain, generally < in damp weather.

Phytolacca - rheumatism: of right frontal region, accompanied by nausea, pain < in morning; of shoulder and arm, pains fly from one part to another, like an electric shock, < at night; of several years? standing, joints of all the fingers badly swollen, very painful, hard and shining; chronic of left hip joint; pain obtuse, heavy, aching, generally < in damp weather; coldness of limb, pain < by warmth; pain in outer and back part of right limb, < at night but never going away entirely, unable to bear any weight on limb or to move it without extreme pain, which is dull, aching and at times lancinating; chronic, of lower extremities, and knee joints with or without effusion; periosteal, with syphilitic taint; enlargement of glands of neck and axilla.

Phytolacca - swelling and redness, with rheumatism.

Phytolacca - syphilitic and mercurial rheumatism; nightly pains in tibia, with nodes and irritable ulcers on lower leg.

Phytolacca - young girl, suffering several weeks; periosteal rheumatism.

Phytolacca - syphilitic bone pains; chronic rheumatism.

Platina - hysteric rheumatism, < sitting or standing, > walking; greatly aggravated at night.

Podophyllum - mercurial rheumatism.

Psorinum - girl, aged 11, light complexion, full face, ruddy cheeks, ill about a week, four years ago had severe rheumatic attacks; rheumatic carditis.

Pulsatilla - fleshy man, brewer, crippled for years; rheumatism.

Pulsatilla - lady, exceedingly mild and gentle disposition, after an attack of influenza; neuralgia rheumatica of leg.

Pulsatilla - man, aged 22, suffering from inflammatory rheumatism; blindness.

Pulsatilla - man, aged 50, quiet disposition; chronic rheumatism.

Pulsatilla - man, plethoric habit, subject to attacks of rheumatic gout; rheumatism in hand.

Pulsatilla - man, stout, full-blooded, suffering ten days; rheumatism in wrist.

Pulsatilla - pains, rheumatic, shifting from one place to another.

Pulsatilla - sophia t, aged 29, suffering three or four years; rheumatism.

Pulsatilla - woman, aged 24, single, hereditary tendency to arthritic affections; rheumatism.

Pulsatilla - woman, aged 25, tailoress, suffering six months; rheumatism.

Pulsatilla - woman, aged 33, single, robust, after getting wet; rheumatism.

Pulsatilla - woman, aged 35, single, mild character, blonde, year ago had rheumatic fever; rheumatic pains.

Pulsatilla - woman, aged 37, maid, single, few weeks ago caught cold, since then suffering; neuralgic rheumatism.

Pulsatilla - woman, aged 40; rheumatism.

Pulsatilla - woman, aged 44, single, suffering two years; rheumatism.

Pulsatilla - woman, aged 50; rheumatism.

Radium bromatum - chronic rheumatic arthritis.

Ranunculus bulb. - rheumatic and arthritic soreness, with stitches over whole body.

Ranunculus bulb. - rheumatic pain < in damp weather, and particularly from change of weather or change of temperature; rheumatic headache.

Ranunculus bulb. - rheumatism of muscles, particularly in muscles about trunk; intercostal rheumatism; muscles sore to touch; feel bruised as if they had been pounded.

Rheum - acute rheumatism, going from joint to joint, right shoulder to hip, left hip to right.

Rhododendron - general rheumatic pains, brought on by damp, cold weather and < during wet.

Rhododendron - man, aged 37, good-humored, well built, seven days ago caught cold, since then suffering; rheumatism.

Rhododendron - man, aged 55, laborer, strong constitution, suffering fourteen days; rheumatism.

Rhododendron - old lady, irritable, suffering six years; rheumatism.

Rhododendron - rheumatic pains especially in all the aponeuroses, < in rest; < at night; pains do not admit of the limbs being at rest; desire to move, and moving relieves; < before change of weather, particularly before a thunderstorm; especially right side; pains < in night, but more toward morning; in hot season.

Rhododendron - rheumatism of cervical and thoracic muscles; rheumatic neuralgia of extremities; pains < at rest and in cloudy and stormy weather.

Rhododendron - woman, aged 22, delivered a short time ago, after an attack of influenza; rheumatism.

Rhododendron - woman, aged 34, working out by the day, suffering six days; rheumatism.

Rhododendron - woman, aged 51, suffering twelve years; rheumatism.

Rhus ven. - man, aged 30, fifteen months ago had rheumatism in shoulders and arms, pain disappeared from these parts and became fixed in heel; chronic rheumatism.

Rumex - joseph h, aged 13, subject to violent attacks of inflammatory rheumatism, heart being implicated; pain in cardiac region.

Rumex - woman, aged 22, feeble constitution, strumous, subject for several years to subacute rheumatism; cough.

Ruta - man aged 53; suffering five weeks; rheumatism.

Sabina - irritability of temper, with sour stomach and great anxiety; hypochondriacal mood; rheumatic subjects.

Sabina - man, aged 42; chronic rheumatism.

Salicylic-acid. - a tall young man, aged 16, suffered from severe acute articular rheumatism; knee joint especially was seat of terrific pain; painful stiffness of neck; excessive perspiration, followed by miliaria; great lassitude; pulse full, soft, very frequent; went out too early and a relapse set in, with same weakening sweats; patient looked anemic and emaciated; hurried pulse, reminding one of heart's beat in beginning of phthisis.

Salicylic-acid. - a teacher suffered from acute articular rheumatism; a relapse followed from carelessness, attack being very severe, with profuse sour-smelling sweats and extensive eruption of miliaria; very nervous, urine showed heavy sediment; desquamation set in just as after scarlet fever in hands and feet; pains first in shoulder and elbow, then in lumbar region, so that the patient could hardly move; during relapse hands greatly swollen, could not be used; sleeplessness or sleep interrupted by frightful dreams, as if his head were squeezed between two beams (stiffness of neck); constipation.

Salicylic-acid. - acute, inflammatory, articular rheumatism attacking one or more joints, especially elbows or knees, with great swelling and redness, high fever and excessive sensitiveness to least jar; motion impossible.

Salicylic-acid. - girl, aged 12; rheumatism.

Salicylic-acid. - man, aged 80, robust, formerly had foot sweats, and since their suppression is more liable to rheumatic pains; sciatica.

Salicylic-acid. - polyarthritis rheumatica, temperature 105; pain intense, tenderness excessive.

Salicylic-acid. - rheumatism after sitting near an open window in a hot room, so that she felt hot on one side and chilly on the other; left ankle and knee joint, elbow and wrist enormously swollen, of a pinkish color, very sensitive, every motion exquisitely painful, pulse 120, high temperature, sweat, etc, even in bed, shocks passed from thigh down to foot so that she had to scream.

Salicylic-acid. - rheumatism: acute articular; chronic; gonorrhoeal; diphtheritic.

Salicylic-acid. - young man, aged 16, tall; rheumatism.

Sanguinaria - young lady, of rheumatic tendency; rheumatism of arm.

Sarsaparilla - mr h, contracted syphilis nine years ago, for which he received large doses of mercury; rheumatism in joints; headache.

Sarsaparilla - rheumatic bone pains after mercury or checked gonorrhoea.

Secale - rheumatism (peliosis rheumatica of schoenlein) generally is found in cachectic individuals, with purpura; affects joints, especially of lower extremities; thrombosis of abdominal vessels.

Sepia - girl, aged 19, sanguine temperament, brunette, rheumatic; headache.

Sepia - rheumatism, chronic cases, or obstinate remains of acute.

Sepia - tailor, aged 37, dark hair, pale, lean; rheumatism.

Sinapis nigra - rheumatalgia.

Spigelia - adapted to anemic, debilitated subjects, of rheumatic diathesis; scrofulous children afflicted with ascarides and lumbrici.

Spigelia - boy, aged 10, three years ago had an attack of rheumatism, a year thereafter another attack, followed by dropsy, six weeks ago a third attack; cardiac disorder.

Spigelia - boy, aged 17, well developed, naturally vigorous and active, dark hair, blue eyes, fair complexion; rheumatic carditis.

Spigelia - girl, aged 14, after acute articular rheumatism; endocarditis.

Spigelia - laborer, aged 36, after rheumatism pericarditis.

Spigelia - man, aged 51, suffering from rheumatic iritis; ciliary neuralgia.

Spigelia - rheumatism attacking heart.

Spongia - rheumatic affections of valves of heart; fibrous deposits upon valves.

Staphisagria - woman, aged 30, rheumatic; prosopalgia.

Sticta - boy, aged 7 to 8, had severe attack year before, followed by heart disease, was under treatment four months, present attack cured in nine days, rheumatism.

Sticta - boy, aged 8; rheumatic bursitis.

Sticta - girl, aged 10, nervous sanguine temperament, medium size, skin pale, transparent, freckled, hair auburn; rheumatism.

Sticta - man, aged 45, rheumatism of arm.

Sticta - man, aged 48, rheumatism.

Sticta - mrs g, aged about 40, suffering three months; rheumatism.

Sticta - woman, aged 41; rheumatic pain in chest.

Sticta - young lady, aged 20, married, nervous sanguine temperament, slightly built, hair deep auburn, suffering six months; rheumatism.

Stillingia - chronic periosteal rheumatism, syphilitic and scrofulous affections.

Stramonium - lady, aged 42, robust, dark complexion, black eyes, subject to rheumatism; headache.

Strontia carb. - chronic sequela of hemorrhages; great forgetfulness; bright colors before eyes; semilateral (r side) affections; rheumatic pains, debility, trembling, emaciation, desire to keep warm; old sprains.

Strontium carb. - rheumatic pains, chronic sprains, stenosis of oesophagus.

Sulphur - girl, aged 10, sanguine-choleric temperament, brunette; rheumatism.

Sulphur - man, aged 40, phlegmatic temperament, strong; rheumatism in shoulder. - man, aged 56; rheumatism. - man, aged 60, gouty; rheumatism.

Sulphur - miss h, aged 50, suffering sixteen years; rheumatic gout.

Sulphur - subacute and chronic rheumatism with profuse sweating.

Sulphur - woman, aged 21; rheumatism of knee.

Sulphuric acid. - man, aged 36, during rheumatic attack; purpura.

Syphilinum - chronic eruptions and rheumatism.

Syphilinum - man, aged 48, robust, weight 250 lbs, height 5 feet 9 inches; rheumatism.

Syphilinum - mrs abc, suffering from diabetes Mellitus, subject to rheumatism in rainy weather; rheumatic ophthalmia.

Syphilinum - pains in limbs every night after midnight, weary, tired pains, making rest impossible, could lie nowhere without suffering in part on which he rested; < in lower limbs; much perspiration which partly relieved - rheumatic fever.

Syphilinum - rheumatic neuralgic pains in all muscles, even in cremaster, not in joints; darting pains in irregular attacks, sometimes lasting a week or two; pains gradually increase and decrease; < in damp and especially in frosty weather; <

at 4 or 5 p m, attain their height at 2 or 3 a m, ceasing about 8 a m (improved).

Syphilinum - rheumatism with sweating of hands, wrists and legs below knees and feet, with great soreness of soles, < at night.

Syphilinum - shifting pains of a rheumatic character obliging a repeated change of position and posture.

Taraxacum - neuralgia and rheumatism during and after typhus.

Tarentula hisp. - weakness of all limbs; rheumatic pains; restlessness; formication; paralysis; spasmodic paralytic affections; neuralgia; rheumatism; nervous diseases where functions of vagi are more or less disturbed.

Taxus - also in gout and chronic rheumatism.

Terebinthinum - atonic gout; rheumatism and gout; asthenic inflammation; passive hemorrhages; purpura haemorrhagica; burns; hospital gangrene; cold. Gangrene; hydrophobia; gangrenous wound from bite of a dog; wounds of skin, tendons and nerves; dissection wounds; old ulcers.

Terebinthinum - joints swollen stiff; pain on motion - rheumatism.

Teucrium - man, barber, thin, sandy complexion; rheumatism.

Thuja - man, aged 30, weight 240, ill seven days; rheumatic fever

Thuja - rheumatic or arthritic pains, especially of a gonorrhoeal nature; arthritis deformans.

Thuja - rheumatism; flesh feels as if beaten off bones.

Trombidium - gentleman of full habits, subject to attacks of rheumatism and congestion of liver; diarrhoea.

Urtica urens - rheumatism attending, following, or alternating with nettlerash.

Vanadium - tuberculosis, chronic rheumatism, diabetes.

Verat-alb. - man, aged 50, suffering from rheumatism and hemorrhoids; affection of throat.

Verat-vir. - acute rheumatism with high fever, full, hard, rapid pulse, pains in joints and muscles; scanty red urine.

Verat-vir. - boy, aged 10, scrofulous; rheumatism.

Verat-vir. - boy, aged 5; rheumatism.

Verat-vir. - inflammatory rheumatism with gastric complications; tongue coated on sides with a red streak through centre; creeping chilliness; aching in all bones, followed by headache and fever; affects especially left shoulder, hip and knee.

Verat-vir. - lady, aged 30; rheumatism.

Verat-vir. - man, aged 35; rheumatism.

Vespa - aged 16, scrofulous since birth, stung by a wasp, carious bones, severe rheumatism, suppurating in hands.

Viola odorata - boy, aged 19; rheumatism.

Viola odorata - man, aged 31, robust, slightly lymphatic; rheumatism.

Viola odorata - man, aged 61; rheumatism.

Viola odorata - mrs —, aged 70; rheumatism.

Viola odorata - woman, aged 29, robust; rheumatism.

Viola tricolor - articular rheumatism, with itch-like eruption around joints.

Zincum met. - general articular rheumatism, with tearing pain, lameness, trembling and crampy pain; twisting in affected limbs, frequent jerking of whole body during sleep, < from being overheated and from exertion.

Zincum met. - rheumatism affecting muscles of sacrum, coccyx, ilium and left hip joint, and leg of left side; soreness of parts upon pressure by ends of fingers, and sore pains from any movement requiring exercise of muscles; when sitting or lying down little or no pain; < rising from chair, from stooping, turning body or bending it backward, drawing a long breath, coughing or sneezing; pains in hip joint and knee, occasionally passing along course of great ischiatic nerve to foot.

Habitual—Diseases that have become habitual

(There are patients rarely found who do not bother for their chronic complaints. It has formed a habit of him. He says it is not a problem or difficulty for him. Rather, he has accepted to live with it and no botheration for him. Examples are: patients with chronic constipation having bowel movement once in three days or so. Those who pass watery stools more than three times and they say it is not a botheration for them).

Remedies having the symptom 'Habitual'

Aletris (Miscarriage, abortion) - habitual tendency to abortion in feeble persons of lax fibre and anaemic condition, even after haemorrhage has set in.

Aletris farinosa - habitual tendency to abortion.

Ant-crud. (Chlorosis) - gastric symptoms predominant, with habitual sensation as if stomach were overloaded, with headache, peevishness.

Ant-crud. (Dyspepsia, weakness of stomach) - habitual sensation in stomach as if overloaded, excessive crossness, even hypochondriasis with suicidal tendencies.

Ant-tart. - man, aged 30, habitual alcohol drinker, got 4 grains of tart emet daily in his liquor; in 15 days he was poisoned.

Apis - a woman, aged 40, with habitual dyspnoea and weak, irregular heartbeats; venous thrombosis with a fatty heart.

Arnica (Erysipelas) - habitual erysipelas running a tedious course.

Ars-alb. (Drunkards, diseases of) - morning vomiting of habitual drunkards.

Asafoetida (Hysteria) - hysteria, the direct sequel of the checking of habitual discharges, after abuse of mercury, after the stoppage of an habitual expectoration with oppression of the chest (amm.).

Aur-mur.-nat. (Miscarriage, abortion) - habitual abortus at the same month of pregnancy depending most frequently on induration of some part of uterus.

Aur-mur.-nat. (Uterus complaints) - habitual abortus or miscarriage, returning constantly at about the same time, caused by indurations in some parts of uterus preventing the natural expansion.

Aurum met. (Chronic catarrh of the head) - habitual nasal tone of voice.

Baryta carb. - habitual colic, with hunger, but food is refused.

Calc-carb. (Jaundice) - habitual constipation.

Caulophyllum (Menses complaints) - habitual cold feet.

Caulophyllum (Miscarriage, abortion) - menstrual irregularities after miscarriage. Habitual abortion from uterine debility with passive haemorrhage.

Caulophyllum - habitual abortion from uterine debility.

Chlorum - j s, aged 52, has suffered from follicular pharyngitis, has had larynx and fauces treated with nitrate of silver, until it became unendurable, has now much pain in throat, habitual cough and expectoration of glairy mucus; spasmodic cough.

Cimicifuga (Miscarriage, abortion) - habitual abortion in women of rheumatic tendencies.

Cuprum ars. (Haemorrhoids) - habitual constipation.

Eup-perf. (Headache) - habitual headaches with bitter vomiting (iris, sour vomiting).

Geranium - habitual sick headaches.

Graphites - adapted to women inclined to obesity, who suffer from habitual constipation, and whose history reveals a tendency to delaying menstruation.

Graphites - dyscrasia, especially when caused by a suppression of habitual secretions and excretions.

Helonias (Miscarriage, abortion) - threatened abortion from atonic conditions, especially in habitual abortion.

Hepar sulph. - temper obstinate and cross, a ferocious spleen which would lead to cold blooded murder even among those habitually gay and benevolent.

Hepar sulph. (Tuberculosis of lungs) - spasmodic cough in paroxysms, with titillation in larynx and efforts of vomiting, or habitual bronchial catarrhs with loud rattling of mucus. as an intercurrent in cases of cheesy pulmonic deposit with strong tendency to suppuration, when the tendency to cicatrize is often interrupted and the expulsion of the caseous material imperfect.

Hydrastis - man, aged 29, after habitual use of purgatives; constipation.

Hydrastis - woman, aged 29, mother of two children, habitually takes castor oil and senna; constipation.

Ignatia - aged women, oversensitive to external impressions; spinal affection (paralysis, fixed pain in spine); habitual constipation; rt. half of body weakest; vertigo.

Iris vers. (Mind symptoms) - habitual headaches from gastric or abdominal causes.

Kali-bich. (Constipation) - habitual constipation, stools scanty, knotty, followed by burning and painful retraction of rectum and anus.

Kali-bich. (Leucorrhoea) - habitual constipation.

Kali-bich. - man, aged 82, lived for thirsty years in india, had fever, dysentery, bronchitis; bowels generally loose, habitual snuff taker; malignant ulceration of nose.

Kali mur. (Insanity) - habitual loss of appetite.

Kali-mur. - habitual loss of appetite; patient absolutely refuses to take food, or imagines he must starve - insanity.

Kali sul. (Duodenitis and duodenal catarrh) - habitual constipation.

Ledum (Arthritis, gout) - habitual gout in the articulations of hands and feet.

Merc-sol. - man, aged 70, always good health, after cessation of an habitual expectoration; typhoid fever.

Merc-sol. - woman, aged 50, after habitual use of blue pills for constipation; ulcers on forehead.

Muriatic-acid. (Dyspepsia, weakness of stomach) - habitual difficult digestion.

Nux vomica - optic nerve atrophy from habitual use of intoxicants.

Nux vomica (Seasickness) - habitual use of tobacco and alcoholic drinks.

Nux vomica (Vagina affections) - good livers, habitual constipation, small stools.

Nux vom. - gout in incipient stage in habitual drinkers; oversensitiveness to pain, constipation; during hard stool, violent pain in affected part; scanty, dark urine; heat mixed with chilliness, especially when moving; perspiration relieves; torticollis.

Phytolacca (Constipation) - habitual costiveness, especially of old people or of those of weak constitutional powers, with weak heart's action, intermittent pulse and general relaxed muscular system. sensation as if the bowels would not move without the aid of laxatives.

Plumb-met. - great depression of spirits; though habitually very temperate had recourse to various stimulants, at first in moderation and openly, but soon immoderately and by stealth; sleeplessness; gloom; despair of her salvation; moody taciturnity; fixed idea that she could only obtain peace and safety through absolution from a priest of the papal church, although she had been a zealous protestant; face nearly of a leaden hue; perpetual movement of lips, as of one smoking, accompanied by a slight sound; very silent, but when spoken to answered rationally; severe pain, starting up from back into head, as if something were working at top of head, with a sense of screwing from behind forward; some flatulence; frequent drowsiness by day, sleeplessness by night; profound melancholy and frequent sighs; brooded over any forbidden thing; would steal from house in servant's cloak and bonnet to obtain stimulants, but from the moment their prohibition was withdrawn ceased to have any desire for them; after being permitted to visit a priest and converse with him ceased to talk and think of the church.

Pulsatilla - disposition mild and gentle, never cross —habitual constipation.

Pulsatilla (Indigestion, gastric derangement) - taciturn, vehement without reason, especially when the patients are habitually of a bland and obliging disposition. (compare dyspepsia.)

Sabina (Haemorrhage from uterus) - plethoric women with habitual menorrhagia, who began to menstruate very early in life, always menstruated freely, and showed more or less a tendency to miscarriage.

Sabina (Hysteria) - habitual threatening abortion in third month.

Silicea - man, aged 32, in good health, a little pale, habitually sad and anxious, having lost his father at the age of 60 from cancer of face; threatened cancer.

Silicea (Dyspepsia, weakness of stomach) - constipation, hard stools, difficult to discharge and crumbling during defaecation. Habitual foot-sweat.

Silicea (Ophthalmia) - amblyopia from suppressed habitual foot-sweat.

Silicea (Varicocele) - suppression of habitual foot-sweat.

Stramonium (Drunkards, diseases of) - suitable to habitual drunkards.

Sulphur (Arthritis, gout) - habitual gout, especially of drunkards and those who indulge in rich food and take but little exercise, red blotches in face, nose habitually red.

Sulphur (Constipation) - habitual constipation, especially in haemorrhoidal and hypochondriac people, complaining of dull feeling in brain, heaviness on top of head, weak, hungry sensation in stomach about noon, burning of the soles of feet at night.

Sulphur (Ophthalmia) - hypopion, cataract, choroiditis and chorioretinitis, if accompanied by darting pains and where the disease is based upon abdominal venosity, stagnation in portal circulation, habitual constipation, cerebral congestion, or upon metastasis of chronic or suppressed skin diseases.

Tabacum (Constipation) - habitual constipation, tympanitic abdomen, strangulated hernia, with nausea, deathly faintness, cold sweat.

Terebinth (Ophthalmia) - iritis rheumatica, from suppression of habitual foot-sweat, or when urinary symptoms are present

Valeriana - a man, aged 50, of florid complexion, almost ruddy, habitual cheerful temper; neuralgia of limbs.

Verat-alb. - young people and women of a sanguine or nervo-sanguine temperament; also people who are habitually cold and deficient in vital reaction; gay dispositions; fitful mood.

Veratrum alb. (Headache) - habitual coldness and deficiency of vital reaction.

Diseases which become a Habit or the patient is used to living with it

(Arthritis, gout) Ledum - low, asthenic cases (maltreated by large doses of Colch.); lancinating, tearing pains; < by motion than by touch and at midnight, when joints feel so hot that he throws off all covering; oedematous swelling of joint, which may feel cold to the touch; affects chiefly left shoulder and right hip-joint; habitual gout in the articulations of hands and feet; ball of great toe swollen and painful; soles very sensitive; tendons stiff; gouty nodosities in joints; fine tearing pains in toes; face bloated; pimples on forehead; after abuse of alcoholic drinks.

(Arthritis, gout) Sulphur - habitual gout, especially of drunkards and those who indulge in rich food and take but little exercise, red blotches in face, nose habitually red; disgust for animal food; dyspnoea with desire to take a deep inspiration; uric acid urine; dull, aching, pressive pain in joints; as soon as he falls asleep the affected limbs jerk and arouse him; pain serratic and leave a sensation of numbness; alternate constipation or diarrhoea, with excessively foetid stools and foetid flatulence; haemorrhoids.

(Chlorosis) Ant-crud. - nymphomania and tenderness over ovarian region after checking menses by a bath; menses commence at an early period, are profuse and cease afterwards, followed by chlorosis; gastric symptoms predominant, with habitual sensation as if stomach were overloaded, with headache, peevishness; irregular stool, lassitude, excessive depression and exhaustion; unrefreshing sleep at night.

(Chronic catarrh of the head) Aurum met. - caries of nasal bones, foetid discharge of greenish-yellow pus; salty-tasting watery discharge through posterior nares; ulcerated, agglutinated, painful nostrils, cannot breathe through nose; loss of smell and discharge of blood through nose; habitual nasal tone of voice; melancholy, with horrible gloom and depression, or even suicidal mood; red, swollen and ulcerated tonsils, with difficult deglutition; caries of palate.

(Constipation) Kali-bich. - habitual constipation, stools scanty, knotty, followed by burning and painful retraction of rectum and anus; periodical costiveness; constipation, debility, coated tongue, headache, cold extremities; sensation of a plug in anus which feels sore, making it very painful to walk.

(Constipation) Phytolacca - habitual costiveness, especially of old people or of those of weak constitutional powers, with weak heart's action, intermittent pulse and general relaxed muscular system. Sensation as if the bowels would not move without the aid of laxatives; feeling of fulness in abdomen before stool, which remains after stool as if all had not passed; continual inclination to stool, but often passes only foetid flatus; torpor of rectum; pains shooting from anus and lower part of rectum along perineum to the middle of penis.

(Constipation) Sulphur - habitual constipation, especially in haemorrhoidal and hypochondriac people, complaining of dull feeling in brain, heaviness on top of head, weak, hungry sensation in stomach about noon, burning of the soles of feet at night; hard, insufficient, difficult stool, with fulness, heat and itching at anus, flat like sheep's dung, first effort so painful that patient stops straining; stool hard and black, as if burnt; constipation of infants; aversion to meat, sleep short and broken, frequent faint spells.

(Constipation) Tabacum - desire for stool without any evacuation; after frequent but ineffectual attempts, a hard stool several hours after the regular time; habitual constipation, tympanitic abdomen, strangulated hernia, with nausea, deathly faintness, cold sweat.

(Drunkards, diseases of) Ars-alb. - morning vomiting of habitual drunkards; chronic gastric irritability; heartburn, as if epigastrium and stomach were being made raw by an acrid corroding substance; fruitless retching, or retching and vomiting; indescribable nausea, loathing and weakness; satiety of life and still fear of death, will not be alone; fear of ghosts, thieves, with desire to hide one's self, trembling of limbs. is morally perfectly upset, what the germans call so pointedly katzenjammer; with cravings for acids and coffee, which relieve.

(Drunkards, diseases of) - Boenninghausen recommends a few drops of Tinctura opii in a cup of coffee for habitual drunkenness, and Ant-crud. As the best antidote for the effects of sour wine. lyons gives ten drops of Tinctura capsici for dipsomania shortly before meals, or whenever depression or craving for alcohol arises. it obviates the morning vomiting, removes the sinking at the pit of the stomach, the intense craving for stimulants, and promotes appetite and digestion. we consider them more reliable for that purpose than the fluid extracts of avena Sativa, or of Erythroxylon coca.

(Drunkards, diseases of) Stramonium - suitable to habitual drunkards; delirium tremens, with frightful hallucinations;

sees strangers and imagines animals are jumping sideways out of the ground or running at him; shy, hides himself, tries to escape; talks incessantly, absurdly; laughs, alternately merry or dejected; epileptic convulsions; red, hot and bloated face; eyes wide open and staring; lockjaw after convulsions; cough of drunkards; convulsive motions of upper extremities, the arms reaching forward and upward with an uncertain, tremulous motion, while the lower extremities feel nearly paralyzed.

(Duodenitis and duodenal catarrh) Kali-sul. - gastro-duodenal catarrh, with yellow-coated tongue and jaundice; indigestion with sensation of pressure as from a load, fulness at pit of stomach and befogged feeling in head; habitual constipation; haemorrhoids.

(Dyspepsia, weakness of stomach) Ant-crud. - overloading the stomach and gastric derangement in children, women and old people; thickly coated white tongue, with anorexia, slow digestion and foetid eructations, often followed by diarrhoea, particularly after acid wines or new beer; habitual sensation in stomach as if overloaded, excessive crossness, even hypochondriasis with suicidal tendencies; dryness of mouth with great thirst, < at night; constipation alternating with diarrhoea; helminthiasis; caused by overeating, hot weather, bathing, during measles; metastasis of gout and rheumatism.

(Dyspepsia, weakness of stomach) Muriatic acid. - habitual difficult digestion; everything tastes sweet; acrid and putrid taste, like rotten eggs, with ptyalism; excessive hunger and thirst, morbid longing for alcoholic drinks, aversion to meat; bitter, putrid eructations; vomiting, with belching, coughing; involuntary swallowing, gulping of contents of stomach into oesophagus, which sometimes go down again; empty sensation in stomach, extending through the whole abdomen; weak feeling in stomach, but no hunger; stool difficult, as from inactivity of bowels; prostration and drowsiness all day, wants to lie about; peevishness.

(Dyspepsia, weakness of stomach) Silicea - canine hunger, with nervous, irritable persons; averse to warm, cooked food, desires only cold things, disgust for meat; small quantities of wine cause ebullitions and thirst; loud, uncontrollable, sour eructations; nausea, with violent palpitations of heart; intense heartburn, sensation of a load in epigastrium, burning or throbbing in pit of stomach; morning nausea and vomiting of viscous matter; after eating, bitter taste, pressure in stomach as from a stone; flow of water in mouth; constipation, hard stools, difficult to discharge and crumbling during defaecation. Habitual foot-sweat.

(Erysipelas) Arnica - habitual erysipelas running a tedious course; phlegmonous erysipelas with extreme tenderness and painfulness on pressure, with tendency to formation of bullae; swelling hot, hard, shining, even deep red; patient nervous, cannot stand pain and feels tired and bruised as after hard work as if beaten.

(Haemorrhage from uterus) Sabina - pain or a feeling of uncomfortableness extending between the sacrum and pubis; flow profuse, intermixed with clots, the blood most frequently of a bright-red color, sometimes dark-red; frequently attended by pains in joints; the slightest motion excites the flow afresh, but very much walking lessens it; excessive, debilitating menses, with abdominal spasms; painless loss of dark-red blood after miscarriage, immediately after parturition; plethoric women with habitual menorrhagia, who began to menstruate very early in life, always menstruated freely, and showed more or less a tendency to miscarriage; great weakness or nervousness in head and extremities; menorrhagia with erethism.

(Haemorrhoids) Cuprum ars. - intense burning itching in anus and thighs, < at night in bed and when undressing, not > by scratching or hard rubbing; scrotum moist and damp; habitual constipation.

(Haemorrhoids) We have also to consider - for anomalies of the haemorrhoidal difficulties and ailments in consequence of the suppression of a habitual haemorrhoidal flow: 1, Nux-v., Sulph.; 2, Cal., Carb-v., Puls.; 3, Aloe, Apis, Mill., Ran.; haemorrhages: 1, Acon., Alum., Bell., Calc., Carb-v., Cham., Collins., Graph., Ham., Ipec., Leptan., Phos., Puls., Sep.; 2, Aesc. Hip., Chin., Sulp.; 3, Amm., Ant., Caps., Cascar., Erig., Fer., Merc., Mill., Mur-ac., Nitr-ac., Nux-v., Trill.

(Headache) Eup-perf. - periodical headache; habitual headaches with bitter vomiting (iris, sour vomiting); bilious sick-headaches in spring; pain in occiput when lying down, with a feeling of a great weight in the head, requiring the hands to lift it; headache better in the house; worse when first going into the open air; relieved by conversation; throbbing headache; darting pain through the temples, with sensation of blood rushing across head; soreness and beating in back part of head; intense headache, throbbing, and great sense of internal soreness in forehead and occiput, with sensation of great weight in occiput; distress and painful soreness in top and back of head; soreness of eyeballs.

(Headache) Veratrum alb. - neuralgia in the head, with indigestion, features sunken; paroxysms in various parts of the brain, partly as if bruised, partly pressure; violent pains drive to despair, great prostration, fainting, with cold sweat and great thirst; cold sensation and pressure on vertex, generally attended by pain in stomach, relieved by pressing on vertex with hand (Meny.); nausea, vomiting and diarrhoea; habitual coldness and deficiency of vital reaction.

(Hysteria) Asafoetida - hysteria, the direct sequel of the checking of habitual discharges, after abuse of mercury, after the stoppage of an habitual expectoration with oppression of the chest (Amm.); globus hystericus, flatus accumulates in abdomen and pressing up against the lung causes oppression of chest; reverse peristaltic action in oesophagus and intestines with sensation as if a ball started in stomach and rose into throat, provoked by over-eating, motion or by anything which excites the nerves; belching of wind of strong rancid taste; food when partially swallowed returns by the mouth; greasy taste in mouth with dryness and burning; flatus passes upward, none downward; nervous palpitation, pulse small, breathing hardly affected; > in fresh air.

(Hysteria) Sabina - very nervous and hysterical; habitual threatening abortion in third month; music is intolerable to her; very tired and lazy; flushes of heat in face, with chilliness all over and coldness of hands and feet; lustreless eyes.

(Indigestion, gastric derangement) Pulsatilla - tongue coated with whitish mucus; foul, pappy, or bitter taste, especially after swallowing; bitter taste of food, especially of bread; bitter, sour or putrid eructations, or tasting of the ingesta; aversion to food, especially warm (boiled food), also to fat and meat, with desire for acids or spirits; acidity of the stomach; excessive mucus in the stomach; regurgitation of the ingesta; excessive nausea, desire to vomit, especially after eating and drinking, or with evening exacerbations; vomiting of food or mucus, or bitter and sour vomiting (especially at night); hard, distended abdomen, with flatulence, rumbling; slow stool, or slimy and bilious diarrhoea; hemicrania, tearing or darting; chilliness, with languor and drawing through the whole body; ill-humor; taciturn, vehement without reason, especially when the patients are habitually of a bland and obliging disposition. (compare dyspepsia.)

(Insanity) Kali-mur. - sad, apathetic, with chilliness in evening; habitual loss of appetite; he absolutely refuses to take food or imagines he must starve; intoxication from the smallest quantity of wine or beer, causing congestion, > from nosebleed.

(Jaundice) Calc-carb. - stitches in liver during or after stooping; cannot bear tight clothing around waist; enlarged liver; habitual constipation; grayish-white faeces; indigestion; pit of stomach swollen out like a saucer turned. bottom up.

(Leucorrhoea) Kali-bich. - yellow, tough, ropy discharge, can be drawn out in long strings (Hydrast.); yellow, stiff leucorrhoea with severe pains and weakness across small of back, and dull, heavy pain in epigastrium; accumulation of thick, tenacious mucus about sexual organs; soreness and rawness in vagina; prolapsus uteri during hot weather; itching at vulva; weakness of digestion; habitual constipation; subinvolution of uterus; especially adapted to fat, light-haired women.

(Mind symptoms) Iris vers. - biliousness, despondency, low-spirited, easily vexed; confusion of mind with mental depression; habitual headaches from gastric or abdominal causes.

(Menses complaints) Caulophyllum - too soon and too scanty; neuralgic and congestive dysmenorrhoea with spasmodic, irregular and very severe pains, especially the first two days of menses; pain in small of back and great aching and soreness of lower limbs, bad breath, bitter taste, vertigo, chilliness. During: scanty flow, blood very light, nausea and vomiting of yellow, bitter water; intermittent uterine pains from retroversion or a relaxed and flabby condition of uterus, with profuse flow; habitual cold feet; intermittent pains in all parts, head, stomach, bladder, upper and lower limbs. after: passive flow, an oozing from the uterine vessels, with tremulous weakness of whole body.

(Miscarriage, abortion) Aletris - habitual tendency to abortion in feeble persons of lax fibre and anaemic condition, even after haemorrhage has set in; weight in uterine region, tendency to prolapsus uteri; general weakness of mind and body; weak from long sickness or defective nutrition.

(Miscarriage, abortion) Aur-mur.-nat. - habitual abortus at the same month of pregnancy depending most frequently on induration of some part of uterus.

(Miscarriage, abortion) Caulophyllum - severe pains in back and loins, threatening abortion, with great want of uterine tonicity; uterine contractions tormenting, irregular, feeble and attended with only slight loss of blood; menstrual irregularities after miscarriage. Habitual abortion from uterine debility with passive haemorrhage.

(Miscarriage, abortion) Cimicifuga - habitual abortion in women of rheumatic tendencies; cold chills and pricking sensations in the mammae; pains fly across the abdomen from side to side, especially from right to left (Lyc.), and seem to double the patient up; subinvolution; abortion following fright; convulsions with the labor-pains.

(Miscarriage, abortion) Helonias - threatened abortion from atonic conditions, especially in habitual abortion; slightest overexertion or irritating emotion tends to cause loss of foetus; useful for many of the sequelae of miscarriage.

(Ophthalmia) Silicea - caries of the orbit; dacryocystitis, swelling, tenderness, pain and lachrymation, patient very sensitive to fresh air; blennorrhoea of lachrymal sac; lachrymal fistula; blepharitis acuta and chronica; crescentic ulcers of cornea with little photophobia or lachrymation; hypopion; sclerochoroiditis ant.; cataract; ciliary neuralgia with darting pains through eyes and head upon any exposure to draught of air or just before a storm; styes filled with pus; suppurating cystic tumors on lids; edges of lids ulcerate; amblyopia from suppressed habitual foot-sweat.

(Ophthalmia) Sulphur - chronic blepharitis in strumous children who are irritable and cross by day and feverish and restless at night; edges redder than natural (graph., paler), < in hot weather and near a hot stove, > in winter; itching, biting, burning, or sensation as if sand were in the eye; lids swollen, red and agglutinated in the morning; cannot bear to have the eyes washed; eczematous affections of lids; blennorrhoea of lachrymal sac, fistula lachrymalis; acute or chronic catarrhal conjunctivitis, with sharp darting pains like pins sticking into the eye, or pressing, tensive, cutting and burning pains; ophthalmia neonatorum, with profuse, thick, yellow discharge, swelling of lids; pustular inflammation of cornea and conjunctiva, with sharp sticking pains as if a splinter or some other foreign body were sticking in the eye; photophobia and profuse lachrymation, considerable redness, especially at angles; discharges acrid, corrosive, or tenacious, lids swollen, burn and smart; chronic scleritis; hypopion, cataract, choroiditis and chorioretinitis, if accompanied by darting pains and where the disease is based upon abdominal venosity, stagnation in portal circulation, habitual constipation, cerebral congestion, or upon metastasis of chronic or suppressed skin diseases.

(Ophthalmia) Terebinth. - iritis rheumatica, from suppression of habitual foot-sweat, or when urinary symptoms are present; ciliary neuralgia with acute conjunctivitis, chemosis or cellulitis of orbit, pain excessive in, around and over eye, sharp, darting, < at night, with severe paroxysms in early morning hours.

(Paralysis) Paralysis in consequence of; habitual drunkenness: Ant-tart., Ars., Calc., Lach., Natr-sulph., Nux-v., Op., Ran., Sep., Sulph.

(Seasickness) Nux vomica - bilious temperament, haemorrhoids; acid vomiting from least motion; gastralgia < from food, > from hot drinks; pressure in epigastrium as from a stone, <

mornings and after meals; vertigo, buzzing in ears, nausea and urging to vomit; hernia; habitual use of tobacco and alcoholic drinks.

(Sore throat) Acute angina: chronic habitual angina: 1, Alum., Bar., Calc., Carb-v., Hep., Kali-mur., Lach., Lyc., Sep., Sulph.; 2, Bell., Chin., Mang., Natr-m., Nitr-ac., Nux-v., Phos., Phyt., Sabad., Seneg., Staph., Thuj.

(Spasmus facialis) Spasmus facialis - tic convulsive when caused by exposure to cold: Bell., Hyosc., Merc.; external injuries: Arn., Hyper.; diseases of bones, decayed teeth: Hecla, Hep., Merc., Sil.; anger: Nux-v.; fright and terror: Hyosc., Ign., Op. constant winking of eyelids: Anac., Bell., Hyosc., Natr-m., stram. habitual hysterical spasm of face: Kali-carb., Sep., Sil. risus sardonicus: Acon., Anac., Alum., Asa., Bell., Bov., Calc., Cic., Con., Croc., Cupr., Hyosc., Natr-m., Nux-v., Phos., Plat., Ran. Scel., Sep., Stram., Veratr., Zinc.

(Tuberculosis of lungs) Hepar sulph. - harsh, dry sounds in bronchi from tumefaction of mucous membrane, moist sounds rare and expectoration not copious; very sensitive to open air, sweats easily from exertion and turns pale, afterwards burning redness of face and heat and dryness of palms of hands; spasmodic cough in paroxysms, with titillation in larynx and efforts of vomiting, or habitual bronchial catarrhs with loud rattling of mucus. as an intercurrent in cases of cheesy pulmonic deposit with strong tendency to suppuration, when the tendency to cicatrize is often interrupted and the expulsion of the caseous material imperfect.

(Uterus complaints) Aur-mur.-nat. - chronic inflammation; induration of some part of uterus; flexions from condensation of uterine tissue, or from softening of the stroma of the neck or body; habitual abortus or miscarriage, returning constantly at about the same time, caused by indurations in some parts of uterus preventing the natural expansion; ulcers of uterus and of vaginal walls, developing themselves from swellings and indurations; cancer mammae et uteri; melancholia.

(Vagina affections) Nux vomica - good livers, habitual constipation, small stools.

(Varicocele) Silicea - sweaty feet; chilblains; suppression of habitual foot-sweat; squeezing pains in testicles; itching humid spots on genitals, mostly on scrotum; sweat on scrotum.

(Vision complaints) As regards external causes, if the weakness should have been caused by fine work, give Bell. or Ruta, or perhaps Carb-v., Calc., Gels., Lachn. and Spigel.; by old age: Aur., Bar-c., Con., Op., Phos., Sec. - after suppression of a habitual bloody discharge, as haemorrhoids, menstruation, etc.: Bell., Calc., Cycl., Lyc., Nux-v., Phos., Puls., Sep., Sulph.

Nutritional disorders

Fever, relapsing - strict hygiene and good nutrition are a necessity, of more importance than medicinal treatment.

Remedies Related to Nutrition

Abies can. (Uterus complaints) - prolapsus from general defective nutrition, with little or no local congestion.

Abies can. - there are peculiar cravings and chilly sensations that are very characteristic; especially for women with uterine displacement, probably due to defective nutrition with debility.

Aletris (Amenorrhoea) - amenia, or delaying menses, in consequence of atony of the womb or ovaries; weariness of mind and body; fulness and distension of abdomen, with bearing-down sensation; night-sweats; constipation from want of muscular action; debility arising from protracted illness; loss of fluid; defective nutrition.

Aletris (Debility) - weariness of mind and body; dizzy when stooping; sleepiness; least food distresses stomach, flatulency and constipation; debility, especially of women from protracted illness or defective nutrition, no organic disease. Debility after diphtheria.

Aletris (Leucorrhoea) - leucorrhoea from loss of fluids or defective nutrition; debility from protracted illness; uterine atony, with heavy, dragging pains about hips; great disposition to miscarriage or early abortion; prolapsus from weakness.

Aletris (Menses complaints) - premature and profuse; discharge dark with coagula; fulness and weight in uterine region, colicky pains in hypogastrium; debility, defective nutrition and assimilation; drowsiness, vertigo, fainting; extreme constipation and prolapsus uteri from muscular atony.

Aletris (Miscarriage, abortion) - habitual tendency to abortion in feeble persons of lax fibre and anaemic condition, even after haemorrhage has set in; weight in uterine region, tendency to prolapsus uteri; general weakness of mind and body; weak from long sickness or defective nutrition.

Aletris (Uterus complaints) - prolapsus uteri from muscular atony; leucorrhoea from loss of fluids or defective nutrition; debility from protracted illness; obstinate indigestion, the least food distresses the stomach; fainting, with vertigo; extreme constipation, great effort being required to discharge faeces; great accumulation of frothy saliva; sterility from uterine atony; heavy, dragging pains about the hips; profuse, painful and premature menses; profuse leucorrhoea.

Aletris (Vertigo, dizziness) - vertigo in cases of debility arising from protracted illness, loss of fluids, defective nutrition; vertigo from mental overexertion, with general debility; excessive nausea with giddiness; frequent attacks of fainting with dizziness.

Alfalfa - disorders characterized by malnutrition are mainly within its therapeutic range, for example, neurasthenia, splanchnic blues, nervousness, insomnia, nervous indigestion, etc.

Alfalfa - from its action on the sympathetic, alfalfa favorably influences nutrition, evidenced in "toning up" the appetite and digestion resulting in greatly improved mental and physical vigor, with gain in weight.

Alnus rubra - it stimulates nutrition, and thus acts favorably upon strumous disorders, enlarged glands, etc.

Arg-nit. (Anaemia) - shortness of breath, without lungs or heart being affected; sallow complexion from defective oxydation of the blood; heart-burn, dyspepsia; irritative flatulent gastralgia; round ulcer of stomach (local failure of nutrition); menses irregular, scanty or copious; spinal irritation, albinuria, tendency to diarrhoea; constant desire for candy or sugar.

Arg-nit. (Chlorosis) - shortness of breath without lung or heart affection; sallow complexion; heartburn, dyspepsia, irritative flatulent garalgia; round ulcer of stomach (local malnutrition); menses irregular, copious or scanty, but clotted; bone-pains; symptoms of spinal irritation, fulgurating pains, with paretic motory and sensory symptoms; albuminaria; tendency to diarrhoea.

Arnica - favors assimilation and increases nutrition. - Gradual loss of weight from impaired nutrition.

Ars-alb. (Sleeplessness.) - blood degeneration, malnutrition, with nervous exhaustion, anguish, driving out of bed, changes to sofa or chair and then back to bed, cannot rest in any place, changes continually, which fatigues him (Iod. has the restlessness, but not the fatigue of Ars.); dyspeptic insomnia; excessive prostration with the restlessness; < after midnight.

Ars-iod. (Chronic catarrh of the head) - malaria; persons with pale, delicate skin, enlarged tonsils, defective nutrition, with tendency to passive oedema, shown by puffiness of the eyelids; tuberculous diathesis; the discharge of the nasal or laryngeal catarrh is generally copious and thin, but sometimes scanty and thick, yellow like yellow honey, or tenacious and frothy. Discharge of very irritating and corrosive watery mucus, burning the nostrils and lip, attended with alternate chills and heat; foetid and corrosive otorrhoea; enlargement of tonsils with tendency to induration.

Berberis aquifolium - hepatic torpor, lassitude and other evidences of incomplete metamorphosis; stimulates all glands and improves nutrition.

Borax (Atrophy of children) - malnutrition and excessive nervousness. Child grows pale, relaxed, flabby, cries; loathes the breast and falls into a heavy sleep; head and palms of hands hot, face pale and clay-colored; hot mouth and aphthae on tongue and cheeks from impaired nutrition, bleeding when rubbed; every attempt to nurse causes screaming; stools light yellow, slimy, green, or painless, as if fermented, thin, brown, smelling like carrion; fear of downward motion; easily startled by the slightest noise; sleeps badly and awakens with screams as if in a fright and clings to something as if afraid of falling.

Calc-carb. - nutrition impaired, with tendency to glandular engorgements.

Calc-carb. (Atrophy of children) - Emaciation more marked in other than adipose tissue; atrophy of muscles, soft bones, retarded teeth (defective nutrition), with deceptive appearance of plumpness from excess of fat. When also the fat wastes, the body dwindles, the pale skin hangs in folds, but abdomen remains disproportionately enlarged; partial sweats; scalp covered with cold sweat, knees clammy, feet damp and cold; crusta lactea, crusts dry or filled with a mild thick pus; ringworms; glands engorged, especially the mesenteric; appetite voracious, yet emaciation persists; morbid appetite for indigestible articles of food; fever and thirst in afternoon; stools green, watery, sour, or pungent, or clay-like, and < in the afternoon, or creamy, foetid, frequent;

urine strong, foetid, clear; vomiting of sour food or of curdled milk; child obstinate, self-willed, cross before stool and faint after; growth retarded, spine weak, it sits stooped, legs curved and bones bent easily, though old enough will not put its feet to the ground; worse by bathing; child craves eggs; thirst at night for cold water.

Calc-carb. (Goitre) - (powdered egg-shell, from which the membrane has been removed.) cystic swellings; painless swelling of glands; granular vegetations, polypi; nutrition faulty with a tendency to glandular enlargements.

Calc-carb. (Mind Symptoms) - malnutrition and malassimilation; fears she will lose her reason and people will observe her mental confusion; feeling of oppression, with heaviness of legs, trembling of body and frequent weeping, < evening and when admonished; grief and complaining about old offences, dread of solitude which is unbearable; dread of being seized by misfortune, on account of her ruined health; loathing of work, with irritability; great tendency to be frightened, the least noise, the most trifling unexpected occurrence fatigues and causes trouble; does not like to talk.

Calc-carb. (Tumors) - leucophlegmasia and malnutrition; polypi, nasal and uterine; fibroid tumors; lipoma, encephaloma; tendency to boils; deficient animal heat, cold feet, perspiration on head and feet; pus copious, putrid, yellowish or white, like milk; worse in cold air or wet weather; better from having the garments loose; pedunculated fibroids (Calc. iod., Calc-ars.).

Calc-carb. - its chief action is centered in the vegetative sphere, impaired nutrition being the keynote of its action, the glands, skin, and bones, being instrumental in the changes wrought.

Calc-phos. - malnutrition and defective cell growth.

Calc-phos. (Rachitis, rickets) - defective nutrition; very sensitive to dampness; child thin, emaciated, with sunken, rather flabby abdomen, predisposed to glandular and osseous diseases; head large, both fontanelles open; cranial bones unnaturally thin and brittle; teeth develop tardily; curvature of spine, which does not support body and child is slow in learning to walk; neck thin, does not support head; persistent vomiting of milk, and colic after every feeding; stools green, slimy, lienteric, accompanied by foetid flatus; craving for bacon and ham; slow mental development, even stupidity. in older children any exposure to dampness and wet causes a general feeling of aching and soreness, especially on motion; every little exposure causes feeling of heat all over body; joints and periosteum irritated and inflamed; hence < from motion; condyles swollen on forearms and lower limbs; nonunion of fractured bones; Spina bifida. It may prevent rachitis and Sil. follows well.

Calc-phos. (Wounds, injuries, sprains, etc) - wounds fail to heal by first intention from impaired nutrition; in fractures it promotes formation of callus; the place of an old injury becomes the seat of new affections.

Calcarea fluorica - a powerful tissue remedy for hard, stony glands, varicose and enlarged veins, and malnutrition of bones.

Carbo-veg. (Gastralgia) - atony of digestion suits old people, the male sex and the haemorrhoidal world; pains in stomach from loss of nutrition; excessive hunger at night, must eat to appease it; painful burning pressure, with anguish, trembling, and aggravation by contact, at night and after a meal, especially after taking flatulent food; spasmodic contractive pain, compelling the patient to bend double, with short breathing and aggravation in a recumbent position; heartburn; nausea; loathing of food, even when merely thinking of it; frequent flatulence, with oppression of chest and constipation, > by belching, eructations sour, rancid; flatulence burning, putrid, moist, offensive; < from debauchery.

Causticum (Scrofulosis) - scrofulous children, though generally emaciated, and particularly about feet, have a large and tumefied abdomen, are slow in learning to walk and stumble when they attempt to walk, from defective nutrition of the whole nervous system; scrofulous ophthalmia, scabs about tarsi; conjunctivae injected, cornea inflamed; constant feeling as of sand beneath the eyelids; eruption on scalp and behind ears; making skin raw and excoriated, with scanty, sticky discharge; purulent otorrhoea.

Cina - great emaciation from impaired nutrition.

Crotalus hor. - very rapid and direct depressing influence on sensorium and medulla oblongata, deranging both circulation and nutrition; after death, in subacute and chronic cases, the cerebrum, cerebellum and medulla are found in a state of engorgement, with dark, fluid, degraded blood, and apparently threatened with softening.

Crotalus hor. - old age nutritional troubles.

Ferr-met. (Debility) - anaemic debility from faulty nutrition and assimilation (Calc.); relaxation and weakness of entire muscular system with emaciation; muscles feeble and easily exhausted from light exertion; pseudoplethora, even tendency to get fat; fainting spells with subsequent weakness; falls asleep when sewing or studying, from weariness and debility; when falling asleep sweat breaks out, which awakens him and keeps him awake till morning; depression of spirits.

Ferrum met. - a cachectic state from faulty nutrition and assimilation.

Glycerinum - it disturbs nutrition in its primary action, and, secondarily, seems to improve the general state of nutrition.

Graphites (Glands, diseases of, adenitis) - scrofulous swelling of cervical glands; swelling and indurations of the lymphatics and glands; rough, harsh, dry skin; deficiency of animal heat, very liable to take cold from the least cold air; improper nutrition, though looking fat, she is not healthy.

Graphites (Insanity) - herpetic constitution; tendency to obesity from faulty nutrition; timidity, fidgety while sitting at work; extreme hesitation, she is unable to make up her mind about anything; very fretful, everything angers and offends him; absent-minded and slow in thoughts, sad, despondent, music makes her weep; solicitude concerning spiritual welfare; full of fear in the morning, feels miserably unhappy; hates work; ailments from grief.

Helonias (Urinary difficulties) - profuse and frequent urination; weariness and feeling of weight in renal region; after micturition some urine will flow out; burning sensation in urethra when urinating; suitable to women who are enervated from indolence and luxury (Alet., weakness from long sickness and defective nutrition).

Hippozaeninum - extrusion of contents overbalances supply of nutrition.

Hydrastis (Cancer) - cancers hard, adherent, skin mottled, puckered, cutting pain like knives and even after ulceration sets in, where it may regulate faulty nutrition; epithelioma; cancer of rectum; cancer of stomach, vomits everything except water with milk; pain in pit of stomach, emaciation.

Hydrastis (Uterus complaints) - ulceration of cervix and vagina, prolapsus uteri; uterine disease, with sympathetic affections of the digestive organs; profuse leucorrhoea, tenacious, ropy, thick, yellow; pruritus vulvae, with sexual excitement;

fibroid tumors, irregular and profuse menses, or scanty and pale from loss of nutrition and assimilation; weakness and faintness in epigastrium, with palpitation of heart.

Ichthyolum - chronic hives. Tuberculosis, aids nutrition.

Ignatia (Chlorosis) - sensitive, nervous and hysteric women, inclined to spasmodic and intermittent complaints, and where the trouble is induced by mental emotions, such as fright, grief, disappointed love; stomach delicate; faulty nutrition from want or other causes.

Lac can. (Gums, diseases of) - Gums swollen, ulcerated, retracted, bleeding, teeth loose, caused by defective nutrition and exposure.

Lac-def. - diseases with faulty nutrition, in consequence of obscure subacute inflammation of stomach or intestines, followed by affections of the nervous centres.

Lac-def. - A remedy for diseases with faulty nutrition; sick headaches, with profuse flow of urine during pain.

Lecithinum - tuberculosis causing marked improvement in nutrition and general improvement.

Lycopodium (Ophthalmia) - disorders of nutrition and function of the deep-seated structures of the eyes; hemeralopia coming on in the early evening; black spots before eyes accompany the night-blindness; ophthalmia neonatorum during the suppurative stage; catarrhal ophthalmia, secretion thick, yellowish, green; arthritic catarrh of the conjunctiva, with accumulation of white matter in the corners; scrofulous conjunctivitis, with yellowish discharge; ciliary blepharitis and hordeola; polypus of external canthus.

Mag-phos. - nutrition and function remedy for the nerve generals, rare-strange-peculiars:

Nutritional disorders

Mag-phos. (Gastric difficulties, colic of infants) - wind colic of small children, with drawing up of legs, with or without diarrhoea; flatus neither passes up nor down; > by warmth and bending double; nutrition not interfered with, though crying day and night.

Natrum mur. (Ophthalmia) - muscular asthenopia, drawing, stiff sensation in the muscles of the eye when moving them; aching in eyes when looking intently; fiery zigzag appearance around all objects; ciliary neuralgia, pain above eye coming on and going off with the sun; blepharitis, ulcers on cornea, with acrid, excoriating discharge, photophobia and spasmodic closure of lids; stricture of lachrymal duct, fistula and blennorrhoea of lachrymal sac; affections of eyes maltreated with lunar caustic; general breakdown, digestion and nutrition slow and imperfect.

Natrum mur. (Sexual complaints) - deficient nutrition and dirty, flaccid, torpid skin; genital organs smell badly and strongly; feeling of weakness in sexual organs; sexual instinct dormant, with retarded emission during an embrace; frequent nocturnal emissions in spite of frequent embraces; after sexual excesses physical weakness, even paralysis; scrotum relaxed, flabby, emission of prostatic fluid without erection when thinking of sexual things; coldness in joints and weakness. Women averse to coitus, which is painful from dryness of vagina; sterility, with too early and too profuse menstruation or too late and scanty; chlorosis and anaemia in young girls.

Oleum-jec. - rheumatism, produced by protracted residence in damp and cold localities; affection confined to joints; gradual exhaustion of strength and impairment of nutrition.

Oleum-jec. - weakness, emaciation and anemia; defective nutrition, especially in children.

Picric-acid. (Debility) - Asthenia from diminished nutrition; weakness of muscles; furunculosis; lame and tired sensation all over the body; > in open air and when at rest.

Picric-acid. (Leucaemia) - perversion of nutrition; great chilliness, followed by cold, clammy sweat; lack of will-power to undertake anything (Sil., the reverse); dull, heavy pains in head and neck, very hungry or no appetite, but thirst for very cold water, oppressive feeling in epigastrium; can get the breath only half way down; weakness and heaviness in limbs, especially left, legs feel as if made of lead; the least exertion exhausts; cold, clammy sweat on hands and feet, in daytime.

Sabal serrulata - promotes nutrition and tissue building.

Silicea (Headache) - headaches from nervous exhaustion; severe pressing or shattering headache, the pain is felt in the nape of the neck, ascends to vertex, and then to supraorbital region, also from the occiput to the eyeball, especially the right one, sharp darting pains and a steady ache, the eyeball being sore and painful when revolving, worse by mental excessive strain, noise, motion, even the jarring of the room by a footstep, and also by light, relief by heat, but not by pressure, blindness after the headache; headache involving nape of neck, occiput, vertex and eyes, when most violent accompanied by nausea and vomiting, and passing away during sleep; obstinate morning headaches, with chilliness and nausea; hemicrania, with loud cries, nausea to fainting, subsequent obscuration of sight > by copious flow of pale, limpid urine; periodical headache every seventh day; vibratory shaking sensation in head when stepping hard, with tension in forehead and eyes; frequent sweat about the head, great sensitiveness of the scalp; falling off of the hair; rheumatic diathesis; great prostration with craving for food and < from abstinence; paralytic weakness from defective nutrition of the nerves themselves, with oversusceptibility to nervous stimuli.

Silicea (Scrofulosis) - decided want of vital heat even when taking exercise; imperfect nutrition, not from want of food, but from imperfect assimilation; canine hunger, in nervous, irritable people; desires only cold things; swelling and induration of parotid and cervical glands; difficult dentition; offensive-smelling sweat of feet and head; headache, > by wrapping head up warmly (Magn-mur.); rachitis; ozaena; swelling and soreness in old cicatricial tissues about neck and throat; curvature of bones; caries of vertebral column with lateral curvature; disposition of skin to ulcerate; tendency to boils, which leave indurations; carbuncles; malignant pustule; eczema, impetigo, herpes; blepharitis; otorrhoea; face pale and bloated; abdomen large and hard; diarrhoea with thin, offensive stools, containing partially digested food. (Calc-fluor. follows well after Sil.)

Silicea (infantile spinal paralysis, progressive muscular atrophy) - paralysis from defective nutrition of the nervous system; over-susceptibility to nervous stimuli; trembling of legs, as if he had lost all power over them.

Silicea (Paralysis) - paralysis from defective nutrition of nervous system, with oversusceptibility to nervous stimuli; brain and spine cannot bear ordinary vibration or concussion; skin tender and sensitive to touch; paralysis as a sequel to convulsions, paralytic difficulty in swallowing, paralysis of left hand, with atrophy and numbness of fingers; paralysis of legs, < mornings, with heaviness of head and ringing in ears; progressive sclerosis of posterior column, sense of great debility, wants to lie down; limbs go to sleep easily, are sore, lame and cold; trembling of legs, as if he had lost all power over them; wandering pains, passing quickly from one part of body to another; spasms or paralysis from checked foot-sweats, depending on alterations in connective tissue in brain and spinal cord; glandular induration; sclerosis of connective tissue; gliomatosis.

Silicea - imperfect assimilation and consequent defective nutrition.

Staphisagria (Dandruff) - painful sensitiveness of scalp, skin peels off, with itching and smarting, < evenings and from getting warm; hair falls out, mostly from occiput and around ears, with humid, foetid eruption or dandruff on the scalp; vexation, disturbed nutrition.

Thyroidinum - thyroid exercises a general regulating influence over the mechanism of the organs of nutrition growth and development.

Zincum met. - debility, especially of females, from protracted illness or defective nutrition; no organic disease.

. Zincum met. - leucorrhoea from loss of fluids or defective nutrition; debility from protracted illness.

Zincum met. - weak digestion, depressed function of nutrition, with cerebral affections; constipation, with affections of liver or flatulent colic; gastric troubles during pregnancy.

Diseases associated with Nutrition

(Amenorrhoea) Aletris - amenia, or delaying menses, in consequence of atony of the womb or ovaries; weariness of mind and body; fulness and distension of abdomen, with bearing-down sensation; night-sweats; constipation from want of muscular action; debility arising from protracted illness; loss of fluid; defective nutrition.

(Anaemia) Arg-nit. - shortness of breath, without lungs or heart being affected; sallow complexion from defective oxydation of the blood; heart-burn, dyspepsia; irritative

Nutritional disorders

flatulent gastralgia; round ulcer of stomach (local failure of nutrition); menses irregular, scanty or copious; spinal irritation, albinuria, tendency to diarrhoea; constant desire for candy or sugar.

(Atrophy of children) Borax - malnutrition and excessive nervousness. Child grows pale, relaxed, flabby, cries; loathes the breast and falls into a heavy sleep; head and palms of hands hot, face pale and clay-colored; hot mouth and aphthae on tongue and cheeks from impaired nutrition, bleeding when rubbed; every attempt to nurse causes screaming; stools light yellow, slimy, green, or painless, as if fermented, thin, brown, smelling like carrion; fear of downward motion; easily startled by the slightest noise; sleeps badly and awakens with screams as if in a fright and clings to something as if afraid of falling.

(Atrophy of children) Calc-carb. - Emaciation more marked in other than adipose tissue; atrophy of muscles, soft bones, retarded teeth (defective nutrition), with deceptive appearance of plumpness from excess of fat. when also the fat wastes, the body dwindles, the pale skin hangs in folds, but abdomen remains disproportionately enlarged; partial sweats; scalp covered with cold sweat, knees clammy, feet damp and cold; crusta lactea, crusts dry or filled with a mild thick pus; ringworms; glands engorged, especially the mesenteric; appetite voracious, yet emaciation persists; morbid appetite for indigestible articles of food; fever and thirst in afternoon; stools green, watery, sour, or pungent, or clay-like, and < in the afternoon, or creamy, foetid, frequent; urine strong, foetid, clear; vomiting of sour food or of curdled milk; child obstinate, self-willed, cross before stool and faint after; growth retarded, spine weak, it sits stooped, legs curved and bones bent easily, though old enough will not put its feet to the ground; worse by bathing; child craves eggs; thirst at night for cold water.

(Cancer) Hydrastis - cancers hard, adherent, skin mottled, puckered, cutting pain like knives and even after ulceration sets in, where it may regulate faulty nutrition; epithelioma; cancer of rectum; cancer of stomach, vomits everything except water with milk; pain in pit of stomach, emaciation.

(Cataract) Cataract from suppression of habitual foot-sweats, disordered nutrition and after inflammation of eyes: Sulph.

(Chlorosis) Arg-nit. - shortness of breath without lung or heart affection; sallow complexion; heartburn, dyspepsia, irritative flatulent gastralgia; round ulcer of stomach (local malnutrition); menses irregular, copious or scanty, but clotted; bone-pains; symptoms of spinal irritation, fulgurating pains, with paretic motory and sensory symptoms; albuminaria; tendency to diarrhoea.

(Chlorosis) Ignatia - sensitive, nervous and hysteric women, inclined to spasmodic and intermittent complaints, and where the trouble is induced by mental emotions, such as fright, grief, disappointed love; stomach delicate; faulty nutrition from want or other causes.

(Chronic catarrh of the head) Ars-iod. - malaria; persons with pale, delicate skin, enlarged tonsils, defective nutrition, with tendency to passive oedema, shown by puffiness of the eyelids; tuberculous diathesis; the discharge of the nasal or laryngeal catarrh is generally copious and thin, but sometimes scanty and thick, yellow like yellow honey, or tenacious and frothy. Discharge of very irritating and corrosive watery mucus, burning the nostrils and lip, attended with alternate chills and heat; foetid and corrosive otorrhoea; enlargement of tonsils with tendency to induration.

(Dandruff) Staphisagria - painful sensitiveness of scalp, skin peels off, with itching and smarting, < evenings and from getting warm; hair falls out, mostly from occiput and around ears, with humid, foetid eruption or dandruff on the scalp; vexation, disturbed nutrition.

(Debility) Aletris - weariness of mind and body; dizzy when stooping; sleepiness; least food distresses stomach, flatulency and constipation; debility, especially of women from protracted illness or defective nutrition, no organic disease. Debility after diphtheria.

(Debility) Ferr-m. - anaemic debility from faulty nutrition and assimilation (Calc.); relaxation and weakness of entire muscular system with emaciation; muscles feeble and easily exhausted from light exertion; pseudoplethora, even tendency to get fat; fainting spells with subsequent weakness; falls asleep when sewing or studying, from weariness and debility; when falling asleep sweat breaks out, which awakens him and keeps him awake till morning; depression of spirits.

(Debility) Pic-acid. - Asthenia from diminished nutrition; weakness of muscles; furunculosis; lame and tired sensation all over the body; > in open air and when at rest.

(Favus, tinea maligna) - A parasitic disease from malnutrition and malhygiene. Constitutional antipsoric treatments are of first choice then give according to indications.

(Fever, relapsing) Fever, relapsing - strict hygiene and good nutrition are a necessity, of more importance than medicinal treatment. According to symptoms we give:

(Gastralgia) Carbo-veg. - atony of digestion suits old people, the male sex and the haemorrhoidal world; pains in stomach from loss of nutrition; excessive hunger at night, must eat to appease it; painful burning pressure, with anguish, trembling, and aggravation by contact, at night and after a meal, especially after taking flatulent food; spasmodic contractive pain, compelling the patient to bend double, with short breathing and aggravation in a recumbent position; heartburn; nausea; loathing of food, even when merely thinking of it; frequent flatulence, with oppression of chest and constipation, > by belching, eructations sour, rancid; flatulence burning, putrid, moist, offensive; < from debauchery.

(Gastric difficulties, colic of infants) Mag-phos. - wind colic of small children, with drawing up of legs, with or without diarrhoea; flatus neither passes up nor down; > by warmth and bending double; nutrition not interfered with, though crying day and night.

(Glands, diseases of, adenitis) Graphites - scrofulous swelling of cervical glands; swelling and indurations of the lymphatics and glands; rough, harsh, dry skin; deficiency of animal heat, very liable to take cold from the least cold air; improper nutrition, though looking fat, she is not healthy.

(Goitre) Calc-carb. - (powdered egg-shell, from which the membrane has been removed.) cystic swellings; painless swelling of glands; granular vegetations, polypi; nutrition faulty with a tendency to glandular enlargements.

(Gums, diseases of) Lac can. - gums swollen, ulcerated, retracted, bleeding, teeth loose, caused by defective nutrition and exposure.

(Headache) Silicea - paralytic weakness from defective nutrition of the nerves themselves, with over susceptibility to nervous stimulii.

(Infantile spinal paralysis, progressive muscular atrophy) Silicea - paralysis from defective nutrition of the nervous system;

Nutritional disorders

over-susceptibility to nervous stimuli; trembling of legs, as if he had lost all power over them.

(Insanity) Graphites - herpetic constitution; tendency to obesity from faulty nutrition; timidity, fidgety while sitting at work; extreme hesitation, she is unable to make up her mind about anything; very fretful, everything angers and offends him; absent-minded and slow in thoughts, sad, despondent, music makes her weep; solicitude concerning spiritual welfare; full of fear in the morning, feels miserably unhappy; hates work; ailments from grief.

(Leucaemia) Picric acid. - perversion of nutrition; great chilliness, followed by cold, clammy sweat; lack of will-power to undertake anything (sil., the reverse); dull, heavy pains in head and neck, very hungry or no appetite, but thirst for very cold water, oppressive feeling in epigastrium; can get the breath only half way down; weakness and heaviness in limbs, especially left, legs feel as if made of lead; the least exertion exhausts; cold, clammy sweat on hands and feet, in daytime.

(Leucorrhoea) Aletris - leucorrhoea from loss of fluids or defective nutrition; debility from protracted illness; uterine atony, with heavy, dragging pains about hips; great disposition to miscarriage or early abortion; prolapsus from weakness.

(Mind Symptoms) Calc-carb. - malnutrition and malassimilation; fears she will lose her reason and people will observe her mental confusion; feeling of oppression, with heaviness of legs, trembling of body and frequent weeping, < evening and when admonished; grief and complaining about old offences, dread of solitude which is unbearable; dread of being seized by misfortune, on account of her ruined health; loathing of work, with irritability; great tendency to be frightened, the least noise, the most trifling unexpected occurrence fatigues and causes trouble; does not like to talk.

(Menses complaints) Aletris - premature and profuse; discharge dark with coagula; fulness and weight in uterine region, colicky pains in hypogastrium; debility, defective nutrition and assimilation; drowsiness, vertigo, fainting; extreme constipation and prolapsus uteri from muscular atony.

(Miscarriage, abortion) Aletris - habitual tendency to abortion in feeble persons of lax fibre and anaemic condition, even after haemorrhage has set in; weight in uterine region, tendency to prolapsus uteri; general weakness of mind and body; weak from long sickness or defective nutrition.

(Ophthalmia) Lycopodium - disorders of nutrition and function of the deep-seated structures of the eyes; hemeralopia coming on in the early evening; black spots before eyes accompany the night-blindness; ophthalmia neonatorum during the suppurative stage; catarrhal ophthalmia, secretion thick, yellowish, green; arthritic catarrh of the conjunctiva, with accumulation of white matter in the corners; scrofulous conjunctivitis, with yellowish discharge; ciliary blepharitis and hordeola; polypus of external canthus.

(Ophthalmia) Natrum mur. - muscular asthenopia, drawing, stiff sensation in the muscles of the eye when moving them; aching in eyes when looking intently; fiery zigzag appearance around all objects; ciliary neuralgia, pain above eye coming on and going off with the sun; blepharitis, ulcers on cornea, with acrid, excoriating discharge, photophobia and spasmodic closure of lids; stricture of lachrymal duct, fistula and blennorrhoea of lachrymal sac; affections of eyes maltreated with lunar caustic; general breakdown, digestion and nutrition slow and imperfect.

(Paralysis) Silicea - paralysis from defective nutrition of nervous system, with oversusceptibility to nervous stimuli; brain and spine cannot bear ordinary vibration or concussion; skin tender and sensitive to touch; paralysis as a sequel to convulsions, paralytic difficulty in swallowing, paralysis of left hand, with atrophy and numbness of fingers; paralysis of legs, < mornings, with heaviness of head and ringing in ears; progressive sclerosis of posterior column, sense of great debility, wants to lie down; limbs go to sleep easily, are sore, lame and cold; trembling of legs, as if he had lost all power over them; wandering pains, passing quickly from one part of body to another; spasms or paralysis from checked foot-sweats, depending on alterations in connective tissue in brain and spinal cord; glandular induration; sclerosis of connective tissue; gliomatosis.

(Rachitis, rickets) Calc-phos. - defective nutrition; very sensitive to dampness; child thin, emaciated, with sunken, rather flabby abdomen, predisposed to glandular and osseous diseases; head large, both fontanelles open; cranial bones unnaturally thin and brittle; teeth develop tardily; curvature of spine, which does not support body and child is slow in learning to walk; neck thin, does not support head; persistent vomiting of milk, and colic after every feeding; stools green, slimy, lienteric, accompanied by foetid flatus; craving for bacon and ham; slow mental development, even stupidity. in older children any exposure to dampness and wet causes a general feeling of aching and soreness, especially on motion; every little exposure causes feeling of heat all over body; joints and periosteum irritated and inflamed; hence < from motion; condyles swollen on forearms and lower limbs; non-union of fractured bones; Spina bifida. it may prevent rachitis and Sil. follows well.

(Scrofulosis) Silicea - decided want of vital heat even when taking exercise; imperfect nutrition, not from want of food, but from imperfect assimilation; canine hunger, in nervous, irritable people; desires only cold things; swelling and induration of parotid and cervical glands; difficult dentition; offensive-smelling sweat of feet and head; headache, > by wrapping head up warmly (Magn. mur.); rachitis; ozaena; swelling and soreness in old cicatricial tissues about neck and throat; curvature of bones; caries of vertebral column with lateral curvature; disposition of skin to ulcerate; tendency to boils, which leave indurations; carbuncles; malignant pustule; eczema, impetigo, herpes; blepharitis; otorrhoea; face pale and bloated; abdomen large and hard; diarrhoea with thin, offensive stools, containing partially digested food. (calc. fluor. follows well after Sil.)

(Scrofulosis) Causticum - scrofulous children, though generally emaciated, and particularly about feet, have a large and tumefied abdomen, are slow in learning to walk and stumble when they attempt to walk, from defective nutrition of the whole nervous system; scrofulous ophthalmia, scabs about tarsi; conjunctivae injected, cornea inflamed; constant feeling as of sand beneath the eyelids; eruption on scalp and behind ears; making skin raw and excoriated, with scanty, sticky discharge; purulent otorrhoea.

(Sexual complaints) Natrum mur. - deficient nutrition and dirty, flaccid, torpid skin; genital organs smell badly and strongly; feeling of weakness in sexual organs; sexual instinct dormant, with retarded emission during an embrace; frequent nocturnal emissions in spite of frequent embraces; after sexual excesses physical weakness, even paralysis; scrotum relaxed, flabby, emission of prostatic fluid without erection when thinking of sexual things; coldness in joints and weakness. Women averse to coitus, which is painful from dryness of vagina; sterility, with too early and too profuse menstruation, or too late and scanty; chlorosis and anaemia in young girls.

(Sleeplessness.) Ars-alb. - blood degeneration, malnutrition, with nervous exhaustion, anguish, driving out of bed, changes to sofa or chair and then back to bed, cannot rest in any place, changes continually, which fatigues him (Iod. has the restlessness, but not the fatigue of Ars.); dyspeptic insomnia; excessive prostration with the restlessness; < after midnight.

(Tumors) Calc-carb. - leucophlegmasia and malnutrition; polypi, nasal and uterine; fibroid tumors; lipoma, encephaloma; tendency to boils; deficient animal heat, cold feet, perspiration on head and feet; pus copious, putrid, yellowish or white, like milk; worse in cold air or wet weather; better from having the garments loose; pedunculated fibroids (Calc-iod., Calc-ars.).

(Urinary difficulties) Helonias - profuse and frequent urination; weariness and feeling of weight in renal region; after micturition some urine will flow out; burning sensation in urethra when urinating; suitable to women who are enervated from indolence and luxury (Alet., weakness from long sickness and defective nutrition).

(Uterus complaints) Abies can. - prolapsus from general defective nutrition, with little or no local congestion.

(Uterus complaints) Aletris - prolapsus uteri from muscular atony; leucorrhoea from loss of fluids or defective nutrition; debility from protracted illness; obstinate indigestion, the least food distresses the stomach; fainting, with vertigo; extreme constipation, great effort being required to discharge faeces; great accumulation of frothy saliva; sterility from uterine atony; heavy, dragging pains about the hips; profuse, painful and premature menses; profuse leucorrhoea.

(Uterus complaints) Hydrastis - ulceration of cervix and vagina, prolapsus uteri; uterine disease, with sympathetic affections of the digestive organs; profuse leucorrhoea, tenacious, ropy, thick, yellow; pruritus vulvae, with sexual excitement;

fibroid tumors, irregular and profuse menses, or scanty and pale from loss of nutrition and assimilation; weakness and faintness in epigastrium, with palpitation of heart.

(Vertigo, dizziness) Aletris - vertigo in cases of debility arising from protracted illness, loss of fluids, defective nutrition; vertigo from mental overexertion, with general debility; excessive nausea with giddiness; frequent attacks of fainting with dizziness.

(Wounds, injuries, sprains, etc.) Calc-phos. - wounds fail to heal by first intention from impaired nutrition; in fractures it promotes formation of callus; the place of an old injury becomes the seat of new affections.

Checked discharges—Suppression of secretions

The above symptom would be of immense help, more particularly in chronic diseases as well as grave acute cases.

Suppression of haemorrhage or habitual depletions or any discharges make the disease travel from less important organs to more important organs. This is the direction of disease. Hence most valuable. If found in a case you cannot afford to ignore them. You may straightaway take it.

IMPORTANT NOTE: Here we must make a mention of 'menopause'.

If the complaint of a female patient starts between the age 42 and 47 and she also continues to get her monthly periods you may think of the rubric MENOPAUSE in the chapter GENITALIA FEMALE in Kent's Repertory. But upon inquiry if you find that her complaints started a few months after complete cessation of monthly menses you should not think of MENOPAUSE but consider the following on page 1006 of Lilienthal:

Suppression of haemorrhage or abandoning habitual depletions: 1, Acon., Bell., Chin., Fer., Nux-v., Puls., Sulph.; 2, Arn., Aur., Bry., Calc., Carb-v., Graph., Hyosc., Lyc., Natr-m., Nitr-ac., Phos., Ran., Rhus, Seneg., Sep., Sil., Spong., Stram.

If a patient tells that his complaints started some time after his bleeding fissure in anus or piles was cured, in such cases too you must take the above rubric.

Suppression of secretions: The principal remedies for the ailments arising from this cause are: 1, Acon., Bell., Bry., Calc., Chin., Lyc., Nux-v., Puls., Sulph.; 2, Ars., Carb-v., Caust., Cham., Dulc., Graph., Kalm., Lyc., Phos., Phos-ac., Rhus, Sep., Sil., Stram.; 3, Amb., Amm., Ant., Arn., Aur., Bar., Cina, Cocc., Cupr., Fer., Hep., Hyosc., Ign., Ipec., Merc., Mur-ac., Natr-m., Nitr-ac., Nux-m., Ran., Seneg., Spong., Veratr., Zinc.

Give more particularly:

After suppression of eruptions and herpes: 1, Ant-tart., Apis, Bell., Bry., Cupr., Dulc., Graph., Helleb., Hep., Ipec., Phos-ac., Puls., Sulph.; 2, Acon., Amb., Ars., Carb-v., Caust., Cham., Lach., Lyc., Merc., Natr-m., Mosch., Phos., Rhus, Sarsap., Sep., Sil., Staph., Thuj., Zinc.

Suppression of ulcers and purulent discharges: 1, Bell., Hep., Lach., Sil., Sulph.; 2, Ars., Carb-v., Lyc., Merc., Natr-m., Phos-ac., Rhus, Sep., Staph.

Suppression of piles: 1, Acon., Calc., Carb-v., Nux-v., Puls., Sulph.; 2, Amb., Amm., Ant., Ars., Bell., Caps., Caust., Chin., Coloc., Graph., Ign., Kalm., Lach., Mur-ac., Nitr-ac., Petr., Rhus-t., Sep., Sil.

Suppression of lochia: 1, Coloc., Hyosc., Nux-v., Plat., Rhus, Sec., Veratr., Zinc.; 2, Bell., Bry., Con., Dulc., Puls., Sep., Sulph.

Suppression of milk: 1, Bell., Bry., Dulc., Puls.; 2, Acon., Calc., Cham., Coff., Merc., Rhus, Sulph.

Suppression of menses: 1, Acon., Bry., Con., Dulc., Graph., Kalm., Lyc., Puls., Sep., Sil., Sulph.; 2, Amm., Ars., Bar., Bell., Calc., Caust., Cham., Chin., Cocc., Cupr., Fer., Iod.,

Checked Discharges—Suppression of Secretions

Merc., Natr-m., Nux-m., Op., Plat., Phos., Rhod; Sabin., Staph., Stram., Val., Veratr., Zinc.

Suppression of catarrh or some other blennorrhoea: 1, Acon., Ars., Bell., Bry., Calc., Chin., Cin., Nux-v., Puls., Sulph.; 2, Amb., Amm., Carb-v., Con., Dulc., Graph., Ipec., Kalm., Lyc., Natr-m., Nitr-ac., Nux-m., Phos., Rhod., Samb., Sulph.

Suppression of sweat: 1, Bell., Bry., Cham., Chin., Dulc., Lach., Sil., Sulph.; 2, Acon., Ars., Calc., Graph., Lyc., Merc., Nux-m., Nux-v., Op., Phos., Puls., Rhus, Sep.

Suppression of foot-sweat: 1, Cupr., Nitr-ac., Puls., Sep., Sil.; 2, Cham., Merc., Natr., Rhus.

(When bleeding is found in a patient, whether haemorrhoidal bleeding or epistaxis or gums bleeding, this has top-most value among generals and you must take this rubric first. See Kent's REPERTORY-Generalities—Haemorrhage).

Diseases Associated with 'Checked Secretions/ Suppression of Discharges'

(Agalactia) Dulcamara - suppression from exposure to cold, damp air.

(Albuminuria) Digitalis - dropsy with suppression of urine.

(Angina pectoris) Asafoetida - nervous palpitation from overexertion or suppression of discharges (in women).

(Aphasia, agraphia) Kali-phos. - aphasia after suppressed sweat from fright or mental emotions, from mental overwork.

(Apoplexy) Pulsatilla - violent palpitation of the heart, almost complete suppression of the pulse, and rattling breathing.

(Arthritis, gout) Abrotanum - ailments after suppressed gout.

(Arthritis, gout) - suppressed gout: Colch., Lith., Natr. Phos., if to the heart.

(Asthma) Ars-alb. - asthma from fatigue, from emotions, from suppressed itch.

(Asthma) Ars-alb. - asthma of senility, after suppressed coryza and coexistence of emphysema and cardiac affections.

(Asthma) For asthma caused by an emotion: Acon., Cham., Coff., Cupr., Gels., Ign., Nux-v., Puls., Veratr. - if caused by a suppressed eruption: 1, Ipec., Puls., Veratr.

(Asthma) Ipecac - threatened suffocation from suddenly suppressed catarrhs.

(Asthma) Thuja - after checked gonorrhoea or removal of fissures or condylomata.

(Back pain–spinal irritation) Sulphur - spinal congestion from suppression of menses or haemorrhoidal flow.

(Blepharophthalmia, blepharitis) Sulphur - blepharitis after the suppression of an eruption or when the patient is covered by eczema, especially in strumous children, who are cross and irritable by day and feverish and restless at night.

(Bone diseases, osteitis, periostitis, exostosis, caries, necrosis, etc.) Dulcamara - scrofulous exostosis on upper and lower limbs, in consequence of suppressed itch.

(Bone diseases, osteitis, periostitis, exostosis, caries, necrosis, etc.) Sarsparilla - bones pain after mercurialization or checked gonorrhoea, < at night, in damp weather, or after taking cold in water and from motion of affected part.

(Bronchitis chronica) Sulphur - sensation as of ice in chest, whenever chilled, or perspiration is checked.

(Cancer) Bromium - scirrhus mammae, great depression of spirits, suppression of menses.

(Cataract) Cataract - after typhoids or suppression of menses, disorders of nutrition in the deep-seated structures of the eyes: Sep.

(Cataract) Cataract - from right to left, after skin affections which were suppressed (psor.), or from general perversion of health: Colch.

(Cataract) Cataract - from suppression of habitual foot-sweats, disordered nutrition and after inflammation of eyes: Sulph.

(Chorea) Causticum - after suppressed eruption on head.

(Chorea) Cimicifuga - < when following rheumatic fever, during menses or after their suppression.

(Chorea) Sulphur - chronic cases, after suppressed eruption or where the skin is full of eruptions, itching < in warmth.

(Chorea) Zincum met. - < from exercise. chorea much affecting the general health, caused by fright or suppressed eruptions.

(Chronic catarrh of the head) Phosphorus - chronic inflammation of the nasal membrane, with suppressed or oversensitive smell

(Cinchona, ill effects of) Calc-carb. - especially when these symptoms are occasioned in consequence of the suppression of fever and ague by large doses of quinine, and Puls. proves insufficient.

(Cinchona, ill effects of) Lachesis - for fever and ague which have been suppressed by large doses of quinine, Puls. being inefficient.

(Cinchona, ill effects of) Pulsatilla - pains in the limbs, after suppression of fever and ague.

(Colic) Nux vomica - colic from suppressed haemorrhoidal flow.

(Constipation) Amm-mur. - piles after suppression of leucorrhoea.

(Constipation) Belladonna - fretful, indolent before stool, contented and cheerful after. From cold or suppressed perspiration, < afternoon and evening.

(Constipation) Belladonna - stools suppressed with bloated abdomen, heat of head and abundant sweat.

(Constipation) China - burning, itching, tingling in anus after stool, < at night, from fruits, milk, checked perspiration. sensation of fulness in abdomen after eating, flatulency, flat taste, vomiting of sour matter.

(Constipation) Pulsatilla - stools hard and large, after suppressed intermittent fever by quinine.

(Convulsions in children) Camphor - spasms from suppressed catarrh of head and chest.

(Convulsions in children) Ipecac - from a suppressed eruption.

(Convulsions in children) Merc-sol. - swelling of gums, profuse ptyalism or from suppressed salivation.

(Convulsions in children) Stramonium - suppression of an eruption, or the exanthem fails to come out.

(Convulsions in children) Sulphur - after suppressed eruptions.

(Convulsions in children) Terebinth. - dentition accompanied by suppression of urine and convulsions.

(Coryza) Belladonna - suppressed catarrh with maddening headache.

(Coryza) Dulcamara - discharge suppressed from least contact with cold, damp air, or from changes from hot to cold weather.

(Coryza) Kali-bich. - suppressed voice.

(Coryza) Silicea - dryness and stoppage after checked foot-sweat.

(Cough) Ars-iod. - frequent, short, suppressed cough, often loose with muco-purulent expectoration, occasionally stringy, especially during night and morning.

(Cough) Benzoic acid. - dry, hacking constant cough after suppressed gonorrhoea, followed by expectoration of green

Checked Discharges—Suppression of Secretions

mucus, oppression of lungs relieved by copious secretion from the bowels.

(Cough) Dulcamara - increased secretion of the mucous membranes and glands, those of the skin being suppressed.

(Cough) Eup-perf. - hectic cough from suppressed intermittent fever.

(Cough) Sulphur - suppressed choking cough.

(Coxalgia, hip-disease) Phos-acid. - the disease originating from suppressed or mismanaged scarlatina or other exanthemata, after abuse of mercury.

(Croup) Cuprum met. - cough with interrupted, almost suppressed breathing.

(Debility) Zincum met. - numbness of feet from suppressed foot-sweat, by getting wet, < from wine.

(Diabetes) Cuprum met. - urine acid, straw-colored, turbid after standing, a reddish, thin sediment adhered to vessel, viscous, offensive, bloody, scanty or suppressed.

(Diabetes) Thuja - diabetes after a long-suppressed gonorrhoea, frequent desire to urinate day and night.

(Diarrhoea of infants) Arg-nit. - urine profuse and watery, or scanty and nearly suppressed.

(Diarrhoea of infants) Lycopodium - thin, brown, faecal, mixed with hard lumps, < after meal, after cold food, after suppressed eruptions (especially scabies).

(Diarrhoea of infants) Silicea - suppressed secretion of urine.

(Diarrhoea) Abrotanum - diarrhoea for several days, stopping suddenly or being checked, followed by rheumatism.

(Diarrhoea) Ant-tart. - diarrhoea of drunkards, or in pneumonia, zymosis, especially if the eruption is suppressed.

(Diarrhoea) Bryonia - diarrhoea from suddenly checked perspiration in hot weather, from indulgence in vegetable food or stewed fruits from getting overheated in summer, from drinking milk, cold drinks, or from anger and chagrin.

(Diarrhoea) Chamomilla - mucous diarrhoea in summer, often caused by checked perspiration or crude food, with abundant griping, < towards evening.

(Diarrhoea) Ferrum phos. - often caused by checked perspiration.

(Diarrhoea) Laurocerasus - skin cold, thready pulse, sallow features, dilated pupils, suppression or retention of urine, no vomiting. Stools discharged involuntarily in bed from paralysis of sphincter ani.

(Diarrhoea) Lobelia inflata - from suppressed cutaneous or mucous discharges.

(Diarrhoea) Lycopodium - diarrhoea after suppression of skin eruptions.

(Diarrhoea) Mezereum - chronic diarrhoea with a psoric anamnesis, after suppression of an eruption of thick crusts covering thick pus. Brown, faecal, fermented, offensive stools with weakness and chilliness.

(Diarrhoea) Stramonium - black, fluid, cadaverous-smelling stools, accompanied by loquacious delirium, violent thirst, pale face, vomiting of mucus and suppression of urine.

(Diarrhoea) Sulphur - after suppressed eruptions. Before: sudden and violent urging, without pain.

(Diarrhoea) Ver-a. - suppression of urine. Diarrhoea from change of water (bad drainage), from emotions, as fright, with cold sweat on forehead and coldness of body.

(Distension of abdomen and flatulence) Sulphur - suppressed skin eruptions.

(Dropsy) Apoc-can. - catching of breath, suppression of urine, great thirst.

(Dropsy) Asclepias cornuti - post-scarlatinal dropsy, or from suppressed perspiration, from renal or cardiac affections. Congestive headaches with dullness and stupidity, scanty urine during headache, profuse after.

(Dropsy) Colchicum - dropsy after scarlatina, with suppression of urine, or urine black, containing alben and destroyed bloodcorpuscles.

(Dropsy) Digitalis - dropsy with suppression of urine nephritis scarlatinosa after desquamation, with anasarca and oedema of lungs.

(Dropsy) Eup-purp. - suppression of urine with severe dyspnoea and oedema all over the body.

(Dropsy) Helleborus - suppression of urine or urine highly albinous with fibrinous casts.

(Dropsy) Sulphur - dropsy after suppressed eruptions, rough skin, bluish spots.

(Dropsy) - dropsy in consequence of suppression of exanthemata: 1, Apis, Apoc-can., Ars., Asclep., Dig., Helleb., Sulph.

(Dropsy) - suppression of intermittent fevers: Ars., Chimaph., Dulc., Fer., Merc., Sol-nig., Sulph.

(Dysentery) Baryta carb. - dysentery after suppression of humid tetters.

(Dysentery) Belladonna - urine profuse or suppressed.

(Dysentery) Cuprum met. - urine scanty or suppressed.

(Dysentery) Erigeron - urination painful or suppressed.

(Dysentery) Ferr-phos. - dysentery from checked perspiration in hot weather.

(Dysentery) Merc-cor. - suppression of secretion or retention of urine.

(Dyspepsia, weakness of stomach) Cuprum met. - nausea and vomiting with brain affections, from suppression of menses.

(Eczema) Clematis - after suppressed gonorrhoea.

(Eczema) Kali-mur. - eczema from suppressed or deranged uterine functions.

(Epilepsy) Agaricus - from suppressed eruptions.

(Epilepsy) Bufo sahytiensis - epileptic aura from uterus to stomach, menses suppressed, or fits worse at times of menses, in sleep, followed by severe paid and pressure on top of head, face bathed in sweat during the fit. severe cases, head drawn to one side, then backward before the fit, with numbness of brain, falls down unconscious, with a wild cry, followed by severe tonic and clonic spasms, distorted facial muscles, grinding of teeth foaming at mouth, ending in loud snoring sleep. angry disposition, occipital compression and stiff neck before paroxysm.

(Epilepsy) Calc-phos. - after suppressed menses from bathing.

(Epilepsy) Camphor - cause: suppressed catarrh of head and chest.

(Epilepsy) Causticum - convulsions with screams, gnashing of teeth and violent movements of limbs, with feverish heat and coldness of hands and feet, involuntary micturition, after fright or after suppression of eruptions, in psoric constitutions, < during new moon.

(Epilepsy) Gelsemium - hysterical epilepsy after suppressed menses.

(Epilepsy) Glonoine - from scanty or suppressed menses, after mental or physical effort, followed by sleepiness and subsequent depression, loss of memory and aphasia. Sunstroke, or too much heat on head and face from any cause.

Checked Discharges—Suppression of Secretions

(Epilepsy) Kali-brom. - the grand remedy to suppress but not to cure the disease.

(Epilepsy) Sulphur - whenever some dyscrasia lurks in the system, or its outward symptoms were suppressed.

(Epistaxis, nosebleed) Conium - nosebleed, with suppressed menses, from taking cold.

(Epistaxis, nosebleed) Nux vomica - epistaxis from suppressed haemorrhoidal flow, < mornings, preceded or accompanied by frontal headache, red cheeks and cephalic congestion.

(Epistaxis, nosebleed) Pulsatilla - nosebleed from suppressed menses, blood partly fluid and partly clotted, intermitting in intensity, < by going into a warm room or in a recumbent position. Nosebleed with dry coryza in anaemic women whose courses are scanty, late or suppressed.

(Excessive Sweat. Night-sweats, etc.) Baryta carb. - checked foot-sweat, followed by lameness, tonsillar angina, etc.

(Excessive Sweat. Night-sweats, etc.) Foot-sweats - suppressed: Apis, Cham., Cupr., Form., Kali-carb., Merc., Natr-carb., Natr-m., Nitr-ac., Puls., Rhus, Sep., Sil., Thuj., Zinc.

(Excessive Sweat. Night-sweats, etc.) Thuja - suppressed foot-sweat.

(Excessive Sweat. Night-sweats, etc.) Zincum met. - paralysis of feet from suppression of foot-sweat.

(Exophthalmic goitre) Ferr-iod. - after suppression of menses protrusion of eyes, enlargement of thyroid gland, palpitation of heart and excessive nervousness.

(Exophthalmic goitre) Ferr-met. - exophthalmic goitre, especially after suppression of menses.

(Gastralgia) Abrotanum - gastralgia after suppressed gout.

(Glands, diseases of, adenitis) Spongia - hardness and swelling of testicles, especially after checked gonorrhoea, < on motion of body and squeezing of clothing.

(Glaucoma) Belladonna - suppression of stool and urine.

(Gonorrhoea) Arg-nit. - excessive burning when urinating, with cutting pains extending to the anus and a discharge of excoriating pus, enlargement and induration of testicles from suppressed gonorrhoea.

(Gonorrhoea) Cantharis - tenesmus vesicae and retention when suppressed by injections.

(Gonorrhoea) Erechthites - orchitis during gonorrhoea or when the discharge was suppressed.

(Gonorrhoea) Gelsemium - orchitis from suppressed gonorrhoea.

(Gonorrhoea) Pulsatilla - scanty urine. Suppressed gonorrhoea causes epididymitis.

(Gonorrhoea) Sarsparilla - rheumatism from suppressed gonorrhoea or when it was checked by exposure to wet or cold weather.

(Gonorrhoea) Sepia - condylomata from suppressing the gonorrhoea with astringent injections.

(Gonorrhoea) Thuja - pointed condylomata. Checked gonorrhoea causes articular rheumatism, Especially knee-joint, prostatitis, sycosis, impotence. Extreme mental depression.

(Gums, diseases of) Calc-carb. - swelling, bleeding, even at night, bleeding of gums after suppressed menses.

(Haematemesis, gastrorrhagia) Phosphorus - haematemesis after suppression of menses.

(Haematemesis, gastrorrhagia) Pulsatilla - vomiting of blood, due to a cold or suppression of menses, with nausea, pale face, chilliness, faintness, blood dark and easily coagulating (Fer.).

(Haematuria, haemorrhage from urinary organs) Ars-hydro. - urine suppressed, followed by vomiting.

(Haematuria, haemorrhage from urinary organs) Erigeron - urination painful or suppressed.

(Haematuria, haemorrhage from urinary organs) Nux vomica - haematuria from suppressed haemorrhoidal flow or menses.

(Haematuria, haemorrhage from urinary organs) Sulphur - haematuria after suppressed cutaneous or haemorrhoidal discharges.

(Haematuria, haemorrhage from urinary organs) Zincum met. - vicarious bleeding through urethra, in consequence of suppressed menses.

(Haemorrhage from the lungs, haemoptysis) Belladonna - suppressed menses.

(Haemorrhage from the lungs, haemoptysis) - suppressed menses: Acon., Ars., Bell., Fer., Mill., Phos., Puls., Senec.

(Haemorrhage from the lungs, haemoptysis) Millefolium - after injuries. Chronic haemorrhages in tuberculosis, menstrual derangement, suppressed haemorrhoids, debauchery. Patient feels unconcerned about his state, and no pain with the bleeding.

(Haemorrhage from the lungs, haemoptysis) Nux vomica - due to debauchery, high living and suppressed haemorrhoids.

(Haemorrhage from the lungs, haemoptysis) Pulsatilla - suppressio mensium followed by obstinate cases of haemoptosis., blood dark, coagulated, coughed out in pieces, < at night, with pain in lower part of chest.

(Haemorrhage from the lungs, haemoptysis) Senecio - haemoptysis in suppressed menstruation.

(Haemorrhage from uterus) Ignatia - great despondency, she seems full of suppressed grief. Menstrual blood black, in clots, of putrid odor.

(Haemorrhages) Ipecac. - < from suppressed eruptions, from having taken peruvian bark at some past time.

(Haemorrhoids) Acetic acid. - haemorrhage from bowels after checked metrorrhagia.

(Haemorrhoids) Aloe - headache over eyes with sensation as if a weight were pressing the eyelids down, > from partially closing the eyelids, dull pressing, followed by difficulty of thinking. haemorrhoids from a suppressed cutaneous eruption.

(Haemorrhoids) Amm-mur. - haemorrhoids sore and smarting after suppressed leucorrhoea.

(Haemorrhoids) Calc-carb. - vertigo, especially when going up stairs, with dullness and heaviness of head from cessation or suppression of haemorrhoidal flow.

(Haemorrhoids) Capsicum - suppressed haemorrhoidal flow, causing melancholy.

(Haemorrhoids) Nux vomica - haematuria from suppressed haemorrhoidal flow or menses.

(Haemorrhoids) Nux vomica - ischuria, suppression of urine.

(Haemorrhoids) Sulphur - suppressed haemorrhoids, with colic, palpitation, congestion of lungs.

(Haemorrhoids) We have also to consider - for anomalies of the haemorrhoidal difficulties and ailments in consequence of the suppression of a habitual haemorrhoidal flow: 1, Nux-v., Sulph.

(Hair falling) - for violent itching of the scalp, especially if in consequence of old suppressed eruptions: graph., Kali-carb., Lyc., Sil., Sulph.

(Headache) Agnus castus - contracting headaches from sexual debility after excesses, > by looking at one point. (Puls., Con., from suppressed sexual excitement.

(Headache) Apis-mel. - suppressed micturition in children.

(Headache) Asclepias cornuti - congestive headache from suppression of sweat or urine and fever.

(Headache) Calc-carb. - headache from suppressed nasal catarrh.

(Headache) Carbo animalis - headache from suppression of menses.

(Headache) Glonoine - bad sequelae of cutting hair. intense congestion of the brain in plethoric constitutions, with persistent sensation of pulsation, from sudden suppression of menses, after anxiety and worry with sleeplessness.

(Headache) Graphites - suppressed herpetic eruptions.

(Headache) Kali-bich. - often caused by the suppression of a chronic catarrh.

(Headache) Lithium carb. - pain from stomach to head, from left temple into left orbit, > while eating and < after eating, after suppression of menses.

(Headache) Mezereum - from suppression of eczema.

(Headache) Nux moschata - worse from getting wet, change of weather, riding in a carriage, after eating, or wine, from suppressed eruptions, before menses, during pregnancy.

(Headache) Sulphur - headache from abdominal plethora, from suppressed skin diseases, or chronic gouty and rheumatic headaches, increased by mental exertion, motion, coughing, sneezing.

(Hearing, defective) Cactus - after otitis from checked sweat.

(Hearing, defective) if by suppression of discharges from the ears or from the nose: 1, Hep., Lach., Led.

(Hearing, defective) - suppression of herpes, or other cutaneous eruptions: 1, Ant., Graph., Sulph.

(Hearing, defective) - suppression of intermittent fever: 1, Calc., Puls.

(Hearing, defective) Ledum - after cutting the hair, after chilling the head, after suppressed coryza or otorrhoea.

(Hearing, defective) Pulsatilla - deafness, as if the ears were stopped up, after suppressed measles, with otorrhoea, from cold after cutting hair (Led.), with hard black cerumen.

(Heart diseases) Ars-alb. - heartbeat too strong, visible to the person standing by and audible to the patient himself, < at night and when lying on back. Endocarditis and pericarditis with restlessness, agony and tingling of fingers of left hand, after suppressed measles or scarlatina.

(Heart diseases) Ars-alb. - palpitation of suppressed herpes or foot-sweat. valvular disease with intermittent pulse, dyspnoea, anasarca, < towards evening and at night, on going upstairs, after deep inspirations or getting angry. general oedema, beginning with puffiness in eyes and swelling of feet. Hydrothorax and hydropericardium, with spells of suffocation, < after midnight and when lying down, skin cool and clammy with internal burning heat.

(Heart diseases) Ars-alb. - pulse sometimes suppressed, with strong beat of the heart.

(Heart diseases) Asafoetida - nervous palpitations, with small pulse from overexertion or suppressed discharge (in women).

(Heart diseases) Calc-carb. - after least exertion, after suppressed eruptions.

(Heart diseases) Tarentula hispp. - rheumatism checked by putting extremities in cold water, followed by panting respiration, anxiety, cramps or twisting pains in heart.

(Hepatic derangements) Berberis vul. - suppression of haemorrhoids.

(Hepatic derangements) Digitalis - dropsy with suppression of urine.

Checked Discharges—Suppression of Secretions

(Herpes) Clematis - eruptions following suppressed gonorrhoea.

(Herpes) Psorinum - moist herpes after suppressed itch, itching intolerably when getting warm, < before midnight and in open air.

(Herpes) Thuja - herpes all over body from suppressed gonorrhoea, itching and burning violently.

(Hydrocephaloid) Arg-nit. - suppression of urine.

(Hydrocephaloid) Carbo-veg. - suppression of urine.

(Hydrocephaloid) Sulphur - urine suppressed.

(Hypochondriasis) Aloe - haemorrhoids from suppressed chronic eruptions.

(Hysteria) Cantharis - previous to the hysterical attack partial or total suppression of urine, followed afterwards by copious micturition, urine deficient in urates.

(Hysteria) Cimicifuga - uterine neuralgia, menses irregular, delayed or suppressed.

(Insanity) Camphor - lochia suppressed with erethism of sexual system, followed by exhaustion and collapse.

(Insanity) Causticum - mental alienation after suppression of eruptions.

(Insanity) Lilium-tig. - has to keep very busy to suppress sexual desire.

(Insanity) Veratrum alb. - despair of her position in society, with suppressed catamenia.

(Iris, affections of) Sulphur - chronic iritis in scrofulous persons, especially after suppression of eruptions.

(Iris, affections of) Terebinth. - rheumatic iritis with intense pains in eye and head, especially if the result of suppressed foot-sweat.

(Labor) Nux moschata - pains slow, feeble or suppressed.

(Laryngitis and laryngeal phthisis) Apis-mel. - laryngeal symptoms accompanying erysipelas, oedema of throat, glottis or larynx or suppression of eruptions.

(Leucaemia) Kali-mur. - menses late or suppressed.

(Leucorrhoea) Agnus castus - suppressed menses.

(Leucorrhoea) Caulophyllum - menses suppressed from nervous causes in young girls or in nervous, debilitated women with relaxed, flabby uterus or displaced and passively congested uterus, especially after miscarriage.

(Leucorrhoea) Erigeron - urination painful or suppressed.

(Leucorrhoea) Pulsatilla - leucorrhoea in young girls about puberty or when menses were suppressed by fright or from exposure to cold and dampness.

(Lienitis) Aranea diad. - swelling of spleen after checked intermittent fever with quinine, < in damp weather and exposure to damp walls.

(Measles) Kali-sul. - suppressed rash which suddenly recedes with harsh and dry skin.

(Meningitis basilaris) Apoc-can. - urine suppressed.

(Meningitis basilaris) Bryonia - suppressed or painful urination with much straining.

(Meningitis basilaris) Lycopodium - suppression of urine.

(Meningitis basilaris) Opium - urine suppressed.

(Meningitis basilaris) Pulsatilla - suppressed otorrhoea.

(Meningitis basilaris) Stramonium - urine suppressed.

(Meningitis basilaris) Sulphur - suppression of a chronic skin disease, or of an otorrhoea, caused the gradual appearance of the disease.

(Meningitis basilaris) Zincum met. - child has not vitality enough to develop the eruption, or it was checked in its appearance.

(Meningitis, cerebro-spinalis) Cantharis - dysuria, retention or suppression of urine.

(Meningitis, encephalitis) Apis-mel. - meningitis from suppression or spread of erysipelas or other exanthemata. Congestion to the head and face, with fullness, burning and throbbing in brain.

(Meningitis, encephalitis) Bryonia - meningitis after suppression of some eruption.

(Meningitis, encephalitis) Cicuta - cerebral diseases following suppressed eruptions.

(Meningitis, encephalitis) Cuprum met. - meningitis the result of suppressed exanthema.

(Meningitis, encephalitis) Helleborus - scanty or suppressed urination, with relief of symptoms when urine passes more freely.

(Meningitis, encephalitis) if caused by suppression of otorrhoea, give Puls. or Sulph.

(Meningitis, encephalitis) - meningitis from suppression of erysipelas, or some other eruption, such as scarlatina, requires: 1, Bell., Rhus.

(Meningitis, encephalitis) Pulsatilla - meningitis from suppressed otorrhoea, or any other discharge.

(Menses complaints) Veratrum vir. - suppressed menses with cerebral congestion.

(Metritis) Belladonna - lochial discharge scanty or suppressed.

(Metritis) Secale - the inflammation seems to be caused by suppression of the lochia or menses.

[Migraine (headache)] Colocynth - hemicrania from anger with indignation, after suppression of menses, pains extending towards forehead and left side of head, with nausea, vomiting or diarrhoea, especially towards evening.

(Miscarriage, abortion) Colocynth - suppression of lochia after abortus, from vexation and anger.

(Myelitis acuta, inflammation of the spinal cord) Colchicum - paralysis after suddenly suppressed sweat, especially foot-sweat, by getting wet.

(Nausea and Vomiting) Nux vomica - haematemesis after suppressed haemorrhoids.

(Nephralgia, renal colic) Erigeron - sharp, stinging pain in left renal region, complete suppression of urine or urging to urinate with emission of only a few burning drops.

(Nephritis) Erigeron - complete suppression of urine, and pain in kidney, followed by urging to urinate, with emission of only a few burning drops.

(Nettlerash, urticaria) Urtica urens - consequences of suppressed nettlerash.

(Neuralgia) Sarsparilla - after mercury or checked gonorrhoea.

(Nightmare) Opium - severe paroxysms, with suppressed breathing, half-opened eyes, open mouth, stertorous breathing, rattling, anxious features, cold sweat, twitchings and convulsive motions of extremities.

(Noises in the ear) - suppressed eruptions: ant., caust., graph., lach., sulph.

(Ophthalmia) - suppression of eruptions: alum., ars., Carb-v., caust., graph., lach., Natr-m., sel., sep., sulph., zinc.

(Ophthalmia) Belladonna - hyperaesthesia and hyperaemia of the optic nerve and retina, apoplexy of retina, with suppressed menses.

(Ophthalmia) Pulsatilla - amblyopia from suppression of any bloody discharge, from gastric derangement, from metastasis of gout or rheumatism.

Checked Discharges—Suppression of Secretions

(Ophthalmia) Pulsatilla - gonorrhoeal ophthalmia, when the gonorrhoea became suddenly suppressed.

(Ophthalmia) Silicea - amblyopia from suppressed habitual foot-sweat.

(Ophthalmia) Sulphur - hypopion, cataract, choroiditis and chorioretinitis, if accompanied by darting pains and where the disease is based upon abdominal venosity, stagnation in portal circulation, habitual constipation, cerebral congestion, or upon metastasis of chronic or suppressed skin diseases.

(Ophthalmia) Terebinth. - iritis rheumatica, from suppression of habitual foot-sweat, or when urinary symptoms are present.

(Orchitis, and other affections of the testicles) Agnus castus - induration of testicles from suppressed gonorrhoea.

(Orchitis, and other affections of the testicles) Ant-tart. - very painful orchitis after checked gonorrhoea.

(Orchitis, and other affections of the testicles) Baryta-mur. hypertrophied testicles after suppressed gonorrhoea, painless or with hard painful stitches.

(Orchitis, and other affections of the testicles) Graphites - herpetic eruption on scrotum, groins or lower extremities preceding or accompanying it, or arising from suppression of a skin disease.

(Orchitis, and other affections of the testicles) Helleborus - hydrocele after suppressed eruptions, either side.

(Orchitis, and other affections of the testicles) Pulsatilla - orchitis or epididymitis from suppressed gonorrhoea.

(Orchitis, and other affections of the testicles) Spongia - testicle swollen, hard, screwing, squeezing pain, with stitches up the cord, throbbing from any motion in bed or clothing, in cases of maltreated orchitis or after checked gonorrhoea.

(Orchitis, and other affections of the testicles) Thuja - checked gonorrhoea causes prostatitis and articular rheumatism. Sycosis.

(Orchitis, and other affections of the testicles) Zincum met. - after checked otorrhoea.

(Otitis and otorrhoea) Cactus - rheumatic otitis from checked perspiration.

(Otitis and otorrhoea) Ledum - sensation of torpor of the integuments, especially after suppressed discharge from ears, eyes, and nose.

(Otitis and otorrhoea) Lobelia infl. - constantly recurring earaches or deafness due to suppressed otorrhoea or to a suppression of an eczema of the meatus of the ear.

(Ovaries, diseases of) Abrotanum - suppression of menses in young girls, followed by nosebleed.

(Paralysis) Apis-mel. - paralysis following devitalizing affections, as diphtheria, typhoids, suppressed eruptions, meningeal affections.

(Paralysis) Causticum - suppressed chronic eruptions.

(Paralysis) Colchicum - lameness after suddenly checked sweat, particularly foot-sweat, by getting wet all over.

(Paralysis) Hepar sulph. - paralysis from suppressed eruptions or after mercurial poisoning.

(Paralysis) Paralysis in consequence of; rheumatism - from suppression or retrocession of an eruption: Caust., Dulc., Hep., Sulph.

(Paralysis) Paralysis in consequence of; rheumatism - suppression of sweat: Colch.

(Paralysis) Silicea - spasms or paralysis from checked foot-sweats, depending on alterations in connective tissue in brain and spinal cord.

(Paralysis) Zincum met. - paralysis from softening of brain, following suppressed footsweat, with vertigo, trembling, numbness and formication, > by friction, < by wine.

(Pemphigus) Bryonia - pemphigus from suddenly checked perspiration.

(Pericarditis) Ars-alb. - pericarditis after suppression of measles or scarlatina, with agony, restlessness, tingling in fingers, especially of left hand.

(Pericarditis) Sulphur - after suppressed itch.

(Peritonitis) Belladonna - drowsiness and stupor, but easily aroused. in complication with metritis, lochia checked or hot in offensively smelling clots, back feels as if broken. in complication with enteritis or typhlitis, clutching as from nails around navel, bloody, slimy diarrhoea, etc.

(Peritonitis) Cantharis - suppressed urine.

(Peritonitis) Colocynth - lochia suppressed from depressing emotions, abdomen painful to touch.

(Pleurisy) Ars-iod. - frequent, short, suppressed cough, often loose.

(Pneumonia) Ferr-phos. - first stage of infantile pneumonia, especially when caused by checked perspiration on a hot summer's day. Pneumonia of adults, as long as no exudation has taken place, pulse full, round and soft, very little thirst.

(Prosopalgia) Natrum mur. - prosopalgia recurring periodically, especially after checked ague.

(Prosopalgia) Stannum - prosopalgia after ague suppressed by quinine.

(Prosopalgia) Thuja - after suppressed gonorrhoea, or eczema of ear.

(Prostate gland, diseases of) Thuja - syphilis and sycosis, especially suppressed or badly treated gonorrhoea.

(Rheumatism) Abrotanum - rheumatism from suddenly checked diarrhoea, cannot move head, arms or legs.

(Rheumatism) Dulcamara - when the weather suddenly changes to damp cold, or gets < on any little exposure to cold, or when rheumatism follows suppression of a cutaneous eruption, or when chronic forms alternate with diarrhoea (Abrot.).

(Rheumatism) Sarsparilla - rheumatic bone pains after mercury or checked gonorrhoea.

(Rheumatism) Tarentula hisp. - rheumatism checked by putting feet in cold water, followed by panting respiration, anxiety, cramps in heart or twisting pains.

(Scabies, itch) Psorinum - repeated outbreak of single pustules or boils after the main eruption seems all gone, or when suppressed, it is an excellent remedy to bring it out again.

(Shock from injuries) Secale - suppression of urine.

(Sleeplessness.) Ignatia - sleeplessness from grief, fright, from suppressed mental suffering.

(Sore throat) Arg-nit. - sore throat following suppressed ulcers of uterus.

(Spasm of glottis or larynx) Ars-alb. - caused by suppressed hives.

(Spasm of glottis or larynx) Belladonna - urine deep yellow or scanty or even suppressed.

(Spasm of glottis or larynx) - suppressed hives: Ars.

(Spasm of glottis or larynx) Sambucus nigra - suppressed perspiration.

(Stricture of urethra) Pulsatilla - stricture of urethra from suppressed gonorrhoea.

(Suppression of secretions) Give more particularly - after suppression of eruptions and herpes: 1, Ant-tart., Apis, Bell., Bry., Cupr., Dulc., Graph., Helleb., Hep., Ipec., Phos-ac., Puls., Sulph.

— Suppression of catarrh or some other blennorrhoea: 1, Acon., Ars., Bell., Bry., Calc., Chin., Cin., Nux-v., Puls., Sulph.; 2, Amb., Amm., Carb-v., Con., Dulc., Graph., Ipec., Kalm., Lyc., Natr-m., Nitr-ac., Nux-m., Phos., Rhod., Samb., Sulph.

— Suppression of sweat: 1, Bell., Bry., Cham., Chin., Dulc., Lach., Sil., Sulph.

— Suppression of haemorrhage or abandoning habitual depletions: 1, Acon., Bell., Chin., Fer., Nux-v., Puls., Sulph.; 2, Arn., Aur., Bry., Calc., Carb-v., Graph., Hyosc., Lyc., Natr-m., Nitr-ac., Phos., Ran., Rhus, Seneg., Sep., Sil., Spong., Stram.

— Suppression of ulcers and purulent discharges: 1, Bell., Hep., Lach., Sil., Sulph.

— Suppression of piles: 1, Acon., Calc., Carb-v., Nux-v., Puls., Sulph.; 2, Amb., Amm., Ant., Ars., Bell., Caps., Caust., Chin., Coloc., Graph., Ign., Kalm., Lach., Mur-ac., Nitr-ac., Petr., Rhus, Sep., Sil. - suppression of lochia: 1, Coloc., Hyosc., Nux-v., Plat., Rhus, Sec., Veratr., Zinc.

— Suppression of sweat: 1, Bell., Bry., Cham., Chin., Dulc., Lach., Sil., Sulph ; 2, Acon., Ars., Calc., Graph., Lyc., Merc., Nux-m., Nux-v., Op., Phos., Puls., Rhus, Sep. - suppression of foot-sweat: 1, Cupr., Nitr-ac., Puls., Sep., Sil.

— Suppression of ulcers and purulent discharges: 1, Bell., Hep., Lach., Sil., Sulph.; 2, Ars., Carb-v., Lyc., Merc., Natr-m., Phos-ac., Rhus, Sep., staph.

— Suppression of piles: 1, Acon., Calc., Carb-v., Nux-v., Puls., Sulph.

(Syphilis and sycosis) Badiaga - chancres suppressed by cautery or mercurial ointment, leaving elevated, discolored cicatrices.

(Syphilis and sycosis) Benzoic acid - warts around anus, appearing after cop. suppressed a chancrous gonorrhoea, with offensive urine.

(Syphilis and sycosis) Medorrhinum - asthma from suppressed gonorrhoea. sycotic children suffering from cholera infantum, emaciation, etc.

(Tonsillitis) Baryta-carb. - liability to quinsy after every cold or suppressed sweat of feet.

(Tuberculosis of lungs) Ars-iod. - frequent, short, suppressed cough, often loose, with muco-purulent expectoration.

(Uraemia) Digitalis - dropsy, with suppression of urine.

(Urinary difficulties) Eup-purp. - suppression of urine in infants.

(Urinary difficulties) Kali-bich. - suppression of urine following cholera.

(Varicocele) Silicea - suppression of habitual foot-sweat.

(Vertigo, dizziness) Conium - suppressed sexual desire or overindulgence, with loss of memory and frequent seminal emissions.

(Vertigo, dizziness) Hydrastis - vertigo from suppression of suppuration.

(Vertigo, dizziness) Senecio - giddiness coming on suddenly several times a day, from suppressed perspiration or menstrual discharge.

(Vision complaints) After suppression of a habitual bloody discharge, as haemorrhoids, menstruation, etc.: Bell., Calc., Cycl., Lyc., Nux-v., Phos., Puls., Sep., Sulph.

after suppression of an exanthemata: Bell., Calc., Caust., Lach., Lyc., Merc., Sil., Stram., Sulph.

(Vision complaints) Belladonna - from a cold, from stoppage of menses, from suppression of exanthemata.

(Vision complaints) - by suppression of a suppuration or mucous discharge: Chin., Euphr., Hep., Lyc., Puls., Sil., Sulph.

(Vision complaints) Chelidonium - dimness of vision and weakness of sight from rheumatic troubles or after suppression of ringworm.

(Vision complaints) Cyclamen - after suppression of menses or an eruption.

(Vision complaints) Pulsatilla - amblyopia from suppression of any bloody discharge.

(Vision complaints) Silicea - dim vision after suppressed foot-sweats, after diphtheria.

(Vision complaints) Sulphur - blindness after suppressed skin diseases.

(Whooping-cough) Allium cepa - hoarse, harsh, dry, ringing, spasmodic cough, causing a raw splitting pain in larynx, so severe that he tries to suppress the cough, worse in a warm room and when lying down.

(Whooping-cough) Sulphur - suppressed cough.

Some useful rubrics of mind

EMOTIONS, Complaints caused by

Abashment: Coloc., Ign., Op,, Ph-ac., Plat., Sep., Staph., Sulph. From
    reproachment: Coloc., Croc., Ign., Op., Ph-ac., Staph.

Ailments of violent anger: Acon., Bry., Cham., Nux-v. **much inclined to anger:** Bry., Phos., Zinc.

    long-lasting ailments from it: Agar., Zinc.

    with mortification: Staph.

    vexation: Cham., Plat., Staph.

    indignation: Coloc., Staph.

    wrath and vehemence: Acon., Ars., Aur-met., Bry., Cham., Grat., Ign., Lyc., Nux-v., Verat.

vexation: Ars., Bell., Caust., Cistus, Kali-c., Lyc., Mez., Nat-m., Nux-v., Petr., Phos., Ph-ac., Rhus, Sep., Sulph.

long-lasting complaints after vexation: Alum., Cham., Lyc., Nat-m., Petr., Puls., Sep.

vexation with indignation: Colch., Ipec., Nux-v., Plat., Staph.

Pride affections from: Lach., Lyc., Pallad., Plat., Staph., Verat.

    egotism: Calc-c., Lyc., Merc., Sil., Sulph.

hateful and vindictive temper: Am-c., Calc-c., Nat-m., Nit-ac.

envy: Ars., Lach., Lyc., Puls., Staph. For

jaundice (after emotions): Cham., Merc., Chin.
convulsions: Bell., Cham., Ign., Hyos., Op., Samb.
tetanic spasms: Bell., Op., Ign.
epileptic attacks: Ign., Op. (Bell., Lach., Caust.)
great **debility with trembling:** Merc., Op., Ph-ac., Verat.
fainting fits: Coff., Op., Verat.
pains **spasmodic**: Coloc.
nervous excitement: Acon., Coff., Magn. arct, Merc., Nux-v.
vascular orgasm: Acon., Coff., Merc.
When there is **fever:** Acon., Bry., Cham., Nux-v.
chills and **shuddering:** Bry., Merc. Puls.
coldness of the body: Op., Puls., Samb., Veratr
heat and **redness** of the cheeks: Acon., Caps., Ign.,
night-sweats: Merc., Ph-ac.
hectic fever: Ign., Ph-ac., Staph.
For **sleeplessness:** Acon., Coff., Caps., Coloc., Merc., Staph.
sopor: Op., Samb. (Ph-ac., Staph.)
melancholy and **sadness:** Aur-met., Ign., Ph-ac., Plat., Staph.
constant **weeping** and **lamenting:** Bell., Hep.
constant **cries:** Bell., Op.
constant **anxiety** and **fear:** Acon., Bell., Cham., Merc., Plat., Staph.
mental derangement: Bell., Hyos., Lach., Op., Stram., Verat.
indifference, dullness, apathy: Hell., Hyos., Ph-ac.
constant **indignation:** Coloc., Staph.
loss of **consciousness** and **stupefaction:** Bell., Hyos., Nux-v., Op.
tendency of blood to the head, and headache: Acon., Bell., Coff., Ign., Nux-v., Op.

hair falling off of the, or when the **hair** turns **gray:** Ph-ac., Staph.

loss of appetite, nausea, vomiting: Bry., Cham., Coloc., Ign., Nux-v., Op., Puls.

bilious ailments: Acon., Bry., Cham., Coloc., Ign., Nux-v.

pains in the **stomach:** Cham., Nux-v., Puls.

colic and **diarrhoea:** Cham., Puls., Verat.

involuntary **stools:** Op., Verat.

pains in the **chest, asthma,** etc.: Aur-met., Bell., Cham., Nux-v., Op., Samb.

violent **palpitation** of the **heart:** Acon., Cham., Hep., Op., Puls.

suicidal disposition, life being a burden: Berb., Caps., Chin., Hep., Lach., Plat., Pod., Psor., Puls., Spig.

by **shooting:** *Aurum-ars.,* Ars., Aur-met., Alum., Ant-c. and Nat-s.

by **drowning:** Bell., Hell., Rhus and Sil.;

great mental depression leads to **suicide:** Cim.

JOY, consequences of: Acon., Caust., Coff., Croc., Cycl., Nat-c., Op., Puls.

startled or struck by it; trembling, crying, weeping, sobbing, or fainting away, even apparent death, particularly children and women; headache after mental exhilaration: *Coff.*

sensation caused by excessive joy, approaching madness, with pallor, headache and confused sight; merry madness, with headache, blindness and pale face: *Croc.*

headache after mental exhilaration: *Coca.* after excessive joy the mouth is suddenly filled with

bright blood: *Cinch.* chilliness and diarrhoea after joyful news: *Gels.* laughing and crying, stunned by joy: *Hyos.* weeping, coughing, trembling; glowing red cheeks:

Hysteria

Abdominal spasms: 1, Ign.; 2, Cocc., Ipec., Nux-v.; 3, Mag-m., Mosch., Stann., Val.; 4, Ars., Bell., Stram., Sulph., Verat.

Mind, affections of the and morbid emotions: Anac., Asaf., Aurmet., Cact., Calc-c., Caust., Con., Gels., Grat., Ign., Nux-m., Nux-v., Phos., Plat., Senec., Sep., Sil., Sul., Viol-o.

Coldness of hands and feet: Bell., Hedeoma

Brooding constant: Ign., Nux-v., Sep.

Constant moaning and lamentations, or persistent silence: Nux-v.

Constant or excessive dread: Acon., Plat., Puls.

Constant troublesome sinking at the stomach: Cim., Gels., Hydrast, Ign.

Fidgety: Val.

Gastric affections: Cham., Cocc., Ign., Mag-c., Nux-v.

Convulsions: Aur-met., Bell., Bry., Calc-c., Caul., Caust., Cham., Cic., Cocc., Coff., Con., Cup-m., Gels., Ign., Ipec., Mag-c., Mag-m., Mosch., Plat., Puls., Sec., Sep., Stann., Stram., Sul., Tarent., Verat., Ver-v.

General increased sensibility: Ign., Cypriped., Sep., Stram.

Anxiety, great: Nux-v., Plat., Puls.

Great nervous debility: Alet, Plat., Ph-ac., Sep., Senec.

Headache: 1, Aur-met., Ign., Iris, Plat., Mosch., Sep.; 2, Bell., Cocc., Hep., Mag-c., Mag-m., Val., Verat.; 3, Bry., Nit-ac., Phos.; 4, Alet., Cact., Gels., Ther., Tarent.

Heightened sensitiveness: Acon., Cocc., Stram., Plat., Puls., Nux-v., Staph.

Illusions: Cim., Val.

Irritability and impatience: Cocc., Cypriped., Gels., Hyos., Nux-v., Puls., Senec., Sep.

Melancholy: Aur-met., Puls., Staph.

Menstrual and uterine difficulties: Alet., Aur-met., Cact., Caul., Cic., Cocc., Con., Hyos., Ign., Mag-m., Mosch., Nat-m., Nux-v., Plat., Puls., Senec., Sep., Stann., Ver-v., Vib.-op.

Oppression of chest: Ign., Mosch.

Shortness of breath: Calc-c., Hedeoma

Sleepiness: Caul., Gels., Mosch.

Sleeplessness: Cypriped., Gels., Ign., Nux-v., Senec.

Spasms in the chest and difficulties of breathing: Acon., Ars., Aur-met., Bell., Coff., Con., Cup-m., Ign. Ipec., Mosch., Nux-m., Nux-v., Phos., Puls., Stann., Stram., Tarent.

Spasms in the throat: Asaf., Caust., Con., Gels., Lyc., Mag-m., Plumb., Senec., Sulph.

Stupid intoxicated feeling: Gels.

Twitching of limbs, tremors: Caul., Cim., Cypriped., Hedeoma, Ign., Mosch., Plat.

Variable disposition: Ign., Mosch., Plat., Puls., Sep., Stram.

Vesical spasms: Asaf., Puls., Sep.

Heart, weakness of: Hydr.-ac., Phos.

Memory Weak, Inability to Think

Ambr., Anac., Arn., Aur-met., Bov., Cal-c., Cann-i., Carb-v., Chin., Con., Dig., Kali-br., Kreos., Lach., Merc., Nat-m., Nux-v., Oleand., Phos., Puls., Rhus, Sil., Staph., Sulph., Syphilin., Ther., Verat., Zinc-picr.

For **weak memory**: Alum., Anac., Bell., Bov., Bry., Calc-c., Cann-i., Con., Cycl., Graph., Hell., Hep., Hyos., Lach., Lyc., Nat-m., Nux-m., Oleand., Petr., Rhus, Sil., Staph.,

Some useful rubrics of mind 459

Stram., Sul., Ther., Verat., Zinc. (See also Absent-minded and Memory, loss of)

For **difficult comprehension:** Amb., Calc., Con., Cycl., Helleb., Ign., Lyc., Merc., Natr., Nat-m., Nux-m., Oleand., Op., Phos.-ac, Rhus., Sep., Staph., Stram., Thuj.

For **slow** flow of ideas: Alum., Am-c., Aur., Calc., Carb-v, Hyos., Lach., Lyc., Nat-m., Nux-m., Nux-v., Op., Petr., Phos-ac, Rhus., Sep., Sil., Staph.

If caused by **debilitating loss of animal fluids:** Chin., Nux-v. and Sulph. (*Compare* Debility.)

If caused by **excessive studying** and **mental labor:** 1, Nux-v. and Sulph.; 2, Aur-met., Cal-c., Lach., Natr., Nat-m., Phos., Puls., Sil. (*Compare* Brain-fag.)

If caused by **external injuries,** as a blow, fall on the head, etc.; Arn., Cic., Merc., Rhus.

If by **abuse of spirits:** Cal-c., Cim., Lach., Merc., Nux-v., Op., Puls., Sulph, (*Compare* Drunkards, Diseases of.)

If caused by **violent emotions, fright, grief, anger,** etc.: Acon., Op., Ph-ac., Staph., etc. (*Compare* Emotions.)

If caused by exposure to **wet or dampness:** Cal-c., Carb-v., Puls., Rhus, Sil., Verat.

If by **congestion** of blood to the head: Chin., Melilot, Merc., Rhus, Sulph.

For general **morbid state of the head:** Acon., Anac., Aur-met., Bell., Calc-c., Caust., Chin., Cocc., Hell., Hep., Hyos., Ign., Lac-c., Lach., Lyc., Merc., Nat-c., Nat-m., Nux-v., Op., Phos., Ph-ac., Plat., Puls., Rhus., Sep., Sil., Staph., Stram., Sul., Verat.

For **loss of memory:** Anac., Bell., Bry., Con., Hep., Hyos., Lac-c., Melilot., Nat-m., Op., Petr., Puls., Rhus., Sil., Stram., Veratr., Sanicula.

—**absentmindedness:** Anac., Caust., Con., Dulc., Lac-c., Lach., Nat-m., Sep.

—loss of memory for **names:** Anac., Bell., Chin-sulph., Chlorof., Croc., Fluor.-ac., Glon., Guaiac., Lyc., Lith., Medorrhin., Merc., Natr-ars., Oleand., Plumb., Puls., Rhus., Syphilin., Stram., Sulph., Tabac.

—**names of objects:** Lyc., Rhus.

—what he **thought or spoke about:** Lac-c., Medorrhin., Nat-m., Rhod.

—when **reading:** Colch., Hydrast., Lach., Lyc., Nat-m., Staph.

—**what he heard:** Hyos., Lach.

—**what he read:** Agn., Amb., Guaiac., Hell., Phos-ac., Staph., Syphilin.

—for **persons:** Croc.

—**orthography** (memory loss for spelling)**:** Lach., Lyc., Melilot.

—for **dates:** Acon., Con., Fl-ac.

—for **words:** Arn., Bapt., Bar., Cann-i., Carb-an. Coca., Colch., Lyc., Nux-m., Sulph., Verat.

—for **places:** Glon., Nux-m., Psor.

—for **his own name:** Kali-bi., Medorrhin., Sulph,

—**loss of ideas:** Alum., Am-c., Caust., Helleb., Hyos., Lach., Nat-c., Nat-m., Nit-ac., Oleand., Staph., Thuj., Veratr.

—**dullness of sense:** Alum., Bell., Cal-c., Colch., Helleb., Hyos., Melilot., Nat-c., Nat-m., Oleand., Op., Phos-ac., Sep., Staph., Stram., Sulph.

—**periodical:** Carb-v.

—**absolute:** Kali-br.
—**sudden:** Calc-sulph.—followed by **liveliness of memory:** Cycl.—followed by **headache:** Kali-c., Viol.

Anguish, paroxysms of

Generally a mere symptom, though sometimes so prominent and distressing that it deserves a special treatment: 1, Acon., Ars., Aur., Bell., Cham., Dig., Merc., Nux-v., Puls., Veratr.; 2, Alum., Anac., Bar-c., Carb-an., Carb-v., Cocc., Cupr., Graph., Hyosc., Ign., Lyc., Nitr., Nitr-ac., Phos., Rhus, Sep., Spig., Spong., Sulph., Tarent., Trill., Vip.

Particular indications:

By **simultaneous affections of the chest:** 1, Acon., Ars., Aur., Ipec., Puls., Veratr.; 2, Cact., Calc., Bry., Carb-v., Dig., Spig.

By **gastric and abdominal affections:** 1, Ars., Calc., Cupr., Natr., Nux-v., Puls., Veratr.; 2, Bell., Cham., Carb-v., Cocc., Laur., Lyc., Natr-m., Stann., Thuj.

By **affections of the heart:** 1, Acon., Ars., Aur., Cact., Dig., Puls., Spig., Spong.; 2, Cham., Cimicif., Gels., Lyc., Nitr-ac., Phos., Sep., Veratr-vir.

By **hypochondriasis:** 1, Acon., Ars., Calc., Dig., Lach., Natr., Nux-v.; 2, Aescul., Alum., Anac., Bell., Caust., Cham., Con., Corn-c., Cyprip., Graph., Hell., Hep., Ign., Iris, Lach., Leptan., Lyc., Merc., Mosch., Nitr-ac., Pod., Puls., Sep., Stram.

By **hysteria:** 1, Acon., Cic., Cocc., Con., Croc., Cyprip., Hyosc., Ign., Mosch., Nux-v.; 2, Alet., Bell., Calc., Caust., Caul., Corn-f., Gels., Hyosc., Magn-mur., Nitr-ac., Nux-m., Phos., Sil., Scutel., Veratr.

By **hyperaesthesia of the brain:** Acon., Bell., Hyosc., Lachn., Merc., Nux-v., Veratr.

Anguish, Agony (A severe pain or distress)

(Note: This rubric is most useful in *acute* diseases, but to be wholly disregarded while treating chronic diseases).

(anguish = severe mental or physical pain or suffering; be very distressed.

agony = extreme physical or mental suffering).

Whenever a patient tells that the pain or suffering is 'intense' 'intolerable' 'horrible' 'unbearable' 'extreme' 'torturing' 'difficult' etc. we must look into the repertory for the word 'anguish' 'agony' 'agonizing' etc.

Anguish and despair: Acon., Amb., Calc-c., Ign., Lach., Lyc., Puls., Sarsap., Val., Verat.

Anguish in children: Acon., Aeth., Ars., Bufo., Nux-v., Samb.,

To describe his pain or suffering whenever a patient uses the word 'difficult', 'difficulty' (PËhÆ) or 'unbearable' 'intolerable' or 'horrible' you must come to this rubric ANGUISH.

Anguish, anxiety: Acon., Arn., Ars., Bell., Bry., Cal-c., Carb-v., Cham., Graph., Ign., Lyc., Merc., Nux-v., Phos., Puls., Rhus., Samb., Spig., Spong., Sulph., Verat.

—fear and apprehensions: Acon., Anac., Ars., Bar-c., Bell., Bry., Cal-c., Caust., Cic., Cocc., Crotal., Graph., Hep., Hyos., Lach., Merc., Nux-v., Op., Sul-ac., Veratr

—uneasiness, as if from a bad conscience: Alum., Am-c., Ars., Aur-met., Carb-v., Caust., Cina, Cocc., Con., Cycl., Dig., Ferr., Graph., Hyos., Merc., Nux-v., Puls., Sil., Stram., Sulph., Verat.

—anxiety, driving one from one place to another: Acon., Ars., Aur-met., Bell., Bry., Canth., Carb-v., Coloc., Cup-m., Dros., Hyos., Lil-t., Merc., Nux-v., Op., Plat., Puls., Sep., Spig., Staph., Stram., Verat.

Remedies for 'Anguish' 'Agonizing' or 'Agony'.

Adrenalinum - the symptom guiding to this is, sensation of thoracic constriction with anguish.

Aethusa - cries of anguish (in a child).

Aethusa - anguish, crying, and expression of uneasiness and discontent, lead to this remedy most frequently in disease in children, during dentition, summer complaint, when, with the diarrhoea, there is marked inability to digest milk, and poor circulation.

Aethusa - vomiting, with sweat and great weakness, accompanied by anguish and distress, followed by sleepiness.

Ambra - anguish and sweat all over at night.

Amm-carb. - anguish as if a crime had been committed.

Amyl-nit. - melancholy without sensation of anguish.

Arnica - violent attacks of anguish. —angina pectoris.

Arsenic alb. - great anguish and restlessness. changes place continually. fears, of death, of being left alone.

Arsenic alb. - great anguish and restlessness. - stricture of oesophagus. - gastralgia. - hematemesis. - colicodynia.

Arsenic alb. - great anguish, tossing about. - colic. - pneumonia. - emphysema. - intermittent.

Arsenic alb. - indescribable anguish, restlessness. - metritis. - pericarditis. - cholera asiatica.

Arsenic alb. - cholera, with intense agony, prostration, and burning thirst.

Arsenic alb. - expression of agony on face.

Aurum met. - anguish of mind and great grief. - headache.

Aurum met. - excessive anguish with palpitation of heart, weariness in all limbs and sleepiness.

Aurum met. - frequent attacks of anguish about heart, with trembling, fearfulness.

Aurum met. - great anguish coming from precordial region, and driving him from place to place, so that he can remain nowhere.

Aurum met. - great anguish increasing unto self-destruction, with spasmodic contraction of abdomen.

Belladonna - anxiety, anguish, trembling, constant restlessness.

Belladonna - cardiac anxiety, with anguish and restlessness.

Belladonna - intolerable anguish during time she is free from rage, with desire to die.

Bismuth - anguish; at times he sits, then walks, then lies down, never long in one place.

Bromium - full of dreams and anguish; jerking and starting during sleep, full of fantasy and illusions; difficult to go to sleep at night, cannot sleep enough in morning; trembling and weak on awaking.

Bufo - great anguish. - meningitis.

Cactus - coldness predominates; cold sweat, with great anguish.

Calc-carb. - despondent and melancholy, in highest degree, with a kind of anguish.

Camphor - was found much excited, screaming loudly, "I shall not faint! I shan't faint, for if I do, I will have fits and never come out of them!" uttered a strange scream, a sort of howl, leaped from bed, apparently in great agony, and bent on something desperate.

Camphor - asiatic cholera, with cramps in calves, coldness of body, anguish, great weakness, collapse, tongue and mouth old.

Carbo-an. - unclouded consciousness and great anguish with sinking of vital forces.

Carbolic acid. - agonizing backache across loins, with dragging down the thighs.

Chamomilla - excessive uneasiness, anxiety, agonizing tossing about, with tearing pains in abdomen.

China-sulph. - anguish and general sweat.

China-sulph. - anguish.

Coca. - feeling of anguish increased with failure of every effort to strive against the weariness; torment only diminishes with perfect rest. –veta.

Coffea cruda - tossing about in anguish. (Acon.)

Coffea cruda - exasperation, tears; tossing about in great anguish.

Coffea cruda - great anguish; cannot be composed; is not able to hold the pen; trembles.

Colocynth - agonizing cutting pain in abdomen causing patient to bend over double, and pressing on the abdomen.

Conium - great anxiety; precordial anguish; superstitious and full of fear, with frequent thoughts of death; loss of memory.

Crotalus hor. - melancholia, with timidity, fear, distress and anguish.

Crotalus hor. - weeping mood, agony and despair.

Cuprum-ars. - intense anguish of mind and body.

Cuprum-met. - loss of spirits; anxiety; fits of anguish and fear of death.

Cuprum-met. - mania with biting, beating, and tearing things to pieces; insane foolish gestures of imitation and mimicry; full of insane spiteful tricks, illusions of imagination, does not recognize his own family; unhappy, apprehensive, anxious, and despairing; precordial anguish, pale, miserable look, general chilliness, not > by heat; attacks en in sweat.

Helleborus - excessive anxiety and anguish < 2 p.m.

Helleborus - melancholy: silent; during puberty; with anguish.

Hepar sulph. - impelled by unaccountable attacks of internal anguish, which sometimes come on quite suddenly, to attempt suicide.

Hepar sulpph. - anguish in the evening and night, with thoughts of suicide.

Hyoscyamus - horrid anguish, fits of anxiety.

Ictodes - troublesome respiration, with sudden feeling of anguish and sweat.

Ignatia - a state of anguish in which she shrieks for help, with suffocating constriction of throat, difficult deglutition; comes out of spasms with deep sighing. —parturition.

Jatropa - anxiety and anguish.

Kali-iod. - torturing feeling of anguish preventing sleep.

Kali-cyanatum - cancer of tongue and agonizing neuralgia have been benefited by this drug.

Kalmia - paroxysms of anguish around heart.

Lactuca vir. - anguish and internal uneasiness.

Lycopodium - anthropophobia (in children); fear of phantoms in evening, with anguish.

Magnesia-carb. - trembling, anguish and fear, as if some accident would happen; all day, > after going to bed.

Merc-sol. - inexpressible pain of soul and body, anxious restlessness, as if some evil impended, < at night, with precordial anguish; sweat of hands and heat of face; disgusted with himself, has not courage to live; constant suspicion, considering everybody his enemy. - melancholia.

Moschus - complains without knowing what ails him, with anguish, palpitation, etc.

Nitric-acid. - after continued loss of sleep, long-lasting anxiety, overexertions of mind and body from nursing the sick, great anguish of mind from loss of his dearest friend.

Ornithogalum - agonizing feeling in chest and stomach, staring from pylorus with flatus that rolls in balls from one side to the other, loss of appetite phlegmy retchings and loss of flesh.

Phosphorus - hypochondriasis; sadness alternating with mirth and laughter; uneasy about one's health; paroxysms of anguish, when alone or in stormy weather, with timorous disposition; told those about him repeatedly that he could not possibly recover, and gave some disjointed directions about his business affairs.

Platina - after anger alternate laughing and weeping, with great anguish and fear of death.

Platina - much anguish; she feels as if she would lose her senses and die soon.

Platina - precordial anguish with palpitation and fear of death and of imaginary forms, ghosts.

Psorinum. - feels the greatest anguish in head, with a whirling before eyes every day, from 5 a. m. until 5 p. m., since two years; walks up and down his room wringing his hands and moaning continually, oh, such anguish! Oh, such anguish! Only when he takes his meals he ceases moaning; appetite is good.

Pulsatilla - anguish in region of heart, sometimes increasing to a desire for suicide.

Raphanus - anguish with dread of death, which is supposed to be near.

Rhus aromatica - incontinence. severe pain at beginning or before urination causing great agony in children.

Secale - great anguish; wild with anxiety.

Spongia - paroxysms of anxiety or anguish. - cardiac troubles.

Stramonium - a peculiar sensation of anxiety; anguish; despair.

Stramonium - downcast and full of anguish, believes herself unworthy of eternal bliss, because she is unable to perform her duties.

Tabacum - becomes quite stupid, loses his senses; precordial anguish, with faintness.

Tarentula hispanica - palpitation; praecordial anguish sensation as if heart twisted and turned around.

Thuja - mental depression, after childbirth, in consequence of being told that there had been a slight rupture of perineum; grows quiet; thinks she must die; cannot sleep; has no appetite; shuns people; does not answer; seems not to understand a question; cannot count; is in constant anguish; wants to jump out of window; does not care for children or her relatives; stares before herself; hydrogenoid constitution.

Thuja - sleeplessness at night; restlessness and tossing about; anguish which does not allow him to sleep; sleep full of dreams and startings.

Verat-alb. - cold sweat on forehead, with anguish and fear of death.

Verat-alb. - anguish in pit of stomach.

Diseases with the Symptom 'Anguish' (or Agony, Agonizing etc.)

(Albuminuria) Apis-mel. - urine suppressed or scanty, high-colored, foetid, containing alben, blood-corpuscles, uriniferous tubes and epithelium. great debility, no anguish or fear of death, as in Ars.

(Amenorrhoea) Colocynth - colicky pains, causing her to draw up double, with great anguish and restlessness.

(Angina pectoris) Ars-alb. - agonizing praecordial pain.

(Angina pectoris) Carbo-veg. - praecordial anguish as though he would die.

(Angina pectoris) Digitalis - indescribable deathly anguish when paroxysms come closer together during progress of disease.

(Angina pectoris) Digitalis - mental anguish, with vertigo and fainting.

(Angina pectoris) Glonoine - great anguish in praecordial region.

(Angina pectoris) Kali-carb. - strong palpitations, anguish, frequent interruptions of the beating of the heart.

(Angina pectoris) Latrodectus - violent praecordial anguish, with sense of impending dissolution.

(Angina pectoris) Naja - sudden agonizing pain in heart.

(Angina pectoris) Veratrum alb. - periodical attacks of contractive, crampy pain in left chest, or cutting pains with excessive agony, arresting breathing and extending to shoulder.

(Apoplexy) Glonoine - during prodromal stage severe headache, hot flashes in head and face, mental exaltation or depression, ill humor, anguish, pulsation of the arteries of the head and neck.

(Asthma) Ambra - oppression in left chest through to the back and between the shoulders, as if emanating from the heart, with palpitations, anguish and loss of breath.

(Asthma) Carbo-veg. - asthma of old or debilitated people, during the fit they look as if they would die, so oppressed are they for breath, suffocative asthma, with blue and cold skin and great anguish about the heart.

(Asthma) Cocculus - anguish and palpitations.

(Asthma) Glonoine - constriction of chest with anguish and much sighing.

(Asthma) Kali-nit. - tightness and constriction in chest, with anguish and shortness of breath, < in the morning when lying, extending from the back into the chest, when attempting to take a deep breath, gasping for air, followed by cough.

(Asthma) Nux vomica - distention, aching pains and anguish in the region of heart and hypochondria.

(Asthma) Opium - tightness of breath and oppression, with great anguish and spasmodic constriction of chest.

(Asthma) Pulsatilla - oppression of chest, loss of breath and suffocative fits, with anguish, palpitations and sensation of fulness and pressure on chest, with internal heat and orgasm of blood.

(Asthma) Stannum - asthma and oppression, especially in the evening or at night when lying down, also in daytime during every exercise, and frequently attended with anguish and desire to detach the clothes.

(Atrophy of children) Veratrum alb. - abdomen bloated, hard, hot, and painful constipation of hard, large stools, or watery, greenish or white diarrhoea, painless and involuntary, with cold sweat on forehead, and anguish.

(Back pain–spinal irritation) Ars-alb. - great prostration with anguish.

(Bone diseases, osteitis, periostitis, exostosis, caries, necrosis, etc.) Mezereum - intolerable nightly burning pains in abscess of antrum highmori, periosteum more affected with dull, crampy pain referred to malar bone, with anguish, pale face, cold sweat and anguish.

(Bronchitis acuta) Cactus - great anguish, suffocation and palpitation of heart.

(Bronchitis chronica) Ammoniacum - bronchorrhoea respiration short, quick, with anguish, especially at night.

(Cancer) Acetic acid. - cancer of stomach, ulcerative gnawing pain at one spot in stomach, with agony and depression, preventing sleep, intense and constant thirst.

(Cancer) Mezereum - violent retching, accompanied with the agony of death.

(Cholera) Camphor - face, hands and feet icy cold, cannot bear to have them covered, great anguish as though he would suffocate, groans and moans in a hoarse, husky voice.

(Cholera) Croton tiglium - anguish, oppression and pressure in stomach.

(Cholera) Cuprum ammoniae sulphuric - changed features full of anguish.

(Cholera) Jatropha - anguish, with coldness of body.

(Cholera) Tabacum - nausea and vomiting, if persistent, after purging yielded, recurring in constant paroxysms, with cold sweat, oppressed stomach, anguish and restlessness, cramp and tearing in limbs, occasional drawing in the calves.

(Cholera) Veratrum alb. - deathly anguish in the features.

(Cholera) Veratrum alb. - great oppressive anguish in the chest giving the patient a desire to escape from the bed.

(Coccygodynia) Lachesis - agonizing pain when rising from his seat.

(Colic) Ars-alb. - violent pains in abdomen, with great anguish, has no rest anywhere, rolls about on the floor and despairs of life.

(Colic) Coffea cruda - anguish and pressure in the epigastrium

(Colic) Piper meth. - agonizing pain, with tossing, twisting and writhing.

(Colic) Plumbum met. - knots in recti muscles: anguish with cold sweat and deathly faintness.

(Croup) Acon. - child is in agony and throws itself about.

(Croup) Carbo-veg. - constant anguish and restlessness, child clings to persons, slightly > by fanning or rapid motion.

(Croup) Lobelia inflata - constant cough and great anguish, with fear of suffocation.

(Debility) Coca - feeling of anguish, increased with failure of every effort to strive against the weariness.

(Debility) Ver-a. - sudden sinking of strength from debilitating (choleraic) losses, with anguish and cold sweat on forehead when he rises.

(Delirium) Cup-met. - restlessness and anguish, tossing about.

(Diabetes insipidus) Phos-acid. - bad effects from grief, anguish, care or disappointed love.

(Diabetes) Phos-acid. - bad effects from grief, anguish, sorrow and care.

(Diabetes) Plb-met. - lowness of spirits, anguish and melancholy.

(Diarrhoea) Ars. - stool preceded by restlessness, anguish and pain in abdomen.

(Diarrhoea) Iodum - restlessness and inclination to change position constantly, but no anguish or tossing.

(Diarrhoea) Raphanus sativus - anguish and dread of death.

(Diarrhoea) Secale. - sinking spells at 3 a. m., but not the restless anguish of Ars., and spasmodic symptoms, fingers spread asunder with tingling in hands and feet, < in childbed, during typhoid fever.

(Dropsy) Apis-mel. - anguish of mind without fear of death.

(Dropsy) Apis-mel. - feeling of dyspnoea with mental anguish as if he could not draw another breath and as if he were going to die. Dropsy of chest with dyspnoea and great restlessness, ascites with great soreness of abdominal walls, cannot get breath except when sitting up, even leaning backward causes suffocative feeling.

(Dropsy) Lactuca virosa - anguish and internal uneasiness. ascites with induration of liver and asthma.

(Dropsy) Merc-sol. - constant short and racking cough, anguish, etc.

(Dysentery) Colchicum - long-lasting agonizing pain in rectum and anus after stool, causing screams and crying.

(Dyspepsia, weakness of stomach) Baptisia - irritation of stomach showing itself by violent pains at short intervals over the whole cardiac region, with anguish and a burning sensation

(Dyspepsia, weakness of stomach) Bovista - tension in temples, mental anguish.

(Dyspepsia, weakness of stomach) Natrum mur. - intermittent palpitations with anguish and faintishness.

(Dyspepsia, weakness of stomach) Phosphorus - cardiac anguish at night with nausea and a peculiar craving for food, relieved by eating.

(Emotions, ill effects of-fear, dread, fright) Alumina - anguish and vague uneasiness, as if he had committed a crime.

(Emotions, ill effects of-fear, dread, fright) Ars-alb. - praecordial anguish with constriction, cold sweat, trembling, prostration.

(Emotions, ill effects of-fear, dread, fright) Lycopodium - forgetfulness, anguish and excitement when alone, with restless moving about.

(Emotions, ill effects of-fear, dread, fright) Pulsatilla - tremulous anguish, as if death were near.

(Emphysema) Opium - great anguish and dread of suffocation.

(Enteritis) Belladonna - anguish, with congestion to the head and dimness of vision.

(Epilepsy) Oenanthe crocata - convulsions with vertigo, madness, nausea, vomiting, heat and agony in stomach, followed by unconsciousness, eyes turned up, pupils dilated, lockjaw.

(Epilepsy) Tarentula hisp. - sensation of dizziness before the fit, followed by convulsions and great praecordial anguish.

(Exophthalmic goitre) Aur-met. - palpitation of heart with cutting pain and feeling of anguish and tremulous fearfulness.

(Fainting) Nux-vom. - and generally when nausea, pale face, scintillations before the eyes or obscuration of sight, pains in the stomach, anguish, trembling, and congestion of blood to the head or chest are present.

(Fainting) Veratrum alb. - the paroxysms set in after the least motion, or are preceded by great anguish or despondency.

(Gall-stones) Calc-carb. - darting pain from right to left, with profuse sweat, abdominal spasms and colic, cutting colic in epigastrium, has to bend double, clench hands, writhe with agony.

(Gastralgia) Ars-alb. - intense heat and burning in stomach and pit of stomach, with anguish, great restlessness and fainting.

(Gastralgia) Burning in stomach, particularly on pressure, when empty, accompanied by dyspnoea and apparent stricture of oesophagus; eructations, with burning pain running into the back, in line of the stomach, with nausea and vomiting, especially of tough mucus; salivation; sensation like a worm creeping up from pit of stomach into throat, causing coughing; vomiting only of frothy, bitter mucus or of food as soon as it reaches the stomach: terrible heartburn after eating sweets, from wine and sour eructations after milk; aversion to meat, fish or sweets, to cooked or warm things. - for pains in the stomach, with great anguish and oppression in the pit and region of the stomach: Anac., Ars., Calc., Carb-v., Cham., Chin., Graph., Guaiac., Laur., Lyc., Natr-m., Nux-v., Op., Puls., Spig., Stann., Stram., Sulph., Thuj., Veratr.

(Gastralgia) Carbo-veg. - painful burning pressure, with anguish, trembling, and aggravation by contact, at night and after a meal, especially after taking flatulent food.

(Gastralgia) Chamomilla - aggravation of the pains after a meal, or at night, with great anguish and restlessness.

(Gastralgia) Silicea - anguish in pit of stomach.

(Gastralgia) Veratrum alb. - pains coming gradually, first in epigastrium, radiating to both sides and upward, reaching to back, between lowest point of scapulae, become agonizing and then gradually subside.

(Gastric catarrh, febris mucosa, biliosa) Belladonna - anguish, restlessness.

(Gastric catarrh, febris mucosa, biliosa) Chamomilla - great anguish, tension and pressure in the region of the stomach, hypochondria, and especially in the pit of the stomach.

(Gastric catarrh, febris mucosa, biliosa) Chelidonium - feeling of anguish in pit of stomach.

(Gastric catarrh, febris mucosa, biliosa) Merc-sol. - painfulness of hypochondria, pit of stomach and around navel < at night, with anguish and restlessness.

(Gastric difficulties, colic of infants) Ars-alb. - anguish and restlessness.

(Gastritis) Arg-nit. - anguish in praecordia.

(Gastritis) Belladonna - difficult breathing, anguish, with congestion of blood to the head, dimness of sight, faintishness, restless and sleepless.

(Gastritis) Veratrum alb. - pains radiating from stomach upward and to both sides, reaching the back between lowest points of scapulae, becomes agonizing and then gradually subsides.

(Gastritis) Veratrum alb. - violent vomiting, with continuous nausea and great prostration, hippocratic face, icy coldness of extremities, anguish in pit of stomach.

(Haematemesis, gastrorrhagia) Veratrum alb. - haematemesis, with continuous nausea, fainting, anguish, vertigo, pale face, profuse cold sweat, prostration and collapse, nausea < on moving or rising.

(Haematuria, haemorrhage from urinary organs) Ars-alb. - anguish and restlessness.

(Haemorrhage from the lungs, haemoptysis) Ergotinum - passive pulmonary haemorrhages, mostly venous, but may be also arterial, usually preceded by sensation of pressure upon the chest, with anguish, faint feeling, weak and small pulse.

(Haemorrhages) Camphor - great anguish.

(Haemorrhages) Carbo-veg. - anguish of heart.

(Headache) Ars-alb. - > by wrapping head up warm, < by lying with head low, before and during windy weather, with anguish, especially when alone.

(Headache) Cantharis - pains deep in the brain, with constant expression of anguish in the face, with eyes closed or without expression when opened.

Some useful rubrics of mind 477

(Headache) Colocynth - aggravation afternoon and evening, with great restlessness and anguish, especially when the sweat smells urinous.

(Headache) Graphites - pain as if head were numb and pithy, as if constricted, especially in occiput, extending to nape of neck, with pains on looking up as if neck were broken. during amenorrhoea frequent congestion to head and chest, dark-red cheeks, oppression and anguish when lying down.

(Headache) Kali cyanatum - agonizing neuralgic pains between temporal region and ciliary arch and maxilla, with screaming and apparent loss of consciousness, recurring daily at same hour, with flushing of affected side of head.

(Headache) Lac felinum - acute pain from vertex down left eye and temple, with so much agony that she has to hold her head firmly with her hands and rush through the house from room to room screaming.

(Headache) Naja - chronic neuralgic headache with agonizing pains, depriving her of sense and memory.

(Headache) Pulsatilla - pale face, whining mood, loss of appetite, no thirst, chilliness, anguish, palpitations.

(Heart diseases) - with anguish and anxiety: Acon., Amm-carb., Ars., Arg-nit., Asa., Calc., Carb-v., Graph., Natr-m., Plat., Puls., Sep.

(Heart diseases) Ars-alb. - heartbeat too strong, visible to the person standing by and audible to the patient himself, < at night and when lying on back. Endocarditis and pericarditis with restlessness, agony and tingling of fingers of left hand, after suppressed measles or scarlatina.

(Heart diseases) Ars-alb. - palpitations with anguish, < after stool, from going up-stairs.

(Heart diseases) Ars-iod - praecordial anguish, dry cough, great pain in cardiac region going through to back.

(Heart diseases) Aur-met. - great anguish, with suicidal tendency and spasmodic contraction of abdomen. Endocarditis with loud endocardial bruits of fluttering action of heart, or sudden jerks through the heart, pulse rapid, compressible and intermittent. in old people attacks of oppression of heart at night with palpitation and great debility. Fatty heart (Arn.), the fat being imbedded around the heart and between the muscular fibres, but without destroying their structure (Ars. and Phos., fatty degeneration of the heart, with destruction of the muscular fibres) atheroma of the heart and bloodvessels with its consequences.

(Heart diseases) Cannabis ind. - pressing pain and anguish at the heart, with dyspnoea the whole night.

(Heart diseases) Carbo-veg. - anguish and great thirst.

(Heart diseases) Carbo-veg. - excessive palpitations for days, after eating, when sitting. Aneurisms, blue varicosities, fine capillary network having a marbled appearance. praecordial anguish as if he would die. Impending paralysis of heart, complete loss of vitality, cyanosis, blood stagnates in capillaries, cold face and limbs, cold sweat, filiform pulse.

(Heart diseases) Cocculus - irregular murmuring action of heart. occasional endocarditic attack after Acon. when there remain great fearfulness and anguish about heart, face of leaden hue.

(Heart diseases) Digitalis - vertigo, delirium, abnormal vision, vomiting, rapidly increasing dyspnoea, spasmodic cough with expectoration, mixed with blood, livid, turgescent face, cannot lie down or be moved without anguish from dyspnoea. Organic diseases of the heart, sensation as if the heart would stop beating if she moved.

(Heart diseases) Kalmia - especially useful when gout or rheumatism, after external applications, shifts from joints to heart sharp, severe pains about heart, taking away the breath and shooting down into stomach and abdomen, with slow pulse (Dig.) and numb feeling in left arm. pericarditis rheumatica, first stage, with tumultuous, rapid and visible beating of the heart, paroxysms of anguish with great dyspnoea, febrile excitement, pains in limbs, stitch in lower part of chest, right-sided face-ache.

(Heart diseases) Phosphorus - anguish about heart with nausea and a peculiar sensation of hunger.

(Heart diseases) Pulsatilla - violent fits of palpitation, often with anguish and obscuration of sight.

(Heart diseases) Sulphur - palpitation of the heart without any apparent cause, without anguish, when lying or during the siesta.

(Heart diseases) Vipera - anguish about heart.

(Hepatic derangements) Belladonna - agonizing, tossing about.

(Hepatic derangements) Pulsatilla - frequent attacks of anguish, especially at night, with diarrhoea.

(Hernia) Ars-alb. - great anguish, restlessness, tossing about, feeling as if the intestines became twisted.

(Hernia) Cuprum met. - intussusception of bowels with singultus, violent colic, faecal vomiting, great agony and anxiety.

(Hernia) Veratrum alb. - intussusception of bowels, great anguish, rushes about bent double, pressing the abdomen.

(Hydrocephaloid) Camphor - great anguish, semi-stupor.

(Hydrophobia) Hyoscyamus - horrid anguish, fits of anxiety.

(Hypochondriasis) Calc-carb. - paroxysms of anguish, with orgasmus sanguinis, palpitation of the heart.

(Hypochondriasis) Ictodes foetida - sudden feeling of anguish, with oppression of breathing and sweat, > after stool.

(Hypochondriasis) Phosphorus - anguish when alone, especially at twilight, or in stormy weather, with timorous disposition. hepatic or renal affections.

(Hypochondriasis) Sabadilla - great anguish about heart.

(Hysteria) Calc-carb. - depression and melancholy, with anguish and palpitations, < as evening approaches.

(Hysteria) Chamomilla - agonizing tossing about with tearing in abdomen.

(Hysteria) Ignatia - anguish, with shrieking for help and suffocating constriction of throat.

(Hysteria) Tarentula hisp. - anguish and oppression of chest, nearly amounting to suffocation.

(Indigestion, gastric derangement) Ars-alb. - colic or burning pains in stomach and abdomen, chilliness and anguish or violent burning pressure at a small spot in stomach.

(Indigestion, gastric derangement) Merc-sol. - painful sensitiveness of the epigastrium and abdomen, especially at night, with anguish and restlessness.

(Insanity) Amm-carb. - great anguish as if he had committed a crime.

(Insanity) Ars-alb. - excessive anguish and irresoluteness.

(Insanity) Aur-met. - religious anguish and longing for death, being unfit for this and the other world, though he prays all the time.

(Insanity) Bismuth - anguish, cannot remain long in one place.

(Insanity) Cannabis ind. - horror of darkness, great anguish and despair.

(Insanity) Chelidonium - horrible anguish by day and by night as if she had killed somebody.

(Insanity) Cina - anguish about heart as if he had committed some evil deed, when walking in open air, chorea, epilepsy.

(Insanity) Cuprum met. - praecordial anguish, pale, miserable look, general chilliness, not relieved by heat.

(Insanity) Iodum - gloomy mood, despondency, anguish, oppression of chest.

(Insanity) Kali iod. - torturing feeling of anguish preventing sleep.

(Insanity) Platina - praecordial anguish, with palpitation and fear of death and of imaginary forms, ghosts.

(Insanity) Secale - great anguish, wild with anxiety.

(Insanity) Veratrum alb. - after short anguish the patient passes from this frenzy into one of deepest melancholy, abject despair of salvation, imbecile taciturnity and complete prostration of mind and body.

(Iris, affections of) Merc-cor. - burning, agonizing pains, excessive photophobia, profuse, excoriating lachrymation.

(Kidney/bladder stone) Arnica - agonizing pains in back and hips from passage of calculi.

(Leucaemia) Natrum sulph. - sycotic pneumonia, inexpressible agony, slowly coagulating blood.

(Mania) Tabacum - proecordial anguish, with faintness.

(Mind symptoms) Alum., Ars., Chel., Cocc., Cycl., Dig., Ign., Merc., Sulph., Veratr.; as if persecuted: Chin., Lach., Sulph., etc. - anguish and despair.

(Mind symptoms) Ars-alb. - burning neuralgia with agony and great restlessness, and this anxiety drives him from one place to another.

(Mind symptoms) Cannabis ind. - anguish, with great oppression, > in fresh air.

(Mind symptoms) Digitalis - anguish, which seems to proceed from epigastrium.

(Mind symptoms) Hepar sulph. - the patient is impelled by unaccountable attacks of internal anguish, which sometimes come on quite suddenly, to attempt suicide (Alum.)

(Mind symptoms) Pulsatilla - anxious dreams with praecordial anguish and ideas of suicide.

(Meningitis, cerebro-spinalis) Cactus - anguish at the heart, and lacerating pains in the nape of the neck.

(Meningitis, cerebro-spinalis) Cannabis ind. - anguish in chest, with great oppression.

(Meningitis, cerebro-spinalis) Tarentula hisp. - deep intense headache, with restlessness, anguish and malaise, the pain flies to forehead and occiput, with photophobia.

(Meningitis, encephalitis) Cantharis - pain deep in brain, with constant expression of anguish on face, resembling a sullen scowl or frown.

(Meningitis, encephalitis) Nux vomica - anguish.

(Menses complaints) Ambra - spasmodic dyspnoea, cardiac anguish and palpitations.

(Menses complaints) Cactus - agonizing uterine spasms, < evenings.

(Menses complaints) Ignatia - headache with heat and heaviness in head, photophobia, anguish, beating of heart, great debility unto fainting

(Menses complaints) Stannum - too early and too profuse. Before: great anguish and melancholy the week previous and ceasing with the appearance of menses.

(Menses complaints) Xanthoxylum - agonizing bearing-down, as if everything would be pushed out.

(Metritis) Ars-alb. - restlessness and anguish, with fear of death
(Migraine) Capsicum - stitching, tearing, drawing pains

with sensation as if the skull would burst, at height of attack nausea, vomiting, anguish, < from motion, stooping, light, > in fresh air, from cold.

(Miscarriage, abortion) Chamomilla - great agony and restlessness.

(Mortification, insults:) Aur-met. - great anguish, coming from praecordial region, driving him from place to place.

(Nausea and Vomiting) Croton tiglium - vomiting immediately after drinking of ingesta, of yellowish-white frothy fluid, with anguish, oppression and pressure in stomach.

(Nephralgia, renal colic) Dioscorea - agonizing pain in small spot over crest of right ilium.

(Nephritis) Belladonna - great anguish and colicky pains.

(Neuralgia) Ars-alb. - great anguish, excessive weakness, has to lie down, affected parts feel cold.

(Neuralgia) Spigelia - fear, anxiety, as if something would happen, praecordial anguish.

(Neurasthenia) Asafoetida - agonizing tightness of chest, as if patient could not breathe.

(Neurasthenia) Coca - feeling of anguish, increased with failure of every effort to strive against this weariness.

(Oesophagus, affections of) Ars-alb. - dryness, thirst, anguish.

(Ovaries, diseases of) Eupion - mental anguish from disappointed hope.

(Ovaries, diseases of) Hamamelis - after a blow, ovary swollen, diffuse, agonizing soreness over whole abdomen.

(Pancreas, diseases of) Carbo-veg. - praecordial anguish.

(Pemphigus) Causticum - large vesicles on chest and back, with anguish in chest and fever.

(Pericarditis) Ars-alb. - pericarditis after suppression of measles or scarlatina, with agony, restlessness, tingling in fingers, especially of left hand.

(Pericarditis) Kalmia - great anguish, dyspnoea, fever, stitches in the heart's region.

(Peritonitis) Cantharis - great anguish and restlessness.

(Prosopalgia) Kali cyanatum - agonizing neuralgic pains between temporal region, ciliary arch and left upper jaw.

(Prosopalgia) Kalmia - right-sided faceache, pains rending, burning, agonizing, stupefying or threatening delirium.

(Prostate gland, diseases of) Apis-mel. - agony in passing urine.

(Purpura) Ars-alb. - unbearable internal heat, dyspnoea, coma, restlessness and anguish, < at night.

(Rabies canina) Hyoscyamus - horrid anguish, fits of anxiety.

(Rheumatism) Actaea spicata - very severe agonizing pain in metacarpal and metatarsal joints, wrists, fingers, ankles and toes, of a tearing, drawing character, < from least motion or touch, at night. Great stiffness of joints after rest.

(Rheumatism) Colchicum - torticollis with paroxysms of anguish, dyspnoea, beating of heart, especially at night

(Rheumatism) Lachesis - intermitting pulse, with irregular action of heart, valvular murmurs, deathly pallor of face, and anguish.

(Seasickness) Ant-tart. - continual nausea, with anguish and oppression in pit of stomach.

(Shock from injuries) Camphor - nervous anguish.

(Shock from injuries) Coffea cruda - mental anguish, afraid of the surgeon, more quiet when left alone.

(Shock from injuries) Hydrocyanic acid - anguish and pressure in chest.

(Shock from injuries) Lachesis - pain in heart and sensation of suffocation, want to tear everything away from throat from anguish, which causes cold sweat to break out.

(Shock from injuries) Laurocerasus - anguish and pressure in chest.

(Shock from injuries) Nitric acid. - anguish after crushing losses of dearest friends.

(Shock from injuries) Nux vomica - cold sweat, anguish and vertigo.

(Sleeplessness) Aranea diad. - sensation of creeping of ants all over chest, anguish and gaping.

(Sleeplessness) Ars-alb. - blood degeneration, malnutrition, with nervous exhaustion, anguish, driving out of bed, changes to sofa or chair and then back to bed, cannot rest in any place, changes continually, which fatigues him (Iod. has the restlessness, but not the fatigue of Ars.).

(Sleeplessness) Belladonna - anguish and restlessness.

(Sleeplessness) Opium - insomnia from sudden shock caused by bad news, with dullness and dazed depression (Acon., agonizing restlessness).

(Smallpox) Hyoscyamus - eruption fails to appear at the proper time, causing great nervous excitement, with rage, anguish, delirium, coming on in paroxysms.

(Sore throat) Capsicum - contraction in the curtain of the palate during deglutition and agonizing pains in ganglions of neck in paroxysms.

(Sore throat) Hyoscyamus - dry, spasmodic cough at night, respiration labored and agonizing.

(Sunstroke) Belladonna - great anguish and restlessness.

(Tetanus and trismus) Veratrum alb. - paroxysms preceded by anguish and despair.

(Tuberculosis of lungs) Ars-alb. - haemoptysis, with anguish, fear of death, burning heat all over body, > by getting up.

(Tuberculosis of lungs) Kali-nit. - lancinating pains in chest, can hardly breathe or lie down, with anguish and extreme prostration.

(Uraemia) Hydrocyanic acid - palpitation, with indescribable anguish and dyspnoea.

(Uterus complaints) Ars-alb. - open cancer of womb, with burning and agonizing pain, and secretion of foetid, brown or blackish ichor.

(Vagina affections) Stannum - great anguish and melancholy a week previous to menses, ceasing as soon as they begin to flow.

(Vertigo, dizziness) Belladonna - accompanied with loss of consciousness and falling, with anguish and luminous vibrations before the eyes.

(Vertigo, dizziness) Thuja - nausea and giddiness when walking in the open air, with heat in the face, anguish and sweat.

(Vision complaints) Capsicum - anguish, capriciousness, homesickness.

(Vision complaints) Hydrocyanic acid - anguish at pit of stomach.

SECTION 3
ACTUAL CASES TREATED

Actual cases treated

In his Lesser Writings Dr. James Tyler Kent points out, "Homoeopathy is slow to win its way because of defective use of books as well as because of defective books".

Following are actual treated cases which are illustrated to guide the selection of the remedy.

Case 1: A patient met with a vehicle accident and his thigh bone was broken. After treatment he was okay but very soon he developed complications and after taking all the necessary tests he was told by the doctors that his kidney (though not injured in the accident) was not functioning and he was put on dialysis. If the practitioner has thorough knowledge of the valuable reference works, he can prescribe the *similimum* in many cases without even seeing the patient (and questioning for 'sensation, modality, concomitants' etc.)

This case is very easy. In all vehicular accidents a victim invariably rolls down either inside the vehicle or on the road and the spinal cord and/or the trunk is twisted (as when we twist a cloth after washing by holding both ends to extract excess water from it).

Now his kidney is not functioning. After road accidents if an organ fails (without any injury to that organ) the only probable cause is that the plexus (bundle of nerves) of that organ is affected and this is not revealed in x-ray or scan report. (*See* ENCYCLOPAEDIA OF DIAGNOSIS AND DIFFERENTIAL DIAGNOSIS FOR HOMOEOPATHIC PRACTITIONERS-12 volumes).

Wilkinson's Materia Medica comes to our help in this case. In this book under the remedy *Eupatorium purpureum* we find the following:

"Through the renal plexus, this remedy has a specific and special action upon the kidneys".

This remedy was given in one single dose in the 10M potency. His kidney started functioning normally and dialysis was stopped. It is now more than two years and the patient is in good health.

Case 2: For outstation patients, I ask them to *write down their symptoms on a paper in their own handwriting* and send it to me. There is lot of difference between writing down in one's own handwriting and typing. The letter of one such patient is given below:

"Respected doctor, I am suffering from chronic sugar for 15 years, and I am taking medicines regularly. I am having ulcer also for the past 10 years and taking medicines only for ulcer then and there and mostly avoiding pain-killer tablets and antibiotics.

Now for the past six months I am having throat pain due to reflux in the stomach irritation. Now throat infection got cured but mouth ulcer started before 2 months. For that also I took Reboflavin daily six tablets and Histac, Pan40 etc. But I am vexed of tablets, tablets, tablets. In the meantime I have seen your valuable books and getting excited. Please kindly guide me".

Finding the remedy—the *similimum* for this patient is simple and very easy. There are two mind symptoms:

1. "I am vexed of tablets, tablets, tablets". For 'vexation' *Kent's Repertory* tells us to see "Irritability"

2. She says that she got excited by seeing my books because she feels they are valuable. For this mind symptom you should not take the rubric 'Excitement, excitable'. The correct rubric for this is 'gay, frolicsome, hilarious'. The equivalent rubric in *Kent's Repertory* (under the chapter 'MIND') is 'Mirth'.

I compared the remedies in top-grade in both the rubrics *viz.*, 'Mirth' and 'Irritability'. Only one remedy *viz.*, *Natrum carb* was found in top-grade in both the lists. As a next step I read the remedy in the MATERIA MEDICA OF MIND SYMPTOMS. (See page 535) Therein we find the following: "exceedingly irritable . . . dyspepsia, with sour belching, waterbrash, retching..." (*see* the patient's letter above. She writes, 'I am vexed of tablets, tablets, tablets'.) Again in Wilkinson's Materia Medica we find the following under Nat-carb.:

> "Irritable, excitable mood . . . Subacute, inflammatory irritation of whole alimentary mucous membrane, from mouth to anus".

Natrum-carb-10M single dose was given. It not only completely cured her of the gastric complaints but also diabetes.

Case 3: I once visited an old friend of mine in Delhi and in the house his pregnant daughter was sitting shedding tears. Upon enquiry her mother told me that the next day is her delivery date and the doctors said that she is very weak and so wouldn't be able to develop any labor pain; therefore, caesarean alone was to be done. In the reference book *The Accoucher's Emergency Manual* by Dr. W.A. Yingling on page 231 we find the following:

> Weak, patient too weak to develop normal pains: Caul., Mur-ac.

Since the remedy *Muriatic acid* has more weakness I started putting questions to the patient. A characteristic symptom in Muriatic acid is "Mouth and anus chiefly affected". (See Boericke's *Materia Medica*). I asked her whether she was having soreness or any complaint in mouth and to this she replied in the affirmative. I further asked if she had similar complaint in her anus and she confirmed this too. I went to a nearby homoeo drug store, bought one dram pills of *Muriatic Acid 200* (they did not have this remedy above the 200th potency) and asked the patient to take one pill every four hours. (Had 10M potency been available then, I would have given that. For example, if you want to give a dose of 10M and if that potency is not available you may give 200th or 1M potency every 4-8 hours, three doses only. Three doses of 200 or 1M would act like a single dose of 10M).

Within minutes of taking a dose of the remedy Muriatic Acid-200 she developed labor pains; was rushed to the hospital and upon entering she took another dose. Within half-an-hour it was a normal and safe delivery.

Case 4: A pregnant lady in a village went to a town (where her sister lived) for delivery. The doctors in a nursing home after examining her, declined to admit her because instead of descending, the uterus was in an upward position. She was then taken to the Govt. hospital. Upon examining her, even they said that a major surgery had to be done and since the senior surgeon was not available they would not admit her. She came home weeping. When I heard this I wanted to find out if homoeopathy could help her and so turned to Yingling. On page 229 we find the following:

> Upward, uterus seems to go: Cimic.

> I gave her *Cimicifuga* (Actaea recemosa)-*10M,* one single dose. Within minutes she felt the uterus coming down to its normal position; and also developed labor pains: so, was rushed to the hospital. This time, upon examining her, the attending doctor said that everything was normal and so admitted her and

it was a safe and normal delivery! Does the reader need any further or better justification for having a copy of Yingling? Every homoeopath should read at least once a month, the *Preface* and *Introduction* in the *Accoucheur's Emergency Manual* by Dr. W. A. Yingling.

Most of the mind symptoms cannot be classified under any specific rubric in the repertory and, therefore, a practitioner will do well by learning them by note. The following cases nos. 5 to 16 would illustrate this point.

Case 5: A renal failure patient under dialysis and waiting for kidney transplant, was under our treatment. We could not find his remedy.

There is no guarantee for kidney transplant, because after a few years, many patients die when the donor kidney stops functioning. After transplant he was heard saying, "Now I feel as if I am released from prison . . . as if I have taken a rebirth". This he said because he is now freed from the torturing and exhausting bi-weekly dialysis, taking rest, body becoming weak etc.

...desire to be released from what seems to be a perpetual burden of sorrow.......

This mental picture clearly indicates Ignatia.

I gave him *Ignatia* and was confident that his other kidney would start functioning and even if the donor kidney fails he would live long.

Case 6: A patient with weeping eczema etc., came to me and said, "Doctor, I am not taking the treatment to live long. But I have an aged daughter to be married and a son who is looking out for a job. Who would come forward to marry my daughter, if I have a weeping eczema? Only because of that, I want to get cured. Before I die, I want to settle things in my family; my daughter getting married and son getting a job. Then I can die peacefully".

Under the homoeopathic remedy *Petroleum* (Boericke's Materia Medica) we find the following:

"feels that death is near and must hurry to settle affairs"

Now, this sentence fits in approximately with the remarks made by the above eczema patient. This remedy was given in single dose and it cured him completely.

Case 7: A peptic ulcer patient's condition worsened day by day and allopathic antacids were giving only temporary relief. At the height of his suffering (hunger pain with burning sensation in the food pipe, temporarily relieved by eating) he was heard saying, "I think that my end is approaching; I must call the lawyer to write the will; that this hotel of mine should go to my wife; money deposited in the bank is for my son. My widowed sister who has been living with me for several years and helping me should take the house which I bought recently".

This mind picture fits with Petroleum. One single dose of Petroleum-10M cured this patient. We do not prescribe on names of disease or pathology but on 'uncommon' symptoms having no connection with pathology.

The above mentioned case 6 and case 7 show the reader that

1. one and the same remedy may be called for different persons with different diseases; also,
2. different persons suffering from one and the same disease may need different remedies.

Case 8: A seventy-year old carpenter was under my treatment for skin complaint. During one of his visits he was accompanied by his 48-year old son. The son was coughing with chest congestion etc. The carpenter told his son; "Why don't you too take treatment from this doctor? See how much I have improved, whereas the other seven doctors to whom I consulted earlier could not do anything in my case".

To this, the son said: "The new house where I shifted has no *raasi*".[3] ('Raasi' in Tamil means luck). In other words the person feels that everything was going wrong ever since he started living in a particular house. So, that house has no raasi. Or, a person feels that ever since he bought and started using a car, nothing went right. He attributes his sufferings, failures, difficulties etc. to that vehicle. I hope the reader would understand this. The son continued, "Even the new work place where I am going daily is not raasi (or has no good luck)".

The other word to describe 'raasi' would be 'sentimental' 'luck'. The carpenter's son was not ready to take treatment from me only because he felt that the house and the work place is the cause of his respiratory complaints.

I gave him one dose of a remedy telling him to take that and he need not pay me any fees. He took it. (Later I learnt that he was completely cured).

Can any homoeopath tell me what remedy I gave the patient?

Read the remedy *Staphisagria* in the chatper *Melancholia* in Lilienthal. (page 701). There we find the following:

> Inwardly gnawing grief and anger, he looks at everything from the darkest side.. disinclination to work and think; dread of the future and dread of being constantly pursued..

The enthusiastic reader would be eager to know how I selected this remedy for the above case.

1. Reproaches others (blaming the house and work place).
2. Sentimental. I write down the remedies common to both the above rubrics (Kent's Repertory—MIND) and read them in the "sorrowfulness ending in paralysis of the intellect"chapter *Melancholia* in Lilienthal. *Staphisagria* suited the symptoms of the case.

Case 9: A lady of forty-two came with a large calculus in her urinary bladder. She said that allopathic doctors advised surgery as the only answer but she declined to undergo it. She continued that she had already undergone two caesarean sections and one appendicectomy; after each one of these surgeries, her general health ran down. Therefore she could not afford deterioration of health any further with another surgery and she had to safeguard her health for the remaining period of her life. Under the remedy Nux vomica (in the *Materia Medica of Mind Symptoms* at the end of this book) we find the following:

Afraid he might not have enough to live on...

Nux-vomica-1M, one single dose was given in the evening. Not only did her general health improve, but also the size of the stone started reducing. (Patient still under treatment)

Case 10: A chronic renal failure patient came to me with a few relatives, all of whom were allopathic doctors. They showed me a file containing the medical papers of the patient. After this, one by one, the relatives went out.

The patient was still sitting. He said, "Doctor, my sons say that I am sick and so I should not ride bicycle, go out and do our business. They say they will do everything and ask me to sit at home taking rest. As my children, they should only tell me that I am alright and would recover soon. But instead of encouraging me for speedy recovery they have branded me as a permanent and incurable patient[3]".

This patient feels that his sons, instead of encouraging, are letting him down. What one requires from his relatives is not money nor help but *moral support*. In this case the patient feels that this is completely missing.

This symptom we find in two remedies. (*See* the *Materia Medica of Mind Symptoms* at the end of this book) They are

"... a feeling of moral deficiency..." - *Kali brom.*

"... despondency, sadness, moral depression and relaxation..." - *Tarentula hisp.*

Tarentula hisp. 10M - single dose was given.

Case 11: A lady of fifty-five, school teacher, was under my treatment for three months for sinusitis with little relief. She lives thirteen kilometers away from my clinic and she works in a school which is near my clinic. Before going to school she would come to me once a month, take medicine and go to school. Seeing no relief inspite of three visits, I told her that a certain acupressure doctor would come and give just 3-minute treatment once only and for this she need not pay any fees and I also assured total relief. Since the acupressure doctor comes to my clinic on Sundays only, I asked her to come on a Sunday. To this she replied, "I have to come all the way... from .. (her residence)".

During the earlier three visits she would come to me in the morning before going to her school which is near to my clinic. Sunday is holiday for school and she feels it an ordeal to come for acupressure treatment all... the... way from her residence thirteen kilometers away.

It is hesitation. I told her that she need not pay any fees for the one-time acupressure and 100% cure was also assured. Therefore, travelling thirteen kilometres won't be a crime. But to do this she has hesitation. Before we show the reader how we selected the remedy on this symptom, let us now see two more cases.

Case 12: A lady allopathic doctor was learning homoeopathy from me every Sunday morning for two hours. She consulted me for her complaints and total relief of her ailments. Once she said, "Doctor, can you give one-dose treatment for my son? Since birth he is having perennial cold; now he is five years and almost every week he has to take drugs". I told her that she must bring her son at least once and I would cure him completely. Bringing her son once (and I am not going to charge her since she is my student) is not an ordeal or something immoral. To this she replied, "For this I have to... bring him all the way from my home" (which is just ten kilometers away).

She hesitates for this small thing of bringing the boy once only to me and for which the boy is going to get total relief permanently.

Only if you actually listen to the patient's reply in person may you understand this. Let me explain and elaborate on this.

Suppose you are asked by your teacher to murder a certain person. What would be your reaction? Immediately you would reply as under: "Sir, I... have to..." (The sentence would be incomplete. Because you have hesitation since doing this job would prick your conscience).

In the above said cases for merely travelling ten kilometres they have lot of hesitation as if I am asking them to do some crime or immoral thing. In other words, they are over conscious of a trivial thing. The apt term would be "Conscientious scruples". This symptom is in the remedy Arsenicum album (see the materia medica of mind symptoms at the end of this book).

One single dose of Arsenicum Album-10M completely cured the above sinusitis patient and even acupressure treatment was not given.

Case 13: This is a cancer patient and after the consultation was over, I asked my fees of six thousand rupees. To this he replied, "Money... is..." (The sentence was incomplete and hesitation was as if they are asked to do some immoral act). He should say that either he has no money or that he would try to borrow from relatives. But he didn't say such thing. Ars. Alb-10M, one single, dose cured him.

The above cases would illustrate the meaning and interpretation of mind symptoms of a patient. In some cases the repertory or software is not useful and you have to learn by rote these uncommon mind symptoms.

The above three cases are quoted here to illustrate that if the practitioner can memorise the symptoms of various remedies given in the *Materia Medica of Mind Symptoms* at the end of this book, he would be able to select the remedy in more than fifty percent of cases that too at the very first attempt.

Case 14: A patient with chronic headache, after spending much money with various doctors, specialists and homoeopaths came to me. After finishing the history of his seven years pain in head, he ended up saying: "Doctor, if you or anyone can cure me of this terrible headache, I won't mind even giving away half of my property (worth three millions) to that doctor".

Doctors of all other systems would simply ignore this statement of the patient.

If a patient is ready to pay 1.5 million.. I thought over this. I took this as a challenge to homoeopathy. I asked him to first pay me ten thousand rupees and also give me two weeks time with a promise that if I do not cure him in one single dose (or a few doses) I would return double the amount paid by him. Also, if he is cured he may pay me another ten thousand rupees. He agreed to this condition and paid ten thousand rupees.

I took a copy of Boericke's Materia Medica and went to a professor of English and requested him to render me a help; that he has to read the lines given only under the chapter 'Mind' in all the remedies in Boerick's Materia Medica and underline if any relevant line is found equivalent to the statement of a person who says that he would pay half of his wealth if his headache is cured. I paid him five thousand rupees (which the professor said is more than sufficient for the work).—It may take a few days, spending two or three hours daily to go through the lines given under the chapter 'Mind' in Boericke's 688-page materia medica.

To another professor of English I gave a copy of *Wilkinson's Materia Medica* and paying him the remaining five thousand rupees requested him to do the job of reading the lines given only under the chapter 'Mind' in all the remedies (and this too would take a few days, working for three hours daily) and to tell me if he finds anything equivalent to the above said statement of the headache patient.

The first professor (using Boericke's) could not find anything apt. But the second professor underlined and pointed out the following lines in the remedy *Stillingia* (under 'Mind' in Wilkinsons).

"Deplorably downhearted; suffering extreme torture from bone pains."

Stillingia 1000, one single dose cured the patient and he paid me another ten thousand rupees. After this case I cured two more patients with *Stillingia*. both of whom said the above words (ready to give his entire wealth to the doctor who cures him).

Diligence and *knowledge of English language,* both to the core, are required to practise homoeopathy.

Case 15: Here is another case of headache. This 55-years old male patient remarked: "Doctor, all these years I have been having these pains; my sufferings are such that no amount of compensation would be equal to it. Even if you make me the President of all the nations in the world that would not be a sufficient compensation". I told him the same condition which I put to the patient in the earlier case. After taking ten thousand rupees I went to the two English professors, one with Boericke and the other with *Wilkinson's Materia Medica*. In this case the professor going through Boericke's Materia Medica could help me. He pointed to the following found under the remedy *Selenium*.

Extreme sadness. Abject despair uncompromising melancholy

Selenium 10M, one dose cured the patient and he paid me ten thousand rupees.

On a later occasion the above said professors asked me what I did by their help and I showed them how I practice homoeopathy. Soon both of them started learning and practicing homoeopathy.

Homoeopathic system of medicine is *exact and accurate. Precision* and *versatility* is its culture.

Case 16: The other day I was sitting by the side of a senior homoeopath in his clinic. A patient entered and asked, "Do you have medicine for diabetes"?

Doctor: Yes, tell me your symptoms.

Patient: (Stretching his hand towards the doctor) & ("see my pulse; give medicine").

(The tone of the patient was in a commanding note similar to a king, who, when anything is required would order, "Bring the head of the thief in two hours").

The doctor turned towards me and said, "See doctor, these patients don't tell symptoms. How can I prescribe"? That doctor always thinks "Sensation, Locality, Modalities, Concomitants. What a wrong teaching"? I took Calvin B. Knerr's REPERTORY to him and showed the following:

MIND, Answers, imperiously: Lycopodium.

Further I showed him the following from Wilkinson's Materia Medica under the remedy Lycopodium:

"Talks with an air of command.. manner stiff and pretentious".

Lycopodium 10M, one single dose, cured diabetes.

Let us reiterate the following:

Homoeopathy is a system where the patient himself (by way of some words or actions or as a reaction to his disease or treatment or attitude towards the doctor) indicates the remedy to us.

Homoeopathy is practical and practical only and there is no place for any theory, imagination, etc.

Case 17: This is an interesting case. A boy of twelve was brought to me for lung tuberculosis. I asked the boy a few questions (no standard questionnaire etc. please) just to make him talk—name of his school, what games he plays etc.

Nothing 'uncommon' or 'rare-strange-peculiar' or 'mind symptom' came out. I got up and went to the cupboard of medicines, took out a bottle and was preparing doses of some medicines.

At this time it occurred to me to consult Lilienthal. I studied all the remedies given under the chapter *PHTHISIS PULMONUM*. While doing so, under the remedy Lycopodium, the words "observing disposition" made me to pause and ponder. I found that the boy was constantly observing me at what all I had been doing, writing on the case sheet, referring to books, preparing the doses etc. I could remember that unlike other patients, he was constantly observing me.

Lycopodium 10M was prescribed. Next month, he was to report but he didn't. Later when I met the boy's father, he said he was perfectly fine. That is why we did not come to you again.

Case 18: A certain breastfed baby was brought to me for constipation. On the symptoms (which I don't remember now), I prescribed one dose of Nux vomica-30. The lady came three days later saying that with the one dose the child passed normal stool the next morning. But constipation relapsed.

It has never been my experience that one dose acted for one day only. I only thought that my selection of Nux-vom was wrong. To select a better (correct) remedy, I looked through all the remedies given under "CONSTIPATION" in the Chapter

"CHILDREN, DISEASES OF" in Lilienthal. I read *Nux-vom.* Also wherein the following words under the remedy caught my attention:

"...the nurse takes too much coffee and lives too high.

On questioning she affirmed that she took seven or eight cups of strong coffee daily.

I gave one dose of *Nux-vomica* 30 to be given to the baby at bedtime and emphatically told the mother that she must (i) either stop coffee or (ii) stop the breast feeding. She agreed to take light coffee 1-2 times only. After the second dose of Nux-vomica there was no relapse of constipation. Without Lilienthal I would only have concluded that my first prescription of *Nux-vom.* was wrong and would have meddled with the case by changing the remedy.

Remember the words of Dr. Samuel Lilienthal: **"Drop a symptom in Lilienthal and you get the remedy". Yes, it is so quick and certain in some cases".**

Selection of the remedy manually with the repertory(ies) is neither difficult nor time-consuming. It is definitely quicker than the computer. What is time-consuming and difficult is *Case Taking* which the computer cannot do even one per cent.

Most homeopaths consider "totality-of-symptoms" and so administer a questionnaire to the patient, but they are not taught that "Totality-of uncommon symptoms" is the correct method. (Section 153 of the *Organon*). In any patient "uncommon, rare, strange or peculiar" symptom is one or, at the most, two only. For referring these one or two symptoms to the repertory takes really less time and less efforts.

Non-homeopathic uses of the homoeo medicine *Phosphorus* to prevent cancer and brain tumor caused by computer radiation effect, television, cell phone and atomic power plants.

This information is for those sitting before the computer for hours together.

Every scientific invention carries a sting on its tail. But we can preserve our health with the help of homoeopathic medicines. *Phosphorus-1000,* one single dose taken once a month is a *must* for our computer and atomic age. More particularly in U.S.A., atomic power plant is everywhere. Though scientists may cheat us, it is an undeniable fact that sooner or later there would be more and more cancer hospitals and hospitals for brain tumour. Atomic power plants, plastics and computers as well as colour televisions constantly emit minute quantity of radiation which, in turn, causes cancer and cell phones cause brain tumour. I do not say this but it is scientists who are telling this and no conscious scientist can deny this. For the side-effects of the above said scientific invention the homoeo medicine Phosphorus-1000 is the best antidote. Take one dose, once a month. That is one of the extended uses of homoeopathy. Loss of vision after lightning is cured by Phosphorus. For bad effects of electric shock, the same Phosphorus.

Case 19: Mr. S. 47 years. He starts, "Doctor, can you give me some homeo medicine for the pain in my anus?"

Myself: "Okay, tell me about it; how long you have this"? Don't put any leading question but just to make him talk till he throws out some 'uncommon' symptom.

Patient: "Doctor, it is a long story... I have been going to a few homoeopaths in the city. I am having boil like eruption with swelling near my anus. I went to a homoeopath who said that he would give medicine to abort it and so gave me Silicea high potency. The swelling and pain reduced. But, after a few weeks it started appearing on yet another nearby place. This homoeopath consulted his senior who said it is better to give Silica-3x, i.e., low potency, to make it suppurate out so that all impurities in the system may be thrown out, so that I may once for all be cured completely and permanently. I took this Silica 3x thrice daily and in a few days it suppurated, opened out and all pus and other things came. Then total relief. I thought that I was cured once for all. But, after a month the same old story; it appeared in yet another place near anus. I now went to the senior homoeopath, who in turn, referred me to the top-most homoeopath who is an eminent practitioner. He listened to me and said that the 'tendency to skin eruption' is to be eradicated and so he gave me one dose of Graphites-10M. This gave lot of relief but after a month I am back to square number one.

Myself: "How long do you have this?" (I ask this to make him talk further).

Patient: Can I tell you from the beginning?

Myself: Yes, tell me. I have time to listen to you.

Patient: "It all began seven years ago. I first got this skin complaint around my mouth. At that time I took allopathic medicine and got cured(?). One and-a-half year after this it appeared here. (shows the left rib.) As allopathic drugs did not help this time I turned to ayurveda and got cured. A year later it appeared on the right hip. I again took ayurveda and got cured. Two years after this it again appeared, this time, on the left nate above anus and that time I was treated with allopathy and got cured. Now it is around the anus."

A few of what we teach to our students are:

1. 'uncommon' symptoms (Section 153 of the Organon) may be one (or two, at the most, in any case) only.
2. 'uncommon symptom' is told by the patient spontaneously and much less is to be inquired into.

In the above case one characteristic is "sides of the body". (Left or right side aggravation or appearance has the least value among symptoms, but since in this case no other more valuable or uncommon symptom or general symptoms are found, we take this as a matter of exception).

The complaint first appeared around mouth. Then on left rib—then right hip; from there to left Nate above anus. Now, it is in anus.

1. Mouth to left rib
2. Left rib to right hip—this is upper left to lower right.
3. Right hip to left Nate—this is upper right to lower left.

The complaint had traveled crosswise, both ways, *i. e.* upper left to lower right and upper right to lower left.

Kent's Repertory: GENERALITIES... SIDE...

Crosswise, left upper and right lower... 62 remedies...

Left lower and right upper: 57 remedies.

Remedies common to both the two lists are: Chel., Euphr., Mur-ac., Nux-v., Rhus-t.

These five remedies were studied in Boericke's Med. Med. While doing so the following lines under the remedy *Muriatic acid* enabled us to confirm it for this case.

"Mouth and anus chiefly affected".

(The complaint first started in his mouth. Now finally it is in the anus).

Muriatic Acid-10M single dose was prescribed. He was completely cured and it is now more than twelve years and there is no relapse. Also, he said that weakness felt by him for a very long time also was cured with my prescription and it is only now that he is now in good health and strength.

The 'left or right side' affinity of a symptom and 'time modality' are considered least important for the selection of a remedy in a chronic disease. But in the above mentioned case, the side affinity has been considered due to the absence of any other more valuable symptom.

Some notes on the use of Boericke Materia Medica may not be out of place here.

1. After selecting one or a few remedies with the aid of the repertory you may read them in Wilkinson's and/or Lilienthal and/or Boericke to confirm the one remedy (or one of the few remedies) selected by you got through repertory.

2. In respect of Boericke Materia Medica we want to say a few things. This is useful to confirm our selection but only the preamble or first para(s) given under each remedy is useful. Also symptoms found under 'Mind' in respect of some remedies. Other things after this such as Head, Eye etc. are not found by us to be useful and so we don't use them. ('Modalities' and 'Relationship of Remedies' given at the end of each remedy is partially useful in some cases. In respect of the latter when the patient is partially cured with one remedy, for follow up, the remedies given under "Remedies follow well" or "Complementary" are quite useful).

In respect of preamble a few more things in Boericke Materia Medica. If your selection of the remedy (with the aid of the repertories) is correct then the symptom or main complaint of the patient would, in most cases, be found

(i) either in the first sentence; if not

(ii) in the second and following sentences, the complaint will either be *preceded by an adjective* or *followed by an adverb.*

In the case of Muratic Acid case mentioned above, in Boericke we find the adverb: "Mouth and anus *chiefly* affected".

In respect of Knerr's we want to say a few things: When a general symptom occurs as a modality or concomitant to another general symptom and if you find a remedy for such a condition in Knerr's it is like the apex court judgment.

Case 20: After finishing my lecture on homoeopathic practice in Bombay to an audience of senior homoeopaths and Professors and Lecturers of homoeopathic colleges, one professor of materia medica asked me whether I can cure his son's epilepsy with one dose. A meeting was arranged and I ordered the boy to be brought to me along with the mother. On arrival the Professor started talking what all remedies he had tried—Cuprum met., Agaricus etc. etc. being chief remedies for epilepsy?

With a gesture of my hand I asked him to keep quiet and turned to his wife (mother of the patient) to tell me about the boy's complaints.

She started narrating what all allopathic diagnosis were done, E.E.G. taken etc. Then history of homoeopathic treatment with no relief etc. etc. We do not note down all these things. We have to note down only 'uncommon', 'mind' and 'general symptoms'. Also family history.

While the patient talks, the practitioner should keep quiet. Any interruption would only break the chain of thought of the narrator... (Section 84 to 87 of *The Organon*)

After the narration was over, after a pause, she leaned forward towards me with wide open eyes, "Doctor, one thing, whenever he sits in the commode for passing bowel movements, he invariably get the convulsions... What is it due to doctor?" At this point the professor interrupted saying that she need not tell all these things as they are of no use.

I took out Knerr's and fortunately I found the following on page... Therein

During stool, convulsions: Art-v.

Apart from 'mind symptoms' and 'uncommon symptoms' equally important are general symptoms. (Generals is different from general symptoms. See Kent's REPERTORY—Preface etc).

Mind or uncommon symptom may misguide us; but with 'general symptoms' they are sure shot. One dose of Artemisia vulgaris-10M was given and from that day the convulsions started reducing gradually and in a week's time completely stopped.

Things are exact and crystal clear. But no homoeopathic practitioner seems to be interested in excellent reference works such as Lilienthal, Knerr etc. With the use of the few above said materia medicas and repertories we have no complaint and no wants in homoeopathic practice.

In the above mentioned reference books everything is in down-to earth language and matter of fact manner.

Case 21: A certain patient with several years of pain in abdomen came to us. He has tried various systems and doctors all in vain. There was a herbal specialist in our city who has never failed in respect of abdominal colic cases. But he too failed in this case. I went through all the remedies under Colic in Lilienthal. Under the remedy *Cuprum met.* I found the following words:

"Lack of reaction".

One dose of this remedy cured the patient completely and permanently. Lilienthal is hundred times worth its weight in gold. Subsequent to this case, whenever a chronic and worse case of colic of years standing come to us after trying various doctors, we first give Cuprum and in most cases it gave good result.

Most cases of fracture of the tibia bone continues to give trouble; does not heal. One singe dose of *Anthracinum* has cured all such cases. (See Calvin B. Knerr's Repertory – page 1148 – Injuries, fractures… of tibia, Anthrac).

Certain symptoms cannot be classified in the repertory under any head. Therefore, it is better to memorise and keep them in your finger-tips.

For the following two cases one and the same remedy cured.

Case 22: A patient consulted me for allergic rash on skin on both upper limbs and chest.

He said, "Doctor, for the last three years I have gone to allopaths, ayurveda, homoeopaths etc. They have treated me for weeks and months with just five per cent relief. If I eat unstrained cooked rice or wheat flour preparation, that afternoon I would get distension of my belly; that evening the rash on skin will start; in the night if I pass flatus freely per ano or have a free bowel movement the rash would disappear".

Case 23: A school boy of twelve was brought by the parents. The mother started talking: "Doctor, he has to leave the house for school at 9.30 in the morning. He gets up at 6.00 a.m. By 7.30 a.m. he becomes so restless—jumps, cries etc. This would last for half-an-hour. Then this disappears; it is followed by 3-4 times loose bowel movement. After that he becomes completely all right and goes to school".

In both the above cases the symptoms that should come to our mind is given below: "Symptoms disposed to appear periodically and in groups.. intermitting . . ".

The above lines are found in the remedy *Cuprum met.* (Boericke's Materia Medica). This remedy cured both the above patients in one single dose in the 200th potency.

CASE 24: A lady, the mother-in-law of a fourth stage cancer patient, came to me asking medicine for cancer. When I asked her to bring the patient she said that he wouldn't come. I asked her to tell me *verbatim* what he had said. She replied, "He does not say anything".

At this stage I asked her whether she did not care to go and see her son-in-law who is said to be in fourth stage cancer. She replied:

"My daughter wrote me a letter stating that doctors have said that he would live for another six months only, and he is not afraid of death, but he wants to live with his family in the same quarters in which he had been living all along and said that he does not want anyone (be it friends or relatives) to visit him".

(Sometimes, we do get valuable symptom from the report of messengers).

Let us now see how to work out this case.

"Does not want anyone to visit him" –Aversion to company "Till death wants to live with family in the same quarters where he had been living all these years" – Homesick

KENT'S REPERTORY was consulted:

Company, aversion to: (several remedies)
Homesickness: (several remedies)

Remedies common to these two rubrics and scoring more points are: Aur.-4, Carb-an.-6, Ign.-5, Nat-m.-5

To confirm one out of the above four remedies, they were studied in the *HOMOEOPATHIC THERAPEUTICS* (By Dr. Samuel Lilienthal). In the chapter "Carcinoma". Under Carb-an. we find the words "cachexia full developed".

Again, in the Materia Medica of mind symptoms at the end of this book under the remedy Carb-an. we find the following words:

"desire for solitude".

Carb-an.10M, single dose was prescribed. Patient is improving.

Case 25: A lady in Chennai asked me if I can give medicine for her brother who complains of partial loss of hearing with ringing in ears; this started at the time of train bomb blast in Bombay (in July 2006) in which he was travelling.

I told her that the patient (if he cannot come to me personally) may *write down his complaints* and send it to me. The lady told me that she would tell all about her brother. It is ringing in ears and partial hearing loss after the train bomb blast. I insisted on the point that *the patient should himself write down his complaints on a paper* and send it to me along with the report of E.N.T. doctor. (E-mail will not serve our purpose, nor telephonic talk). Anyway, the lady brought a printout of e-mail from her brother that read as under:

> "I am giving the details of how I am feeling after the incident. On that day I was practically deaf and could not hear anything. There was a constant ringing in my ears and I was feeling very confused. At that time I did not feel anything, but after reaching home and what I saw on TV, only then I felt very scared. I had some bruises on my arm and my hair was completely filled with black powder.The ringing sound has not stopped yet. It becomes louder in the evening. Now also as I am writing this, the sound is there.
>
> I got my audiometry test done and it was diagnosed as low to moderate hearing loss in my left ear and moderate hearing loss in my right ear. There is no rupture in ear drums. Now-a-days I feel very scared if I have to enter local train. The thoughts about the blast keeps recurring and I am never normal while travelling. I must have received some body blows during the blast on my back and neck. My right wrist hurts if I have to clamp something with it. Both my arms ache. All sorts of negative feelings come in my mind and I have become a nervous wreck".

We now turn to *HOMOEOPATHIC THERAPEUTICS* by Dr. Samuel Lilienthal, the above three remedies (Bell., Calc., Lyc.) alone are read under the chapter "EMOTIONS, Ill Effects of – Fear, Dread, Fright (page 377-378)". The following words are found in the remedy Calc-carb.

....< evening...grief and complaining about old offences... great tendency to be frightened....
(portions relevant to our case alone are quoted here).

Calcarea-Carb. 10M, was prescribed in one single dose. Taking bath would stop the action of Calc-carb. (see Kent's *Lectures on Homoeopathic Materia Medica*). Patient was advised not to take bath for a few days. Patient is improving.

Case 26: (Sometimes it is the past health history that helps us to find the remedy for a patient). Baby Lakshmi, four years (Referred to me by an allopath for 'muscular dystrophy').

When you don't have sufficient valuable symptoms in the present state of the patient, you may ask for the past health history. If the past history has more valuable symptoms you may work out the case on those. The allopath was present and he pointed out that lower limbs alone are mostly affected and the child is freely using both the upper limbs. When the child was shown to me she started crying and the father said that the child was afraid of strangers.

Since the father did not say any further symptoms I asked him a general question as to what all diseases the child had since birth (for which they had gone to a doctor and got treatment). The father replied that the child had

1. frequent fever with running nose;
2. discharge from ears;
3. frequent diarrhoea.

(Sometimes it is the past health history of the patient that may help us find the remedy).

Let us now learn what is an artistic method of working out a case.

A correct interpretation of the above three symptoms for homeo prescribing is as under. Ponder on the above three (past history) symptoms and you get the following:

1. rhinitis (frequent fever with running nose is rhinitis)

2. otitis media (discharge from ear)
3. gastro-enteritis (frequent diarrhoea)

The suffix '-itis' appears in the above three symptoms. 'Inflammation of any part is denoted by the suffix '-itis'.

Therefore we look into KENT'S REPERTORY GENERALITIES: INFLAMMATION... internally; Acon., Ars., Bell., Bry., Canth., Echi., Gels., Iod., Lach., Merc., Nux-v., Phos., Plb., Puls., Sec., Ter. (Top-grade remedies alone are taken)

The child is afraid of strangers. For this we should not take "Fear of strangers" but it is 'timidity'

KENT'S REPERTORY: (Page 88-89) MIND: TIMIDITY: plus above list = Phos., Plb.

We have to do the analysis. Now, at this stage, that is, after having selected the remedies (on available symptoms) through the Repertory, we have to apply our knowledge of materia medica. By looking at the above two remedies we find that the remedy *Plumbum met.* has more spinal symptoms (the reader must note that only lower limbs are affected while upper limbs are intact, which means affection of spinal cord). In reference to Plumbum met. in Boericke Materia Medica the following words in the preamble agree with the case:

...paralysis is chiefly of extensors... partial anaesthesia ...Progressive muscular atrophy. Infantile paralysis. Excessive and rapid emaciation. ...Important in peripheral affections... (The parent told me that they noted that its lower limbs were weak only when she was one year old).

(As far as homoeopathy is concerned, there is not much difference between atrophy/dystrophy/emaciation etc. etc).

Plumbum met. 10M, single dose, was prescribed and the child is making rapid recovery.

Case 27: Aswin, aged four, is brought by her mother for constant and chronic running nose (fluent coryza). I do not ask any question

While I was going through Dr. Calvin B. Knerr's *Repertory*, the boy's mother breaks in, "Doctor, he is very angry at times". (At this stage I simply note in the case-sheet the word *anger*). I copy on the case-sheet the following portions from Knerr's Repertory (page 248).

NOSE, Coryza, chronic: Calc., Canth., Colch, Cycl., Sil., Spig.

MIND, Anger (plus above list); Calc.

At this stage, the lady tells: "Doctor, whenever he is at home on holidays, running nose is not there. But whenever he goes to school, on those days, it is worse". To classify this last symptom is a somewhat difficult job.

I now turned to Lilienthal.

At this stage, after a pause, the lady continues, "Doctor, two years ago he was diagnosed to be suffering from primary complex and we gave a course of allopathic treatment".

To classify the symptom (aggravation on the days of going to school) is a difficult task. For "primary complex' the equivalent rubric in homoeopathy is *phthisis* (prodromal stage).

I just glanced through Lilienthal and under the chapter PHTHISIS PULMONUM (page 858) the following lines under *Calcarea Carb*. caught my attention. ..very susceptible to external influences, currents of air, cold, heat, noise, excitement".

(When he goes to school he is exposed to air, noise, excitement and therefore the above quoted line confirmed my selection of *Calc. Carb).*

I gave this in 10M potency in single dose and the patient is improving.

Case 28: Mr. N. 55 years reported: "Doctor, daily morning I get headache; in the afternoon after lunch I have distension of abdomen, gastric troubles. In the night I get terrible pain in the leg…"

You cannot 'repertorise' this case. The case is very simple. His symptom is to be classified as under:

"Aggravation of head symptoms in the morning; abdomen in the afternoon and legs in the night"

In Boericke's *Materia Medica* under the remedy *Ammonium Mur.* we read as under:

"Its periods of aggravations are peculiarly divided as to the bodily region affected; thus the head and chest symptoms are worse mornings, the abdominal in the afternoon, the pains in the limbs, the skin and febrile symptoms, in the evenings".

It may not be out of place if we write here that the above patient had been to so-called leading, experienced, and classical and Hahnemannian homoeopaths who had treated him with various medicine for months without relief.

Let us reiterate the following:

HOMOEOPATHY IS A SYSTEM WHERE THE PATIENT HIMSELF (BY SOME WORDS OR ACTIONS OR AS A REACTION TO HIS DISEASE OR TREATMENT OR ATTITUDE TOWARDS THE DOCTOR) *indicates the remedy to us.*

Case 29: A mentally deranged patient, 32 years, unmarried, stopped going to work from his twenty-fifth year. The father reported: "He does not take bath daily; just sits at home; never goes out and meets his friends; smokes cigarettes continuously and sees porns in the T.V…. Doctor, one more thing … after passing daily bowel movement, he takes little feces in hand and rubs it on his head. It is quite disgusting… I read the remedies given on page no. 620 to 634 of Lilienthal under the chapter Insanity and the following extracts from the remedy *Merc-sol.* agreed with the case:

"homesickness… senseless, disgusting actions"

Merc-sol. 10M one single dose cured him.

Case 30: A beginner in homoeopathy, one of my students, asked me over phone as to how to proceed in a case of bleeding from the uterus of a 60-days pregnant lady.

My: Did the patient go to a lady doctor?

Student: Yes.

My: What did she say?

Student: After examining the patient, the lady doctor told that the child is okay and the patient need not worry about bleeding.

I asked my student to see the reference books in the order given below:

Calvin B. Knerr's Repertory — Genitalia — Female — Pregnancy — Hemorrhage: Cocc., Rhus-t., Sec., **Trill.**

Lilienthal — Miscarriage — To read all the above four remedies. In the remedy *Trillium* we find the words 'third month'.

Boericke Materia Medica — Trillium (The very first sentence reads:) "A general haemorrhagic medicine.".

Case 31: A primipara (first pregnancy lady) was having morning sickness from her third month till the sixth month. After taking full meals when she gets up to wash the hands she would vomit what all she had taken in the reverse order. As the patient was in a far away place she was asked to write down in her symptoms in her own handwriting as if she is telling her friend about her complaints. Her letter is given below.

"After full meals as I get up I get vomiting. So after eating, I wash my hands in the plate and lie down. After half-an-hour or so only I get up.

I also feel foetus' kicking pain in a particular spot. When a heavy truck goes on the road making a thunder noise, I feel that noise hitting in that place in my belly where the kick of the child causes pain.

Case repertorisation:

Boericke's Repertory (last chapter) MODALITIES (p.970)—AGGRAVATION:

Jar—Ars., *Bell.,* Berb. v., *Bry., Cic.,* Crot., Glon., Ign., Nux-v., *Spig.,* Ther.

Noise—Acon., Asar., *Bell., Bar., Calad.,* Cham., Cinch., Cocc., *Coff., Colch.,* Ferr., Glon., *Ign.,* Lyc., Mag. m., Med., Nux-m., *Nux-v.,* Onosom., Phos., Solan-lyc., *Spig.,* Tar-h., *Ther.*

The six remedies *viz.,* Bell., Glon., Ign., Nux-v., Spig., and Ther. are common to the above two lists. All these six remedies were studied in Boericke's Mat. Medica.

The remedy *Theridion* was selected because of the following found therein.

Sensitive to noise; it penetrates the body.. Noises seem to strike on painful spots over the body.

Theridion-30, single dose completely stopped the vomiting and pain < by noise.

Case 32: A boy of ten years was brought by the father. The latter described:

"He is having less concentration in studies".

Myself: What is the report of the class teacher about him.

Father: He says that my son is intelligent, but lacks concentration. He is a capable boy and only if he concentrates can he shine well. He was scoring 95 marks in earlier classes. He has become dull in the last two years. (I then asked general questions about his food habits, appetite, sleep etc).

Father: One point. He goes to bed at 9 p.m. and immediately will sleep. Morning we have to wake him up and even at 6 o'clock on waking, he is not fresh or active. He goes to drum classes. That teacher says he is excellent in his performance on certain days only. I asked the boy some questions asking him to tell me about his difficulties and he says 'Nothing'. To some questions he nods his head or answers in single words.

Kent's Repertory — MIND — Answers, shortly, curtly ANSWERS, refuses to. In the above case, there are two generals *viz.,* (1) Sleep, unrefreshing; and (2) plethora.

Earlier he was scoring 95% marks. The drums teacher tells that (on some days) he is excellent. First ranking and centum-scoring boys are plethoric individuals.

Kent's Repertory — SLEEP — UNREFRESHING.. GENERALITIES: PLETHORA—

'Sleep' is a general symptom and 'Un-refreshing sleep' is rare-strange-peculiar; good sleep should refresh any healthy person in the morning. The remedy *Phosphorus* alone is common in top-grade in both the above rubrics. This remedy is also found in Kent's Repertory under MIND — 'Answers, shortly, curtly' and 'Answers, refuses to'.

The remedy was read in *Materia Medica of Mind Symptoms* given at the end of this book and the following symptoms under Phosphorus agreed with the case;

Softening of brain.. slow in replies.. weakness..

Case 33: In some cases it is possible to treat a patient by letter. Such a letter from a patient is given below:

Respected Doctor,

I've been suffering from cold and bad throat for quite a long time now. It occurs during the change of season. I also have sinusitis which is hereditary (paternal uncle - Chacha).

I've a tendency of sneezing a lot early in the morning and also if there's dust around. My bowels do not get cleared properly and I feel constipated. I'm probably associating constipation with the lack of a proper eating and sleeping schedule as I'm in 12th std and unable to regulate it.

Also, I have a severe pain in the lower abdomen and lower back during the onset on menstrual cycle which lasts for the first 2 days. Managing it without a hot water bag is difficult. So I usually end up taking doses of DYSMIN (suggested by the physician) in accordance with the pain. The period of cycle is 5-7 days. Menstural cycle occurs every 28-30 days.

The problem of acne started not long back and it has gotten worse over the past few months. Pimples have also developed on the upper arms, shoulder blades as well as on the upper chest.

Regards.

Case Repertorisation: The following portions from the above letter are valuable for selecting the remedy:

"Change of season agg".

'Dust allergy'. (All allergies are syphilitic affections).

'Menses lasts 5-7 days' (Beyond 3 days is haemorrhage)

There are no 'mind' symptoms in this case. We must note here that in his *Lectures on Materia medica* Kent has said that in many remedies mind symptoms have not been fully brought out in proving. But equally valuable are 'general' symptoms. There are three generals in this case *viz.*

1. Syphilis (dust allergy; more than one person in the family has sinusitis).
2. Haemorrhage
3. Change of weather agg.

Haemorrhage—wherever found in any case should be considered first. Whether it is gum bleeding or uterus haemorrhage or bleeding piles, do not look for Metrorrhagia etc. Dr. Kent has said that the best cures are made by working out cases on 'generals'. Therefore wherever may be the bleeding, go to the list of remedies against 'Haemorrhage' in the last chapter GENERALITIES in Kent's Repertory.

Kent's Repertory—GENERALITIES—HAEMORRAGE
28 remedies are in top-grade (Let us call this List 'A')
SYPHILIS—15 remedies in top grade (List 'B').
CHANGE OF WEATHER agg. (List 'C')
In the above three lists we do not find any remedy (remedies) in top-grade in all the three lists.

What is to be done? Let us, as an exercise, take the remedies found common to all the three lists irrespective of grades and compare and find out those remedies scoring more points. (Remedies in bold type - 3 points, italics - 2 points, ordinary type - 1 point)

Remedy name	Haemorr-hage	Syphilis	Change of weather agg.	Total scores
Ars.	2	2	1	5
Lach	3	2	2	7
Merc.	3	3	1	7
Nit-ac.	3	3	1	7
Ph-ac.	2	2	2	6
Phos.	3	2	3	8
Sil.	2	3	3	8
Sul.	3	2	2	7

A beginner would rush to say that we should select either *Phosphorus* or *Silicea*. That is what the so-called authors on repertorisation are teaching.

The correct method is something different. You must arrange the valuable symptoms (be it mind or general or uncommon) *in order of their grade or importance*. See the table above. We have arranged the three symptoms from left to right in order of their importance or grade. Life threatening symptoms are of the highest value. So also, haemorrhage. Next comes broad general *Syphilis*. 'Change of weather' is only a modality (though a general) comes last in the order of importance.

Now, how to make use of the table? Do not merely add-up the points. You write the number (of scores) one after the other. Look at the remedy *Ars*. Do not add $2 + 2 + 1 = 5$, but it should be read as 221 (Two hundred and twenty-one). If this is done for all the remedies we get as under.

Ars. — 221 Lach. — 322 Merc. — 331

Nit. ac. 331 Ph-ac. — 222 Phos. — 323

Sil — 233 Sul. — 322

If you merely add all the three digits, together, of course, Phosphrous and Silicea gets 8 each. But if you look at the above, you find that Merc., and Nit-ac. get 331, each (Three hundred and thirty-one) whereas Phos. is 323 (Three hundred and twenty-three only).

So we must consider Merc. and Nit-ac. only. Under Nit-ac. in the chapter DYSPEPSIA (Lilienthal) we find the following:

Intestinal dyspepsia due to syphilitic cachexia. Again, in Lilienthal under MENSTRUATION, in Nit-ac. We find the following:

Pains in hypogastrium and sides.

In Boericke's Materia Medica under Nit-ac. we find the following.

Excessive physical heritability (dust allergy).. Cachexia due to syphilis.

Nit-ac. 10M, one single dose cured her.

Note: In any case if there is haemorrhage you must give top-priority to it. Wherever may be the bleeding, you should not go to the chapter for the part affected, but you must take the top-grade remedies under HAEMORRHAGE.

Case 34: A patient came in with pain in the femoral part of urethra and backache. It was worse while riding the two-wheeler. He showed his medical file (given by allopathic hospital) and therefrom we noted the following points:
1. hydroureteronephrosis—Left kidney;
2. pain in femoral part of urethra,
3. pain in sacral region.

His complaint (pathology) is in ureter but he has pain in femoral part of urethra and sacrum. This is something rare-strange-peculiar. Both these painful places are at the same distance from the seat of affection—ureter.

Under the remedy Belladonna (Wilkinson's Materia Medica) we find the following: "Inflammation of internal organs... The inflammation... runs in radii as it extends to adjacent parts".

(Femoral part of urethra and sacrum are more or less at equal distance from his left ureter). Belladonna-10M, single dose, cured him.

Case 35: Two years after the above case, a lady came to me for cervical spondylitis. These patients get pain normally in the neck extending to head or one upper limb. Strangely this patient complained of unbearable pain in both shoulder tips. (Both shoulder tips are at the same distance away from the cervical vertebra). Belladonna-10M, single dose cured her.

Case 36: Let us now examine what uncommon symptoms mean: Some of the most useful uncommon physical symptoms *cannot be classified* under any head in the repertory or homoeo software and so it is better to memorise them.

For example, under the remedy *Ignatia* we find the words *great contradictions*. (Boericke Materia Medica) A haemorrhoid patient said at the end of the consultation: [Remember, in most cases, after the narration is over and after a pause, the patient leans forward towards you and with wide open eyes (exclaims)]

"Doctor... one thing. Everyone says that pain, bleeding etc. in piles would increase while straining when constipated; but my case is different. I do not get pain or bleeding whenever I strain during constipation. But during loose bowel movement I get both burning and bleeding".

The contradictory symptom is both ways. Hence Dr. William Boericke writes in plural: "Great contradictions". *Ignatia-1M,* single dose cured this patient.

Case 37: A school boy of twelve was brought by the parents. The mother started talking: "Doctor, he has to leave the house for school at 9.30 in the morning. He gets up at 6.00 a.m. By 7.30 a.m. he becomes so restless—jumps, cries etc. This would **last for half-an-hour. Then this disappears; it is followed by 3-4 times loose bowel movement.** After that he becomes completely all right and goes to school". In this case the following should come to our mind: "Symptoms disposed to appear periodically and in groups.".

The above lines are found in the remedy *Cuprum met.* (Boericke's Materia Medica). This remedy cured the patient in one single dose in the 200th potency.

Among pharmacologically-oriented system of therapeutics homoeopathy is thorough, exhaustive and accurate.

Some of the uncommon-rare-strange-peculiar symptoms cannot be classified under any rubric and therefore, the reader would do well by learning them by note as the following cases 38 and 39 would show.

Case 38: A patient consulted me for constipation. Laxatives and purgatives were said to be of no use. He further said that for several years he had been taking daily anticonvulsant drug for epilepsy and if he stops it, he would get convulsions.

The following symptom under the remedy *Opium* (in Wilkinson's Materia Medica) agrees with this case: "...Increased excitability and action in voluntary muscles, with diminution of it in involuntary muscles..."

When the intestine is full with faeces, urge is not felt (involuntary muscles). In the instant case these muscles are not functioning. Movement of limbs is controlled by voluntary muscles and he gets convulsions in them (increased irritability and action).

Opium-10M, given in one single dose, cured his constipation and he was asked to stop anticonvulsant drugs; he did so and to his surprise convulsions did not appear.

Case 39: A patient showed his right leg with ulcer. He got injury a few months earlier but so far it did not heal in spite of best medical treatment. After a pause, the patient continued, "Doctor, ever since the accident I feel numbness in my right upper arm and I am unable to use it freely. Has this non-healing of wound in my leg anything to do with numbness in my arm? But my arm was not hurt in the accident".

We say that homoeopathy is a system of medicine where the patient tells or indicates the remedy to us. In Wilkinson's Materia Medica the following sentence under the remedy *Pulsatilla* agrees with this case: ... *depression of vital power on one side and increased irritability on the other; Pulsatilla-10M,* one single dose, cured both the ulcer on the leg and numbness in the arm.

Case 40: While I was sitting in the clinic of a homoeopath a certain patient walked in and complaining of terrible itching he removed his shirt and started rolling on the floor scratching the itching places on the floor. The doctor told me that every time the patient behaved like this and he tried Psorinum, Sulphur, Graphites and even high potencies failed.

No skin patient would behave like the above patient to demonstrate the violent itching. The word 'unreasonable' fitted in well with this case. I asked the doctor to give one single dose of

Amm-carb. and in five minutes the itching came down and in the next week it was complete cure. Therefore, you may take a note of this: When a skin patient does not find relief anywhere all over the world and if his behaviour or attitude is 'unreasonable' you can be sure of curing him with one single dose of Amm-carb.

Case 41: Lady, forty-five, around menopause. For a year she had been under my treatment for burnt hands. Once I was asked to visit this patient. She was in bed and her daughter told me that her mother was having excess bleeding from uterus. When I entered the house, the patient asked the daughter (in this case the attendant of the patient) to get out of the room; after she left, the patient asked me in an irritable tone, "I have profuse and excess bleeding (menses). Is it because of the remedies (that you have given me) that caused this bleeding?"

I recalled that she never talked before in such a harsh tone.

Kent's Repertory — IRRITABILITY: several remedies.

I read the remedies listed under "HAEMORRHAGE FROM UTERUS" (Lilienthal). In the remedy Chamomilla I found among other symptoms the word 'irascibility'. Again in the chapter "MENSTRUATION AND ITS AILMENTS" under the remedy Chamomilla I found the following:

"... great irritability and crossness all the time, though unnatural to her when well".

Chamomilla-10M single dose arrested the excess bleeding and also she calmed down. When I saw her a month later, lot of improvement in the burnt areas in her body.

When patient is irritable, cross and unmanageable, and there is not much of other valuable (uncommon, rare-strange-peculiar) symptom the two remedies which should come to our mind are Chamomilla and Nux-vom.

One important note: In Nux-vomica the picture is slightly different. Chamomilla patient shows crossness in words; Nux-v. patient in action.

Case 42: Long ago a patient went abroad to consult a popular homoeopath. That doctor was about to leave his clinic after a day's hectic practice. When this patient entered and started telling his symptom, the doctor asked his assistant to give the patient Nux-vomica. The patient, having come from abroad, took the doctor by his collar and said, "I have come such a long way not to get snap-shot prescribing. I learnt that you take down the symptoms of patient, then work out the case. Do it in my case also".

The doctor sat down, took his symptoms, worked out the case and Nux-vomica came out.

Case 43: A patient consulted me for impotency. I noted down the case. After he finished talking, I told him that I would give him remedies for one month. At that point he got up and said in a snappish manner, "I read in your books that you cure patients completely with one dose. I want you to do that". To this I replied that it is possible in some cases, but his case requires many remedies. He took away the case sheet from my table and went away saying "In that case I don't want your treatment".

Sometimes you get the symptom after you have prescribed! I phoned up the doctor who referred that patient to me to give him Nux-vom.

The attitude of the above said two Nux-vom. patients is aptly described by Boericke in his Materia Medica in the preamble.

"Fiery, zealous temperament".

CASE 44: Ms. Ponnulaxmi, 69 years, reports: "Doctor I have pain in back and hips... cannot walk even up to bus stand from home... I have to engage an auto for this..."

After noting down the date, I ask her name and age and write down this on the case sheet.

To make her talk, I ask a general question. "How long you are having this pain?" She replies, "Doctor, it is not even pain, more of stiffness. I have this for nineteen years". I ask her about the date of menopause and she replies, "Doctor, it stopped around the 50th year and only after this I developed this pain and stiffness".

I just look over the case sheet. Her complaints started immediately after menopause. For complaints around menopause, before complete cessation of menses, you may go to the rubric Menopause under the chapter Female in Kent's Repertory. But for long lasting complaints that dates back to menopause the rubric that you should take, is as follows:

Checked discharges: (Suppression of Secretions)

—Suppression of haemorrhage or abandoning habitual depletions: 1, Acon., Bell., Chin., Ferr-m., Nux-v., Puls., Sulph.; 2, Arn., Aur., Bry., Calc., Carb-v., Graph., Hyos., Lyc., Natr-m., Nitr-ac., Phos., Ran., Rhus, Seneg., Sep., Sil., Spong., Stram. (See Lilienthal p. 1006)

While I was looking at the above list, I was considering whether I can take the rubric 'old people' (Under Generalities in Kent's Repertory). At this time she continues, "Doctor... one thing... I have constipation... ineffectual urging and it is incomplete... Also I get the urge to pass urine quickly but if I go and sit I am not able to pass completely. If the bowel movements and urination is free, on those days I am free from the pain and stiffness. So, at least, give me medicine for my bowel movement and scanty urination.

Checking the habitual secretions (stool and urine) also aggravates her condition of back pain and stiffness. For this too, the above rubric is indicated.

She continues, "Doctor, because of pain I do not get good sleep... it is much disturbed".

Kent's Repertory: Sleepless: I check what all top-grade remedies under Sleeplessness (in Kent) are also found in the list of remedies given against "Suppression of haemorrhage or abandoning habitual depletions". They are as under:

Bell., Bry., Chin., Hyos., Nux-v., Phos., Puls., Sep., Sil., Sul.

To confirm one out of the above ten remedies, I read them in Lilienthal under Rheumatism. The following words found under Phosphorus made me to select this remedy for the patient.

"Rheumatic stiffness,... especially when coming on in old age;

back pains... impending all motion; stiffness of knees..."

The reader may easily recall that the patient said that it was more of stiffness and because of this she could not walk even one furlong and has to sit down.

Phosphorus-1M single dose gave lot of relief. Patient is still under treatment. I read Phosphorus in Wilkinson's Mat. Medica and the first sentence was Emaciation; extreme, rapid; is reduced almost to a skeleton. I looked once again at the patient and found this description exactly fitting her!

Case 45: Letter from Dr. X., 33 years, is given below.

"Respected sir, This is Dr. ... These are the following things all my complaints.

1. Loss of libido (lack of sexual desire). Since 1 year, my U.T.A. and stricture problem started. My sexual life very limited. Now we are trying for kids. But I am not much active sexual life. Please do the needful.

2. Three months ago suffered with severe cough. That I had pneumonia patch in right midzone (of lung). No cough

subsided but on an off pain is coming right posterior chest wall where pneumonia patch was there previously.
3. Hypertension. My blood pressure sometime touching 150/100. If I take twice (BP tablet) daily dose. Then it will be controlled.
4. Overweight. I observed I am putting more weight. My food intake also seems increased. I am fond of sweets and junk food. My present weight is 118 kg. Please do the needful".

Let us know how to work out this case. We are going to learn something new and unique out of this case. Every case is, of course, unique. There is difference between a symptom-coverer and a true homoeopathic physician. Any average practitioner would work out this case on the following symptoms:

❖ Impotency
❖ Hypertension
❖ Obesity

What a patient tells is just and mere cotton. No one can wear cotton as such. We have to make thread out of cotton, then weave cloth with the thread; and stitch a shirt out of that cloth. Then only, it is ready for wearing. So also, out of the symptoms told by the patient we have to conceive and derive many things. In the above case, the practitioner must work out the case as under:

The age of the patient is 33.

Point No. 1: He has (a) impotency, and (b) hypertension. These two symptoms, put together, should be viewed from a different angle. These two normally appears in old age, *i.e.* above sixty years of age. But we find this in a person of 33 years. Therefore, the term *pre-senility* should at once come to our mind.

Point No. 2: He is already an allopathic doctor and the medicines he had taken fail to bring down the blood pressure. Therefore, the term 'lack of reaction' should also come to our mind.

The above two symptoms are 'general symptoms'. Wherever possible we must always work out cases on 'general symptoms'. Craving for sweets, increased intake of food are secondary.

SAMUEL LILIENTHAL'S HOMOEOPATHIC THERAPEUTICS: Constitution, Age...(page 233-234) –For old people—aged persons get very fleshy: Kali-carb., Aur-met., Op., Sec., Amm-carb., Fluor-ac. (We take this because, though the patient is just 33 years old, he has pre-senility).

These six remedies were studied in *Boericke's Materia Medica*. Only the first para or preamble under various remedies are useful for confirming one out of the several remedies selected through the repertory:

The remedy *Ammonium carb.* was selected because of the following words found under that in Boericke Materia. Medica.

The diseased conditions met by this remedy are such as we find often in rather stout . . . have a slow reaction generally, . . . Mucous membranes of the respiratory organs are especially affected. Fat patients with weak heart . . .

HOW TO CONFIRM A REMEDY WITH BOERICKE.

If the remedy selected by you is correct—the similimum, then the symptom appears in the first sentence of that remedy in Boericke. Or, if the symptom appears in the subsequent sentences, it is either given in italics; or, it is preceded by an adjective or followed by an adverb.

Again, let us read Amm-carb. in the MATERIA MEDICA OF MIND SYMPTOMS on page 539; and there we find the following to further confirm our selection:

...makes frequent mistakes in speaking and writing; ... gloomy, depressed...(If the reader carefully reads the letter of the patient, he can notice the glaring grammatical mistakes made by the patient. For this reason alone we have reproduced his letter *in verbatim* without correcting the spelling and other mistakes).

Amm-carb. 10M, one single dose and placebo. Patient shows much progress and is under treatment.

Case 46: Letter from patient (Mrs. V. 30 years)

"I am under your treatment for persistent urinary tract infection problem. Before starting my treatment with you and before my most recent episode of urinary tract infection, I used to feel a kind of burning sensation/mild spasm every time my bladder filled up or when I had to urge to pass urine. This problem is considerably reduced now, but I still experience it sometimes. Also, earlier I used to feel burning sensation when I start passing urine and also towards the end. Now, I notice that the burning sensation at the end has reduced. But sometimes, I experience a sharp pain in my abdomen or lower back which goes away on its own after some 10-20 seconds.

"I got my monthly periods from 24th Sept. to 27th Sep. and even though the medicines have helped in controlling my problem, I felt that for some 3-4 days after my periods, the symptoms were aggravated.

"Kindly advise further medicines. Thanking you".

This case is very easy. No need to work with repertories. This case should at once bring to our mind the following:

"Rapid change of symptoms—pain change in regard to place and character...**Hepatic, and rheumatic affections, particularly with urinary, haemorrhoidal and menstrual complaints**".

The above symptoms are in the first para under the remedy *Berberis vulgaris*, in Boericke's Materia Medica. Berberis vul. 10M, one single dose cured the patient.

Section 4
Materia Medica

Materia medica of valuable and uncommon mind symptoms

Abrotanum—Great anxiety and depression, good-humored, happy or gloomy and desponding (abdominal); ill-natured, irritable and peevish, feels as if she would do something cruel; no humanity; indolence and aversion to physical exercise; head weak, can hardly hold it up; face wrinkled, old, pale.

Dementia; feebleness and dullness of mind; no capacity for thinking, as if all mental and bodily powers were gone; easily tired out by conversation or mental effort.

Aconite—Great fear and anxiety, with nervous excitability; agoraphobia, afraid to go out-doors, to cross the street, especially a narrow one, or to be in a crowd; anxiety and fear about recovery, predicts the day of death; afraid in the dark; remote effects of fright (Op., immediate effects); fainting, turns deathly pale when sitting up; suffocation with violent pains in stomach and scrobiculum; threatened abortion; amenorrhoea.

Great mental anxiety and physical tension; ailments from fright, anger, chagrin; gloomy, taciturn; afraid of a crowd or of crossing a busy street; fear of ghosts; apprehensive of the future and of approaching death; restless, agonizing tossing about; mental and bodily oversensitiveness; mood peevish, irritable, malicious; delirium, patient weeping and laughing alternately; music unbearable, makes her quite mad.

Annoyances which fret and worry, causing fear and anxiety, even after reproaches from trifling causes; congestions, palpitations, fever.

Fitful mood, changing from one thing to another, now full of mirth and in a few moments disposed to weep; ecstasy, inclined to be gay, to dance and sing, loquacity, speech hurried.

Vertigo on rising from a recumbent position; she dreads too much activity about her; complains much of her head; amenorrhoea during puberty; sharp, shooting pains in sexual organs, abdomen very sensitive.

Aethusa cyn.—Idiocy, in some cases alternating with furor; cannot retain any idea; hallucinations; good-natured forenoon, ill-humored and sad afternoon.

Agaricus—Dementia from mental palsy; cryptomania; fancy excited, makes verses, sings, talks, but does not answer questions; constant talking and laughing, considers himself immensely wealthy and happy (second stage of dementia paralytica); mischievous melancholy, trying to do injury or damage from inward restlessness and anxiety; confusion of head, cannot find the right words and wants to be let alone; frequently caused by mental overexcitement and worry; epilepsy.

Fearless frenzy, with intoxication, accompanied by bold, vindictive designs; menacing, mischievous rage, directing it even against herself, with great strength; shy mania; excess of fancy, ecstasy, prophecy, makes verses; very marked choreic twitchings; extraordinary heaviness and languor in the lower extremities, pain all along the spine, which in several spots is tender to touch; cyanosis; breath, flatus and stool foetid (sclerosis of the hemispheres of the brain).

Agnus castus—Sexual melancholia; atonic condition of sexual organs; hopelessness; patient thinks there is no use to do anything, as death is sure to come soon.

Puerperal insanity with suicidal tendencies, aversion to husband, babe and to all sexual intercourse, dissatisfied with herself and incapable of any mental or bodily exertion; absent-minded, cannot recollect things; anxious, fear and weakness.

Hysteria with maniacal lasciviousness; despairing sadness, peevish, inclined to be angry, sometimes on account of her sterility; nervous weakness; lethargy, frenzy; sleeplessness or starting up frightened in her sleep.

Ailanthus—Low-spirited, continued sighing, restlessness, confusion of ideas; electrical thrill, starting from the brain, running to the extremities; perfect indifference to what might happen.

Alcohol—Dementia paralytica; insanity of drunkards, weak and loitering gait, limp and uncertain movements of the whole body; tremulousness of lips and tongue, thickness and hesitancy of speech; uncertain expression of eyes; transcendent notions of wealth and power; tremors and muscular twitching; hemi-anaesthesia, paraplegia, amaurosis, epilepsy.

Aletris far.—Vertigo with vomiting; weariness of body and mind; sterility, amenorrhoea or delayed menses from uterine atony, abdomen distended, bearing down.

Aloe—Hypochondriasis, < in cloudy weather; hates and repels every one, life is a burden; dissatisfied and angry when he is constipated; diarrhoea and constipation alternating; haemorrhoids from suppressed chronic eruptions.

Alumina—Intolerable ennui; depressed and lachrymose; sad thoughts in the morning, feels joyless and comfortless in the morning on waking; dread of death, with thoughts of suicide; seeing blood on a knife, she has ideas of killing herself, though she abhors the thought; no desire to do anything, especially something serious.

Consciousness of his personal identity confused, apprehensive of losing his reason; evil ideas force themselves on him against his will; low spirits, trifling things appear insurmountable, desire to cut his throat, but fears death; time passes too slowly; variable mood, at one time confident, at another timid; peevish and whining, with heat in the earlobes, cannot retain his urine; mental symptoms < mornings when awaking; hypochondriasis.

Fear of losing his mind, of not recovering, of impending evils; anguish and vague uneasiness, as if he had committed a crime.

Full of apprehension and fear that he will go crazy; lassitude and indifference to labor or work; pain in back as if a hot iron were thrust into the spine.

Ambra gris.—Melancholy, sits for days weeping, with great weakness, loss of muscular power and pain in small of back; constipation, sadness; sleeplessness after business embarrassment; the presence of other people makes her feel worse; slow comprehension of old people, feel stupid.

Spasmodic twitching of facial muscles; choking and vomiting when hawking up phlegm; frequent micturition of pale, watery urine; sexual excitation and irritation of genitals; tendency to sanguinous flow on the least provocation during menstrual intervals; sensation of coldness in abdomen (*Aeth., Cist., Petr.*); frequent tenesmus, whatever be the character of the stool; nymphomania, often with discharge of bluish-white mucus; spasms and twitches in muscular parts; < evening and night, with anxious flushes of heat. Fear of getting crazy.

Ammonium carb.—Great anguish as if he had committed a crime; loathing of life; makes frequent mistakes in speaking and writing; ill-humored during wet stormy weather; great aversion to water, cannot bear to touch it; hearing others talk or talking himself affects him; gloomy, depressed, with sensation of coldness.

Great excitement of sexual organs; cholera-like symptoms at the beginning of catamenia; acrid leucorrhoea, with sensation of excoriation and ulceration in vulva; swelling, itching and burning of pudenda; listless and lethargy, talking affects her; headache as if head would burst; vehement palpitation of heart and great praecordial distress, followed by fainting, inclination to stretch limbs; hysteria with symptoms simulating organic affections.

Ammonium mur.—Despondency; grief or irritable peevishness of fat, bloated and lax persons who are indolent and sluggish; body often large and fat, while legs are too thin; consequence of grief.

Melancholy and anxious, as if laboring under some grief or sorrow; apprehensive and gloomy, like from internal grief; falling out of hair; very pale of face; ebullitions with anxiety and weakness, as if paralyzed; full of grief, but cannot weep; ill humor.

Anacardium occid.—Paralysis with imbecility; loss of will, cannot control the voluntary muscles; does not know his surroundings; weak memory; head falls forward, difficult to keep it up; utters only unintelligible words; drinks run out of his mouth; respiration free, pulse slow, moderately full; body cool.

Anacardium orient.—Everything appears as in a dream; excessive forgetfulness, even of recent events; fixed idea that mind and body are separated, that strange forms accompany him; a slight offense makes him very angry, curses and swears, breaks out into personal violence; want of moral feeling; depravity; ungodliness; inhumanity; feels as if he had two wills, one commanding to do what the other forbids; he is separated from the whole world; and having lost all confidence in himself he despairs of accomplishing anything. Melancholia after childbed.

Fearfulness about the future with presentment of approaching misfortune and supposition that he is surrounded by enemies; despair, with a silly, helpless state of mind and extremely sluggish, awkward movements; inaptitude for work; tendency towards suicide by shooting (*Ant.-crud.*), imagines he hears voices of people who are far away; fixed ideas and hallucinations; laughs at serious things and is serious in the presence of ludicrous things; want of moral and religious sentiment; cowardice and loss of will power, a slight offense makes him vehement, angry, malicious, wicked, cruel. Anthropophobia. Dementia of old people, with rapid loss of memory and mental vigor; mental fatigue and brain-fag from overexertion; syphilitic mental debility.

Melancholy and loss of memory in consequence of fright or mortification; he takes everything in bad part and becomes violent, uses profane language; continual babbling of nonsense.

A great deal of foolish talk and foolish imaginations; which makes him irritable and quarrelsome; acts stupidly and childish.

Anxious and hypochondriac, shuns people; fear of impending misfortune and paralysis, of approaching death; despairs of getting well; loss of all will-power.

Mental depression, he is silly and clumsy in his behaviour, desires to be alone; fear of the future; always hungry, > while eating, < after eating and in forenoon; constipation; piles.

Restlessness, must be in constant motion, use of profane language; great forgetfulness, itching and soreness of pudenda; constant desire to urinate, urine as clear as water.

Anantherum mur.—Idiotic monomania for doing the same thing and frequenting the same places; laughs and sings, and sheds tears just as easily; ungovernable jealousy (*Hyos., Lach.*); blunted intellect and loss of memory.

Antimonium crud.—Loathing of life, suicide by shooting; great sadness and weeping; moonstruck and ecstatic love, sentimental and distrustful; gastricismus.

Sorrowful and irritable, ecstasy and exalted love, with great anxiety about his fate; < when walking in moonlight; sexual desire and erections when getting warm in bed.

Anxious reflections about himself, his present and future fate, disposition to shoot himself in the night; continued state of exalted love and ecstatic longing for some ideal female; more in the fresh air than in the room. Satyriasis.

Antimonium tart.—Apathy and indifference, even death would be welcomed; hopeless and despondent, inclined to violence; children get angry, weep and cry.

Gaiety and fury; senseless frenzy, with inclination to suicide; mental lassitude and weakness of mind; timid restlessness; walks constantly about; contradiction between mind and will.

Apis-mel.l.—Irresistible desire to run and jump, has delusion that he cannot walk (*Helleb.*); full of jealousy, insanity from sexual causes in women with great irritability of temper (the widow's remedy); nymphomania; eccentric cheerfulness or despondency; fickle and inconsistent behaviour; great desire for milk, which relieves; pain, tenderness and dropsy of the ovaries, especially right one; scanty micturition; fear of death.

Fidgetiness, restlessness, excitability, ill-timed laughing, fickleness at work; girls are awkward, dropping things and then laughing in a silly way at their clumsiness; sexual desire increased and given to jealousy (*Hyos.*); pains in ovaries, < during coition. At the age of puberty hysteria during amenorrhoea, they are nervous and awkward from incoordination of muscles; flushes in face.

Jealousy with anger and desire to kill, torments others, running about, < in daytime (mostly women).

Fear of being poisoned; dread of death with sensation as if she would not be able to breathe again.

Argentum nit.—Loss of memory; lies with closed eyes, shunning light and conversation; he cannot find the right word, hence falters in speech; feels that all his undertakings must fail, is lost beyond hope for this world, is neglected and despised by his own family; all desire for labor lost; objects to whatever is proposed, he seems utterly bereft of all power of will; agoraphobia and hypochondriasis.

Sycosis; incompetent to undertake either mental or bodily exertion, with fixed delusions and illusions, fixes day of his death, when walking fears he will have a fit and die; awakens wife so that he can talk to somebody; always hurried, must walk very fast, afraid of being too late; suicidal sadness, but lacks courage; fear and excitement bring on diarrhoea (*Gels.*).

General appearance imbecile, talk very childish; does not work, as he thinks it will do him harm and that he is not able to stand it; thoughts of having an incurable disease drive him almost to despair; and sets the time when he will die; frequent turns of anxiety, is nervous, impulsive, must walk very fast, but has to stop, as he tires easily; always hurried in everything.

Patient hardly dare remain alone lest he harm himself; fears and anxiety compel him to move about; he fears to go upon a high bridge or lofty place lest he throw himself down (*Anac.*).

Arnica—Traumatic insanity, as after concussions of the brain; forgetful, absent-minded, thoughts wander from their objects and dwell on images and fancies; does not speak a word, spiteful and ill-tempered; indifferent and hopeless; great heat in head, body cool; awakes from heat and fears to sleep again.

Arsenicum—Profound exhaustion after long *wasting diseases;* physical disease and consequent exhaustion lead to self-mutilation and suicidal ideas; gloomy disposition of mind with religious apprehensions; attacks of anxiousness, especially at night, or in the evening in bed, obliging one to rise, with oppression and difficulty of breathing; anxiousness at the heart, with fainting and trembling; **conscientious scruples,** as if having offended everybody and could not be happy; dread of being alone; great dread of death and still inclination to commit suicide; sensation as if warm air were coursing up the spine into the head; burning neuralgia with agony and great restlessness, and this anxiety drives him from one place to another.

Insanity *due to physical disease and consequent exhaustion;* excessive anguish and *irresoluteness;* fear of ghosts, thieves, vermin and solitude, with desire to hide; hallucinations of smell of pitch and sulphur everywhere and anticipate consignment to sheol, and suicidal tendency especially by hanging; religious melancholia, hopelessness and despair; attacks of anxiety, driving him out of bed at night; restlessness, moves from place to place, wants to go from one bed to another; rage to mutilate himself or others. Chronic effects of food poisoning.

Dread of death when alone or going to bed; excessive anxiety and restlessness, < after midnight; great anxiety, jumps out of bed and hides himself; praecordial anguish with constriction, cold sweat, trembling, prostration.

Grieving after a faithless lover (*Calc-phos., Hyosc., Ign., Phosac.*): talks wildly, weeps and whines; impatient and restless.

Hysterical asthma at every little excitement; screaming from pains, < after midnight; she cannot lie down for fear of suffocation, wants some water every few minutes; sudden arrest of breathing when walking against the wind.

Mental derangement, averse to meeting acquaintances, imagines he formerly offended them, though he knows not how; sad, tearful, anxious mood; exhaustion from slightest exertion.

Asafoetida—Anxious sadness and apprehension of dying, is afraid to be alone; unsteady and fickle, cannot persevere in anything, wants one thing and then another; walks from one place to another; physical and mental oversensitiveness; globus hystericus, nymphomania.

Hysteria, the direct sequel of the checking of habitual discharges, after abuse of mercury, after the stoppage of an habitual expectoration with oppression of the chest (*Amm.*); globus hystericus, flatus accumulates in abdomen and pressing up against the lung causes oppression of chest; reverse peristaltic action in oesophagus and intestines with sensation as if a ball started in stomach and rose into throat, provoked by overeating, motion or by anything which excites the nerves; belching of wind of strong rancid taste; food when partially swallowed returns by the mouth; greasy taste in mouth with dryness and burning; flatus passes upward, none downward; nervous palpitation, pulse small, breathing hardly affected; > in fresh air.

Asterias rubens—Hystero-epilepsy, full of hallucinations; very emotional, cannot bear contradiction, pale face; great epigastric tenderness; debility; convulsive motions of limbs, froth at mouth, shocks through extremities; great excitement of venereal appetite; fear of impending misfortune; relief from tears.

Aurum fol.—Ailments from fright, anger, contradiction, mortification or vexation, with dread, fear and quarrelsome disposition; anxious palpitations and desire to commit suicide; mental labor fatigues; fear of thieves (*Con., Ign.*).

Aurum met.—Woefulness and dejection, with longing for solitude; solicitude in regard to the loss of love and respect of others, with deep grief and weeping; religious solicitude, with weeping and praying, has no confidence in himself; great longing for death, as he thinks himself unsuited in this world, weeps in the evening and wishes to die; feels hateful and quarrelsome, without hope; staring, dreary look; wavering, uncertain gait; insomnia, when he falls asleep, erotic dreams, erections and emissions; in the morning offensive breath, reddish tongue and copious salivation; loss of taste, diarrhoea and constipation alternate; rush of blood to head, roaring in ears; motes and sparks before eyes; all symptoms > in fresh air. Hepatic and testicular (atrophy) disorders, syphilo-mercurialism; spasmodic asthma; climaxis; puerperal melancholia.

Ailments from fright, anger, contradiction, mortification or vexation, with dread, fear and quarrelsome disposition;

anxious palpitations and desire to commit suicide; mental labor fatigues; fear of thieves (*Con., Ign.*).

Suicidal ideas and insanity from depressing emotional troubles; religious mania from hepatic disorders; syphilitic or syphilomercurial hypochondriasis; with quiet demeanor he is in a sly (sly = skilful) way persistent on suicide; hallucinations of sight; from mortification and vexation, with dread, fear, reserved displeasure or vehemence; religious anguish and longing for death, being unfit for this and the other world, though he prays all the time; has no confidence in himself and thinks others have none, and still disposed to grumble and to be quarrelsome, cannot bear sympathy or contradiction; restless sleep, broken by frightful dreams; often asks questions, jumping from one thing to another, without waiting for a reply. Rush of blood to head, palpitations, pollutions, otherwise patient in fair physical health, and > in fresh air and out-door exercise.

Looks at the dark side, weeps, prays and considers herself unfit for the world; desire for solitude; ailments from grief, disappointed love; anxious palpitations.

Great anguish, coming from praecordial region, driving him from place to place; has no confidence in himself and thinks others have none; deep tearing headache, abating in the fresh air; oversensitiveness of the senses; immoderate appetite and thirst for milk, wine, coffee; aversion to meat; palpitation.

Great restlessness, dread of death, whining mood; painful, anxious state of mind; inability to reflect, with headache after making the least mental exertion, as if the brain were dashed to pieces; quarrelsome disposition; suicidal tendency; poor digestion, < after eating, after wine; hypochondriasis in pining, low-spirited boys, whose testicles are mere pendent shreds, on the verge of atrophy, or from hepatic or syphilitic disorders.

Remarkable changeability of mind; impulsive, rash, merry; sad and anxious, longing for death after a merry laugh; pressing in eyes as from acrid dust; fine eruptions on lips, face, forehead; palpitations; afraid to open a window.

Unhappy love; disposed to weep; desires to take his life; despair; sudden anger; quarrelsome or melancholy, with longing for death; alternately joyful or sorrowful; congestion of blood to the head; sparks before the eyes; rushing in the ears; putrid odor from the mouth; excessive hunger and thirst; congestion of blood to the chest and anxious beating of the heart.

Baptisia—Melancholia attonita, mental fag; stupor with profound and rapid physical degeneration, often delusion that their bodies are scattered and that they cannot hold them together; uneasy, gloomy, cast down, head feels very heavy; perfect indifference, does not care to do anything, inability to fix the mind to anything, weak mind, want of power to think.

Melancholia cum stupor; mentally restless, but too lifeless to move; indisposed to give vent to his thoughts, want of power and perfect indifference to do anything, inability to fix the mind on any work; mind wanders as soon as his eyes are closed: marked changes of the vital fluids; degeneration of tissues; high temperature; anxious, frightened look; foul breath; dry, parched tongue; head heavy as if he could not sit up.

Baryta carb.—Senile dementia, mental and physical debility; mental weakness and timidity of dwarfish children with undeveloped brain, who learn with difficulty because they cannot remember; forgetful, in the midst of a speech the most familiar words fail him; loss of memory, especially for recent events, groaning and murmuring, pusillanimous; peculiar dread of men, imagines she is laughed at, which frightens her; full of anxiety and evil forebodings about the most trivial affairs; no self-confidence, fears to undertake anything; full of delusions, thinks his legs are cut off, and that he walks on his knees; aversion to strangers, fear of and in the presence of others.

Perfect irresoluteness; all self-confidence has disappeared; angry on account of trifles, when he may even commit crimes; sudden, excessive, but transient burst of anger.

Baryta mur.—Mania with increased sexual desire, dejection and dread of men; nymphomania from uterine and ovarian disorders, even in idiotic women.

Belladonna—Dejected and discouraged; disgust of life, < in open air, with inclination to drown himself; continual moaning and sighing, even during sleep, and restlessness drives him out of bed; anxiety and great anxiousness, < evening, headache, red face, bitter taste, sweat and longing for death; dread and tendency to start easily, with mistrust and tearfulness; solicitude about sudden death, of putrifying while yet alive, of being poisoned and everlastingly damned; suicidal tendencies in patients suffering from acute violent alcoholism; persistent insomnia, leaving the mind extremely dull, stupid, slow to act, indifferent and pathetic; nothing produces an impression.

Patient wishes others to destroy him, will beg physicians and attendants to do so, hence suicide by drowning; he will sit quietly and break pins, paper, etc., between his fingers into very short pieces; disinclination to talk or very fast talking; mania, at one time merry, again would spit and bite at those around him; froth and foam at the mouth; burning thirst, but aversion to drink on account of difficult deglutition (*Lyssa.*); sees ghosts, animals, insects and hideous faces; is afraid of imagining things and tries to hide himself; memory lively, remembers things long gone by; foolish gesticulations, wild eyes, with fixed furious look, starting and twitching; very excitable mood; drinks hastily, tears his breast to work off his overexcited nervous state; worse at midnight, and at 3 p.m.

Derangement of the will faculty; amorous mania, with sexual excitement; senseless talk, with staring, protruding eyes; merry craziness; gives offense without any cause; wants to touch every one and everything; foolish gesticulations; irritable, curses horribly, wants to strike and bite; wants to drown himself, or that somebody else should kill him; despondency and indifference.

Hysteria with melancholic mood, starts in affright at the approach of others; weeping, irritable mood; excessive nervous excitability, with exalted sensibility, the least noise, the least light is annoying; headache with dizziness, < when stooping, when leaning forward, > when bending backward; nymphomania, mania puerperalis; aversion to work, cannot stay long in one position, too restless.

Long-remaining anxiousness; talks confusedly as if insane; tries to escape from imaginary phantoms, wishes to hide himself; aversion to noise and company; pain going through neck up into head; face burning hot or pale and moist.

Oversensitiveness of mind and body; weeping and vexation about trifles, with headache and pressure in forehead, and great dryness of mouth; sleepless and restless.

Berberis—Everything looks twice its natural size (*Plat.*, everything looks small); melancholy and inclination to weep; mental labor very difficult, the least interruption breaks the chain of thoughts; hepatic and arthritic complaints, affections of urinary organs, menstrual derangements.

Bismuth—Anguish, at times he sits, then walks, then lies down, never long in one place, he is morose and discontented with his condition and complains about it; solitude is unbearable; pressure like a load in the stomach; great debility, languor, prostration; restless, unrefreshing sleep.

Desire for company, solitude is unbearable; anguish, cannot remain long in one place; headache, < in winter season; gastric troubles with languor and prostration.

Great fears and forgetfulness when alone.

Borax—Infant at the breast, starts when anyone clears his throat or sneezes; dread of any downward motion; fright, he starts in all his limbs on hearing an anxious cry; excessive fear of thunder.

Bovista—Sensation as if the head were enormously increased in size; great irritability; everything affects him unpleasantly; awkward, lets everything drop; tired of life in the morning, pleasant in the evening.

Bromium—Great despondency, looks constantly in one direction without saying anything; she does not feel as she generally does, and does not know why; fullness in head and chest; much pain in left hypogastric and iliac regions, especially before menses; carcinoma mammae; swelling of testicles.

Constriction of chest; anxious feeling about heart; aversion to work, even to reading; does not feel or act like herself; great despondency; fulness in head and chest, with difficult respiration and a queer feeling all over, which makes her despondent.

Bryonia—Great depression and anxiety, with fright, fear and apprehension of future trouble and misfortune; irritability, weeping and moroseness; mental exhaustion and confusion of mind; sticking, jerking, throbbing headache; marked inactivity of liver or rheumatic diathesis.

Melancholy, with fear for the future in his domestic or business affairs, even at night he dreams of business; great depression and morose mood, perhaps from some hepatic affection; irritable mood, wishes to be left alone, has no desire to move, although he feels better out-doors; great forgetfulness.

Bad effects from mortification, violence and anger; morose, everything puts him out of humor; after getting angry, chilly or a red face and heat in head.

Peevish and fretful, apprehensive in the room, > in fresh air; fear of death, which he thinks is near; vertigo and confusion of head on slightest motion, < after a meal, when stooping; offensive breath; desire for unusual things; slow digestion, constipation.

Uneasiness and dread on account of the future, < in room, > in fresh air; fears not to have wherewithal to live; despair of recovery; anxious, peevish and hasty disposition.

Cactus grand.—Melancholia, particularly in women, with sensation of stricture around heart; unconquerable sadness, fear of death (*Acon.*); cries without cause, but < from sympathy; often awakes in a fright, but cannot tell the cause of alarm.

Great and unconquerable sadness; hypochondria and melancholy; irresistible desire to weep, does not like to talk; constant and great fear of death; irritable, wants people to keep their consolations for themselves; frequent palpitations of the heart, with a corresponding palpitation, so to speak, in the top of the head.

Hysteralgia, sadness, crying without reason, consolation aggravates; love of solitude; fear of death; constriction of uterus; whole body feels as if caged in wires, pains everywhere, darting, springing like chain lightning, terminating with a sharp, viselike grip, only to commence again a moment afterwards, with restlessness and groaning; menses with most horrible pains, causing her to cry aloud and weep; constrictive sensation around heart and uterine region, < from least touch; pulsating pains in uterus and ovaries.

Calcarea arsen.—Mind much depressed with great anxiety about still greater evils in the future; the slightest emotion causes palpitation of heart (*Lith.*); dull, stupefying headache in different parts of head, but especially above and behind ears; desire for wine and liquors.

Calcarea carb.—Insanity of drunkards, from repulsion of skin diseases; great emaciation or obesity; anxious, timid, full of fear, cannot bear to be alone in the dark, < at twilight and during night, delusions of murder, hallucinations of fire, rats and mice; fear of losing reason or that people would observe her confusion of mind; apprehensive mood of some impending misfortune, and every emotional excitement causes anxious perspiration, especially nocturnal sweat about the head and flying heat through body; ill-humor, obstinacy, restlessness, trembling of limbs; is fearfully affected by tales of cruelty, causing nightmare; < by close application of mind and in the evening, easily chilled and takes cold easily.

Malnutrition and malassimilation; fears she will lose her reason and people will observe her mental confusion; feeling of oppression, with heaviness of legs, trembling of body and frequent weeping, < evening and when admonished; grief and complaining about old offences, dread of solitude which is unbearable; dread of being seized by misfortune, on account of her ruined health; loathing of work, with irritability; great tendency to be frightened, the least noise, the most trifling unexpected occurrence fatigues and causes trouble; does not like to talk.

Many spasms during the day; depression and melancholy, with anguish and palpitations, < as evening approaches; icy coldness in and on head, one-sided; stupefying headache; twitching and trembling of body; cold, damp feet; cannot go to sleep, her mind turning on the same thought all the time; hysterical spasms from nervous excitement, sudden arrest of breathing when walking against the wind; nymphomania, violent itching and soreness of pudenda; sterility.

Fears those about her perceive her distraction of mind; concerns herself about imaginary things which might happen to her; apprehension about present and future, < as evening comes on.

Lowness of spirits, with disposition to weep; paroxysms of anguish, with orgasmus sanguinis, palpitation of the heart; shocks in the region of the heart; despair about one's health; apprehensions of illness, misfortune, infectious diseases, insanity, etc.; dread of death; excessive sensitiveness of all the organs of sense; malaise, aversion to work, inability to think or to perform any mental labor, etc. Compare *Sulph.*

Calcarea fluor.—Great depression of spirit, avarice, feeling of anxiety about money, thinks he will come to want; sharp, lancinating pains in hepatic region, < when lying on painful side or sitting, > walking; bleeding piles.

Unusual tendency to look at the dark side of everything; feeling of unnecessary anxiety about everything; disposition to set a higher value on money than natural to him; avarice (*Lyc.*), thinks he will come to want or would soon be running financially behind hand.

Calcarea phos.—Dementia in young persons or in masturbators; total loss of memory, writes wrong words; wishes to be at home, and when there, wants to go out, from place to place; does not want to do what he has to do; easily frightened and depressed.

Ailments from grief and disappointed love; depressed after vexation.

Camphora—Puerperal rage, uses indecent language, strikes and bites; always in haste, strips herself and wants to jump out of the window; dread of being alone in the dark; lochia suppressed with erethism of sexual system, followed by exhaustion and collapse; < at night, from motion and from cold.

Mania to dispute; acts and talks too hastily; feels insulted about everything; oversensitiveness; food has a strong taste; all objects appear bright and shining; amorous desires, with weakness of the sexual organs.

Cannabis ind.—Hallucinations and imaginations constantly changing; great exhaltation of mind, at times with enthusiastic language; full of fun and mischief; incoherent talking, very absent-minded; laughs indiscriminately at every word; inability to recall any thought or event on account of different thoughts crowding his mind; exaggeration of the duration of time and extent of space; horror of darkness, great anguish and despair; moaning and crying; great fear of approaching death, or of becoming insane; voices, including her own, seem to come from a distance; forgets when speaking what she is going to say; feels at times as if she were somebody else; seems to be in a dream, as if things were not real; puerperal mania, with visions and phantoms which do not frighten her.

Overestimation of time and space; nervous depression and distressing fear of an imaginary character, amounting nearly to hallucinations and illusions, from overworking a delicate nervous organization; horror of darkness, moaning and crying; anguish, with great oppression, > in fresh air.

Exaltation of spirits, with great gaiety and disposition to laugh at the merest trifle, is full of fun and mischief; excessive loquacity; pleasant hallucination of sight and hearing; a perfect horror of darkness; constant fear to become insane.

Great restlessness, obliging him to move constantly; uneasiness day and night, with hot head; strange ideas crowd on him against his will; noisy, insolent and contradicting; unbounded frantic sexual desire.

Cantharis—Hallucinations, especially at night; delirium of people long dead; fits of rage, with crying, barking and striking, renewed by the sight of bright, dazzling objects; worse when touching the larynx, or when trying to drink water; amorous frenzy; intense erethism of sexual organs, impelling him to seek immediate physical gratification; masturbation; scanty urine or frequent micturition; strangury.

Soreness in throat on waking, with relief after expectoration of a little reddish mucus; previous to the hysterical attack partial or total suppression of urine, followed afterwards by copious micturition, urine deficient in urates; more or less troublesome irritation of the mucous membrane of the genitals; burning in soles of feet.

Capsicum—Homesickness, with a disposition to suicide, with redness of cheeks, sleeplessness; he is taciturn, peevish and restless, easily offended, takes everything in bad part; obstinacy; cloudiness of intellect; children become clumsy, awkward, even idiotic.

Whimsical and sensitive; frequent weeping; headache as if bursting when moving; redness of cheeks; heat in fauces; thirst and chilliness; disposed to take a deep breath; sleepy in daytime, sleepless at night; averse to moving and to fresh air; violent cough evenings and nights; haunted by a disposition to suicide in spite of his phlegmatic temperament; hectic fever, disposed to take a deep breath, short, hacking morning cough.

Carbo an.—Sorrowful feeling of dereliction, faintheartedness, desire for solitude, sad thoughts and great tearfulness; despair day and night; timidity and tendency to start.

Sorrowful feeling as if left alone, cannot be consoled; fearful in the dark; easily frightened and low-spirited, especially mornings.

Carbo-veg.—Indigestion and dyspepsia of drunkards, leading to confusion of the head; nightly fear of ghosts, stupor and finally dementia; indifference, hears everything without feeling pleasantly or unpleasantly about it; irritable and despondent, wants to blow his brains out; periodical want of memory with confusion of head; frightful hallucinations in the dark.

Anxiety causes him to tremble all over, as if he had committed a crime; feels oppressed, with heat of face, evenings after lying down, when awaking.

Caulophyllum—Melancholia following long-continued menstrual irregularities and uterine disorders; weakness of mind and memory; fretful and irritable; insomnia and restlessness during menses; tremulous weakness felt over entire body.

Menstrual and uterine epilepsy; hysterical convulsions during dysmenorrhoea; severe pain, by spells, in the temples, as if they would be crushed together; spasmodic intermittent pains in bladder, stomach, broad ligaments (*Groins*), even chest and limbs; profuse, slimy whites; moth spots on forehead; anaemia, general debility; exhaustion.

Causticum—Frightful hallucinations as soon as he closes his eyes; melancholy from care, grief and sorrow, she looks upon the dark side of everything; full of timorous fancies at twilight, child fears to go to bed alone; mental alienation after suppression of eruptions; great anxiety of conscience and at the heart, as if she had committed a bad action, or as if some misfortune impended; irritable and provoked at trifles; absence of mind, indolence, lassitude, great heat of skin, dryness of mouth and fauces; constipation. Chorea, epilepsy, hysteria; sensation as if there were an empty space between the brain and skull.

Mental ailments from long-lasting grief and sorrow; excessive sympathy for others, always afraid others might take harm, no desire for life on account of that constant dread and anxiety; timidity about the future or as if he had committed a crime; great sadness, with weeping on the slightest provocation; looks at the dark side of everything, especially before and during menstruation, which flows only in daytime, none at night; deep yellow complexion, sour sweat.

Anxious, uneasy mood, unfitting him for every work, feels worried about the heart; timorous anxiety and depression, child fears to go to bed alone, fear of death; anxiety after night-watching, cares and troubles.

Cannot keep her upper eyelids up; thinking of her troubles aggravates them, especially the piles, which are made almost intolerable by walking; enuresis nocturna; intolerable uneasiness in the limbs in the evening; cannot get a quiet position at night, or lie still a minute; jerking mostly on right side of body.

Mental and other ailments, chronic headache, neuralgia, chorea, from long-lasting grief and sorrow, pains < from mental exertion; taciturn and listless; hopeless; thinking of complaints aggravates them, especially haemorrhoids.

Cedron—Fits come on regularly twice a day, morning and evening at same hours; intense pain in forehead, bloated face with pupils much dilated; giddiness and falling down in convulsions, difficult breathing, irregular pulse and heart's action; fit lasts six to eight minutes, on recovering consciousness feels very weak and discharges a large quantity of watery urine; menstrual epileptoid convulsions; choreic attack after coition.

Chamomilla—A morbidly sensitive nervous system; melancholia, with constant moaning and muttering to herself; walks all the time, looking down; is disinclined to talk and angry if any one speaks to her, tries to get away from her friends if they seek to comfort her; sleepless at night and uneasy during the day.

Deeply-felt mortification, with irresistible, impatient, feverish mood; cross against others; faintness and prostration; bitter taste; hot, bilious diarrhoea.

Great anxiety, feels excited in all the senses; peevish, fretful.

Peevish disposition, nothing pleases; full of anxiety with great uteasiness; agonizing tossing about with tearing in abdomen; jerking and twitching in sleep; profuse menses smell offensive, with laborlike pains before and during the flow.

Chelidonium—Anxiety, allowing no rest at any employment, as if she had committed a crime; fear of getting crazy, with restlessness and heat; distaste for mental exertion or conversation; forgets what she wants to do or has done.

Horrible anguish by day and by night as if she had killed somebody; anxiety takes away all pleasure for her labor; pit of stomach and left hypochondrium sore to touch; no appetite or thirst; bitter taste; stools hard, whitish-yellow; often vertigo as if she would fall forward; flushes of heat in face; palpitation, with oppression in chest.

China—Fixed idea that he is unhappy, compelled to jump out of bed, wants to destroy himself but lacks courage; dislike to all mental or physical exertion; indifference, apathy, taciturnity, inclined to reproach and vex others; alternate condition of cheerfulness and gloominess; nervous irritation with slowness of ideas; hallucinations on closing eyes which disappear when eyes are opened.

Mental depression as a reflex of general lowered vitality; low-spirited, despondent and tired of life, with suicidal tendencies; great sensitiveness; easily moved to tears by the least contradiction; indifference and apathy with obstinate taciturnity; weakness and exhaustion after the least exertion, > in the evening and at night; nocturnal dread of dogs and other animals; desire for solitude.

Languor; mental dullness, or excessive sensitiveness of all the organs of sense; mental distress, discouragement, fixed idea that he is unhappy and persecuted by enemies; headache, or boring pain in the vertex; weak digestion, with distention of the abdomen, ill-humor, indolence after eating; sleeplessness on account of ideas crowding upon his mind, or rest-less, unrefreshing sleep, with anxious dreams, tormenting the patient even after he wakes, etc.

Chloralum—Violent hysterical fits, lies in a state resembling catalepsy; extraordinary depression of nervous system; heart's action feeble, pulse weak; sense of sinking and oppression at pit of stomach, cold limbs; slow breathing; great muscular prostration; sleeplessness; severe spasmodic pains in and about uterus.

Chloroformum—Neurosis of sexual organs, hysterical condition dependent on irritability and spasms of the cervix; sudden jerking and trembling of every muscle of the body, without waking him from sleep.

Cicuta—Anxious thoughts about the future, feels sad; excessively affected by sad stories; weeping, moaning and howling; fondness of solitude; great dislike to society; indifference and apathy; disposition to be frightened; mistrust and shunning of the male sex (*Bar-c.*).

Attacks of inability to collect his senses, with thoughtless, staring fixed look and vanishing of sight; indifference to everything, confounds the present with the past; everything about him appears strange and frightful; childish humor, in which he finds everything lovely and attractive like a toy; insane dancing, laughing and clapping of hands at night, with violent heat and redness of face; quiet disposition, contented, happy; easily affected by sad stories.

Crazy delirium; funny gesticulations, with redness of face and heat of body; confounds things of the present with those of the past; is afraid of society and wants to be alone. Epilepsy; after concussion of brain.

Great fearfulness whenever the door is opened and at every word, though not loudly spoken; she feels, from fright, shooting pains in left side of head; old men fear a long spell of sickness before dying; anxious thoughts of the future; is afraid of society, wants to be alone.

Hysterical spasms, she feels a blow deep in epigastrium, which passes like lightning up the back and forces her to throw herself backward in the midst of most tormenting pains; during intervals head falls back if she attempts to raise herself, with violent spasmodic pains; body and extremities hard as wood; great weakness and prostration after fit; complete sleeplessness or while asleep jerking, starting and biting tongue; periodical ecstacy; coccygodynia during menses.

Cimicifuga—Deep melancholy, with sleeplessness; a heavy black cloud has settled over her, so that all is darkness and confusion, while at the same time it weighs like lead upon her heart; perfect indifference; taciturnity; takes no interest in household affairs; sighs and moans and is suspicious of everybody; brain feels too large for the cranium, a pressing from within outward; sensation of enlargement of the eyeballs, which feel as if they would be pressed out of the orbits; foul breath; faintness and goneness in the epigastrium; prolapsus uteri; nervous exhaustion from the least exertion; chorea, puerperal melancholia.

Epileptic insanity; remarkable heat in the back of the head, extending down the back; sensation as if a heavy black cloud and settled all over her and enveloped her head, so that all was darkness and confusion, while at the same time it weighed like lead on her head; desire for solitude or to wander from place to place, answers questions hurriedly and evasively; frequent sighing; indifferent, taciturn, takes no interest in anything; fear of death and still suicidal mood; suspicious of everything, will not take her medicine; hysteria and melancholia, with frequent changes of heat and cold in different parts of the body; sleeplessness on account of frightful dreams leading to sudden starting up in sleep; great anxiety about one's self without knowing why; alternate empty and full feeling in head; nervous tremors, like a chill, without actually feeling cold; prickling in the fingers; small, quick irregular pulse, frequently icy-cold hands and feet; mental depression, amounting to even suicidal tendency; mania puerperalis; mania following disappearance of neuralgia; from business failure or disappointed love;

after abortion or confinement, after drunken sprees; dizzy when rising in the morning with pain over eyes; nausea and occasional vomiting; delirium tremens; insomnia, incessant talking with constant change of subject, must move about despite the intense prostration.

After going to bed jerking, commencing on side on which she is lying, compelling change of position; nervous shuddering and chills, feels as if top of head would fly (ther., as if she could lift it off); delirium with jumping from subject to subject, sees strange objects; great apprehensiveness; pains darting into the eyeballs, through to occiput; sleepless and restless; fear of death; uterine neuralgia, menses irregular, delayed or suppressed.

Cina—Optical illusions in bright colors, sees imaginary things, screams and talks hurriedly; easily offended from slightest joke; anguish about heart as if he had committed some evil deed, when walking in open air, chorea, epilepsy; < at night.

Cinnamum—Anxiety and oppression in cardiac region, causing constriction of chest; head severely affected with great stupor, < when talking; each attack subsides with eructations or vomiting, but soon returns; profound sleep and insensibility with each hysterical attack; anaemia and chlorosis from chronic uterine haemorrhages.

Clematis erect.—Ailments from homesickness or contrition of spirit; low-spirited and fear of approaching misfortune; fear of being alone, but disinclined to meet even agreeable company; great debility; vibratory sensation through the whole body, after lying down; uneasy sleep, dreaming and tossing about.

Coca—Melancholy from nervous exhaustion; bashful, timid, ill at ease in society; peevish; delights in solitude and obscurity.

Mental and physical lack of will to do anything; excessively phlegmatic and apathetic; slow in finding the words to express himself; mood changeable, mostly very morose; unbridled passion for brandy.

Cocculus—Suits especially bookworms and sensitive romantic girls, with irregular menstruation, also onanists, rakes and other debilitated persons; melancholy and sadness, with weeping and constant profound absorption in sorrowful thought; great apprehensive anxiety of conscience and at the heart as after committing a wicked deed, with propensity to escape; joylessness and discouragement; tearful chagrin about the least trifle; changeable humor, frequent lively contentment, talkativeness, with witty joking; spasms and convulsions, extreme weakness, even to fainting, worse from sleeping (*Lach.*), from wine, smoking, riding in a carriage; great dread of the cold open air; time passes too quickly (can.ind., time passes too slowly); ill effects of disappointed ambition, of anger and grief, indulges in sad reveries, is sensitive to slights, insults and disappointment.

Great sorrowfulness, with constant inclination to sit in a corner buried in thought, and to take no notice of anything about him; discontented with himself and still easily offended; great anxiousness as if he had committed a crime; confused feeling in the head, especially after eating and drinking; vertigo, with flushed hot head and face; seasickness; uterine spasms and dysmenorrhœa; excessive prostration, as if it were impossible to make any exertion.

Hyperaesthesia of all the senses, the least jar is painful, noise and light unbearable; choking constriction in the upper part of fauces, with difficult breathing and indisposition to cough; retarded menses, which finally appear, with great weakness and nausea, even to faintness; roaring in ears; great lassitude of whole body; hysteric complaints, with sadness; hysteric palsy; sudden spasms from non-appearance or sudden checking of menses; spasm < about midnight.

Coffea—Oversensitiveness of all the senses; crying, howling and getting beside himself; fainting.

Colchicum—Arthritic melancholia with suicidal thoughts; peevish and dissatisfied; want of memory.

Gouty diathesis; alternately excited or depressed; loss of memory; great desire for mental and bodily rest; intense melancholia, peevish and dissatisfied.

Fear of being unable to bear suffering; external impressions, light, noise, strong smells, contact, etc., disturb his temper.

Colocynthis—Absence of religious sentiments; apathy with lassitude, cannot bear the society of persons he is intimate with; laconic mode of expression; no disposition to talk; dissatisfied with everything; consequences from indignation and internal gnawing grief over his imaginary or real troubles.

Depressed and joyless, disposition to cry and weep, disinclined to talk, to answer and see friends; bad effects from anger and indignation.

Disposition to cry and weep; anger with indignation; extreme irritability; violent abdominal pains; diarrhoea and vomiting every time food is taken; pain in hips, extending from renal region down to upper part of thighs; cramps in calves; sleeplessness.

Conium— The great inhibitory remedy of the sexual passions; excessive nervous prostration, with vertigo when lying down and when turning over in bed; great concern about little things, and becomes easily excited; dreads being alone, and still avoids society; praecordial anguish; superstitious and full of fear, with frequent thoughts of death; loss of memory; alternate fits of silent depression and quarrelsome liveliness; mood serious; unsympathizing, from indolence and want of proper will-power; confused feeling in head, often sits lost in thought.

Senile dementia, ailments of old maids and widows from ungratified sexual desire; *folie circulaire,* alternate excitement and depression; cannot endure any kind of excitement, it brings on physical and mental depression, weakness; inability to sustain any mental effort, excessive difficulty to recollect things, especially dates; desire for solitude and unsympathizing insensibility from indolence; aversion to company and yet averse to being alone, is inclined to abuse company, scolds and will not bear contradiction; chilliness, frequent spasmodic motions; weak sexual power and frequent pollutions; anaemia of brain.

Hypochondriasis starting from sexual organs, often in connection with enforced abstinence from sexual intercourse; weakness with great sexual erethism, amatory thoughts occurring and even emissions by the mere presence of women; spermatorrhoea from long-lasting abuse of genital organs, face pale and sunken, with blue rings around eyes; dread of company, yet does not want to be alone.

Vertigo in a recumbent position; globus hystericus; during micturition her urine alternately flows and stops; the breasts swell, become hard and painful before the menses, when the hysterical symptoms increase, dislike to society and yet dreads to be alone; craves coffee, salt and sour things; aversion to bread.

Crocus sat—Extravagant ideas and great loquacity, jumping, dancing, laughing, whistling; very affectionate, wants to kiss everybody; witty, uncommon mirth and cheerfulness; alternation of excessive happiness, affectionate tenderness and great ill-humor and rage, quarrelsome mood with great repentance, great timidity, haemorrhages; sleepiness, great prostration, with dilated pupils and obstruction of sight; obstinate constipation, caused by stagnation in portal system.

Fearful, apprehensive sorrowfulness, even of a religious kind; is not fit to live; takes everything in anger and suddenly repents having injured others; restless, anxious, timid; gay extravagance and liveliness alternate with sorrowful dejection.

Hysteria, with excessive mirth and cheerfulness alternating with melancholia; childish follies; pleasant dementia, with paleness and headache; alternation of affectionate tenderness and rage; spasmodic jerking of single sets of muscles; vertigo in room, > in fresh air; music affects her (*Tarent.*).

Hysteria; excessive mirth and cheerfulness alternating with melancholy; immoderate laughter.

Crotalus cascavella.—Insomnia, great sadness; her thoughts dwell on death continually, especially when alone; dreams about the dead, when she falls asleep.

Crotalus horridus—Timidity, fear, anxiety; weeping or snappish temper, cross; irritable, infuriated by the least annoyance; sadness; her thoughts dwell on death continually; twitching and nervous agitation; lethargy, loss of co-ordination; incipient stage of senile dementia.

Incipient stage of senile dementia; mental delusions, such as mistakes in keeping accounts or writing letters, forgetfulness in figures, names and places; awaking at night struggling with imaginary foes; thinks he is the prey of enemies or of hideous animals; dislike to members of his own family; marked indifference and apathy, seems only half alive; fits of drowsiness or coma; apoplexy in broken-down constitutions or inebriates.

Croton tigl.—Melancholia attonita; feeling as if one cannot think outside of himself, feels all pent up inside and no chance for the thoughts to flow outside; feeling of anxiety as if some misfortune would befall him; morose, dissatisfied.

Cuprum. met.—Mania, with biting and tearing things to pieces; insane foolish gestures of imitation and mimicry; full of insane spiteful tricks, illusions of imagination, does not recognize his own family; unhappy, apprehensive anxiety and despair; absence of thought and weakness of memory; stupidity and insensible prostration in a corner; patient shrinks with fear, drawing himself away from every one who approaches him; praecordial anguish, pale, miserable look, general chilliness, not relieved by heat; decrease of brain functions.

Mental and bodily prostration after overexertion of mind and loss of sleep; anxiety, fear of persecution, is in despair, with very difficult breathing and faint feeling; skin cool, covered with cold sweat; unconquerable sadness and restlessness, as if some misfortune were approaching; weeps often, shuns the sight of people, seeks and loves solitude; anxious concerning death, which she believes near and inevitable.

A kind of fear of vigorously walking, he must tread lightly in order to avoid doing harm or disturbing those in the room with him; child afraid of falling, shrinking away from every one who approaches him, clinging tightly to nurse; won't stay in bed, but in lap; restless tossing about.

Cyclamen—Mental derangement at climaxis; vertigo with pain in head and nausea, < in right temple, but extending all over head; answers incoherently; disposition to weep; fear of death; faeces and urine pass unconsciously and involuntarily; ailments from inward grief and terrors of conscience.

Digitalis—Great anxiety, depression and dread of the future, with sadness and weeping, < about 6 P. M. and by music; morose, irritable and gloomy; weakness of memory, mind dull and confused; sleep unrefreshing, with frequent waking; anguish, which seems to proceed from epigastrium; weakness and exhaustion; slow pulse; relief of stupor by weeping.

Profound great melancholy, worse by music, with frequent sighing and weeping, which bring relief; gloomy, morose, ill-humor, great fear of the future; insane obstinacy and disobedience, with desire to escape; patient dull and lethargic, pupils widely dilated and all sensibility to light and touch seems lost; chronic heart disease; pulse full, regular or but slightly intermittent and very slow. When rallying from his stupor the patient moans greatly and his eyes are all afloat in tears, with relief from the lachrymation.

Fear of death; great anxiety, like from troubled conscience.

Drosera—Fear of being poisoned; of being persecuted on all sides; dread of ghosts, < when alone in evening or when awaking at night.

Dulcamara.—Imbecility more frequent than insanity; mental confusion, cannot concentrate his thoughts; inclination to scold without being angry; asks for one thing or another to reject it when offered; hasty speech and hasty drinking.

Elaps coral.—Excessive horror of rain; dread of being alone, as if something would happen; violent headache when the desire for food is not immediately satisfied, < from fruits or cold drinks; irregular menses, weight in vagina with violent itching; weakness and trembling.

Eupatorium purp.—Feels homesick when at home with her family; sighing; sick-headache; choking fulness of throat, must swallow often; bowels loose; constant desire to urinate; restless and moaning, weak, tired and faint, with urinary symptoms.

Eugenia jambos.—Desire for solitude, mental depression, loss of memory; his mind seems to brighten up after urinating, feels depressed before and shivering after urination.

Euphorbium—Temporary attacks of craziness, insists upon saying his prayers at the tail of his horse; knows his freaks and wants to be by himself and in silence; imagines he sees the same man walking after him that he sees walking before him; vertigo when standing or walking in open air.

Ferrum met.—Mind exceedingly oppressed; great solicitude about those belonging to him, with constant thoughts of death; anxiety as after committing a crime; from slightest cause anxiety, with throbbing in pit of stomach; excited by slightest opposition, everything irritates and oppresses her; anaemia and debility with congestion to head and chest.

Ferrum phos.—Transitory mania depending upon hyperaemia of the brain; severe headache, soreness in vertex, general soreness of scalp, great nervousness at night; blinding headache, < on stooping.

Fluoric acid.—Aversion to his own family, bordering on insanity, but knows enough to behave well to strangers; discontent and excessive ill-humor followed by indifference and forgetfulness, and finally by perfect contentment and uncommonly gay disposition of mind.

Gelsemium—Melancholia stupida during its early stages, after protracted work and anxiety, after night-watching with loss of sleep, after excesses in alcohol; after grief; depression of spirits, hates consolation, wants to be let alone and brood over real or imaginary loss; inability to attend to anything requiring mental effort; great lack of courage and fear of death; dull heavy pains in head and neck; intense prostration of muscular system.

Fear of lightning (*Bor.:* fear of thunder); incessant screaming after a heavy thunderclap; nervous dread of appearing in public of singers and speakers; bad effects from fright and fear; great want of courage; diarrhoea and abortion after fright.

Hysterical convulsions, with spasms of the glottis; hysterical epilepsy; excessive irritability of mind and body, with vascular excitement; semi-stupor, with languor and prostration; nervous headaches commencing in the neck and spreading over whole head; migraine, dysmenorrhoea, of a neuralgic or spasmodic character.

Glonoinum—Acute dementia, religious mania; well-known streets seem strange, forgets where she lives, attempts to run away; fear of death, of being poisoned; disinclined to speak, would hardly answer; bad effects from mental excitement, fright, fear, mechanical contusions; congestion alternately to head and heart; head hot, body and feet cold; head feels larger and throbs.

Graphites—Herpetic constitution; gloomy and low-spirited; great inclination to grief, even to despair, propensity to feel himself unhappy, with thoughts of deep grief and weeping; timid restlessness, < mornings; oppression about heart, with uneasiness in stomach, great anxiousness as if after the commission of a crime or as if a misfortune impended, with hot face and cold extremities; anxiety when seated at work; repugnance to labor; venous persons, with disposition to obesity.

Timidity; fidgety while sitting at work; extreme hesitation, she is unable to make up her mind about anything; very fretful, everything angers and offends him; absent-minded and slow in thoughts, sad, despondent, music makes her weep; solicitude concerning spiritual welfare; full of fear in the morning, feels miserably unhappy; hates work; ailments from grief.

Full of fear in the morning, as if his end were near or the greatest misfortune were impending, with inclination to weep.

Gratiola—Fretful, angry outbreaks, misanthropic, with solicitude about his own health, no desire to talk or move; wants to be alone; dullness in head while standing or walking, > when lying down; offensive breath in the morning when awaking; aversion to eat and to smoke; feeling of flatulency; watery diarrhoea more than constipation.

Hamamelis—Wants "the respect due to me" shown.

Helleborus—Quiet, placid melancholy, with sighing, moaning and dread of dying; feels unhappy in presence of cheerful faces; ameliorated by vomiting; slow comprehension; obstinate silence; homesickness. Repercussion of exanthemata. Acute idiocy as well as chronic idiocy and cretinismus; diminished power of mind over body, cannot fix ideas, slow in answering, stares unintelligently; muscles fail to act properly if will is not strongly fixed upon their action; depression of sensory and obtuseness of intellectual faculties; stubborn silence; fixed delusions and hallucinations, especially towards morning; demoniac melancholy, sees spirits at night; woeful despairing mood, with tendency to drown himself; irritable, easily made angry, < from consolation; homesickness; anxiousness about heart, which prevents him from resting anywhere; want of bodily irritability; cold hands and feet, coldness of whole body, can bear neither heat nor cold; pale, sallow complexion.

Helonias—Mind exceedingly dull and inactive; desires solitude; irritable, faultfinding, cannot bear the least contradiction, all conversation is unpleasant; pressure from within upward to the vertex, aggravated by looking steadily at any fixed point; atonic condition of the sexual organs.

Profound melancholy, restlessness, wants to be continually moving about, is fault-finding from a sensation of undefined soreness and weight in the uterus, a consciousness of a womb; she feels better when her mind is engaged and she is doing something; dragging weakness in small of back, prolapsus uteri, or dislocation (*Murex.*).

Hepar sulph.—The patient is impelled by unaccountable attacks of internal anguish, which sometimes come on quite suddenly, to attempt suicide (*Alum.*); chronic abdominal affections; excessive nervousness from abuse of mercury; dejected, sad, fearful; repulsive mood and desire to be left alone; (dementia, with stupidity, sits silent and speechless in a corner); violent outbursts of passion, so that he does not wish to see the members of his own family; hasty speech and hasty drinking.

Hyperaesthesia, maniacal paroxysms, with quick, hasty speech; extreme discontent, indisposition to everything; wrathful irritability, even to the most extreme violence, threatening to end in murder and arson; terrific visions of dead persons;

Hydrocyanic acid.—Anxious feeling and fretfulness; uneasy confusion of head; hysterical spasms; semiconsciousness; limbs and jaws rigid; eyes fixed; the beat of the heart very irregular and feeble.

Hydrophobinum.—See Lyssin.

Hyoscyamus.—Acute mania with extreme excitation of sensorium and abnormal impulses; impatience, precipitate liveliness, talkativeness, tells everything; great inclination to laugh; lascivious shamelessness and going about naked (pruritus pudendi, pruritus of the skin, > by the cooling fresh air); insulting, shouting, brawling, ungovernable rage, with exhibition of unusual strength and great muscular activity; all objects appear larger, a straw looks like a beam, etc.; senseless apathy and indolence, refuses to speak, makes no complaints and has no wants; morose dejection, despair, fear of being poisoned and refuses food, or of being bitten by animals; epileptoid spasms, rush of blood to head with sparkling eyes and fixed look; spasms of pharynx and dread of drinks; face only slightly flushed, pupils dilated; restless sleep, he lies awake for hours, every little noise disturbs him; debility and great prostration on every attempt to move, < after eating, though bulimy might be present; unfortunate disappointed love, with jealousy and excited sexual desires.

Nervous irritability without hyperaemia; melancholy with despair and propensity to drown himself (*Bell.*) and total indifference to food and drink; reproaches of conscience; dread of being sold, poisoned, bitten by animals; syphilophobia; jealousy with attempt to murder, aversion to mankind, mistrust and indolence; hyperaesthesia cutanea, wants to go naked, with loss of all shame; constant absurd talking or muttering to himself.

Restless, jumps out of bed; fright, followed by convulsions; disposition to escape in the night (*Bell., Merc.*).

Indomitable rage, wants to kill somebody or himself; horrid anguish; complains of being poisoned; thinks he will be bit by animals and wants to drown himself; fantastic craziness; converses with people who are not present; looks at men as hogs; considers the stove a tree and wants to climb up;

loves smutty talk; wants to go naked (hyperaesthesia of the skin). Erotomania; very little rush of blood to head; restless sleep; dizziness; muscular twitchings; dry mouth and dilated pupils; no appetite or bulimy, but eating aggravates all symptoms.

Jerking and twitching in the spasms; alternate convulsions of upper and lower limbs; jerks of single muscles or sets of muscles; she is disposed to uncover herself and to go naked from hyperaesthesia of the skin; much silly laughter and foolish actions. Irritable uterus; irregular menses; head falls from side to side; full of suspicion and jealousy; refuses food and medicine.

Unfortunate love, with rage and incoherent speech; lascivious mania; uncovers body, especially sexual organs; sings amorous songs; jealous and vehement; talks confusedly; hectic fever.

Hypericum—Mental depression following nerve injuries; convulsions, spinal affections, trismus and tetanus, following wounds of nerves or a blow on head; irritable and despondent; sees spirits and spectres; tympanitis; spasmodic jerking of lower limbs.

Ignatia—contradictory state of concomitants; Emotional instability, rapid alternation between hilarity and desire to weep; inward grief from disappointed love or mortification, loves solitude; senseless staring at one object with sighing and moaning; remorse about imaginary crimes, intolerance to noise, sensitive mood and delicate conscientiousness; great tendency to have fixed ideas, but she hides her grief and her delusions from others.

Tears wept inwardly; suicidal **desire to be released from what seems to be a perpetual burden of sorrow;** desire for solitude so that he may still nourish his inward grief;

great anxiousness at night or when awakening in the morning, with taciturnity; fear of thieves on waking after midnight; timidity and fear of contracting disease; aversion to any amusement; no desire to eat or drink; weak memory; heaviness of head, losing hair on one side; voice low, trembling; staggering walk; general weakness; cold feet, mostly evening; sexual desire with impotence; menses scanty, black, of a putrid odor; increased stool and urine; recent cases.

Brooding over imaginary troubles, prefers to be alone, sits quietly and gazes into vacancy; face distorted, deathly pale and sunken; no desire for nourishment; voice trembling; staggering walk; pain in left hypochondrium, worse from pressure; late sleep and restlessness; cold feet, more in the evening.

Effects of disappointed love, with silent grief and delicate conscientiousness; affectionate disposition, with very clear consciousness.

Grief and sorrow with shame; suppressed internal vexation which continues, especially when of recent origin; night-sweats from sheer exhaustion; anorexia, sensation as of a heavy pressure on top of head, as if a gread load lay there; face flushes at every motion; broods over imaginary troubles, with relief from weeping; vertigo and amenorrhoea.

He fears every trifle, especially objects approaching him; fear of thieves; frequent profuse passage of watery urine; painless diarrhoea.

Longing after his friends; flat, watery taste of all food; gone feeling in stomach, not relieved by eating; brooding in solitude over her imaginary griefs and disappointments.

Perversion of the co-ordinations of functions; clavus hystericus; disposition to grieve, to brood in melancholic sadness over real or imaginary sorrows; anguish, with shrieking for help and suffocating constriction of throat; difficult deglutition; emptiness in pit of stomach, with frequent sighing and much despondency and grief; mental symptoms change often, cheerfullness with great despondency; sensation as if stomach were hanging on a thread (*Val.*, nausea and sensation as if a thread were handing in throat); feels as if she must be in a hurry; irritability, impatience and quarrelsomeness alternating with undue hilarity or silent melancholy.

Indigo—Patient feels very gloomy, taciturn, timid, is tired of life, spends his nights crying; epileptic convulsions; flushes of heat from abdomen to head; sensation as if the head were tightly bandaged around forehead; the epileptic fit always commencing with dizziness; undulating sensation through the whole head from behind forward.

Iodum—Melancholy, must keep in motion day and night; brain feels as if it were stirred up, feels as if going crazy; shunning and fear when any one comes near, particularly the physician; excessive excitability and sensitiveness; expects an accident from every trifle.

Great fear of people, restless moving about from place to place; gloomy mood, despondency, anguish, oppression of chest; excessive nervous irritability; violent orgasm of blood, with uneasy trembling, extending from stomach to all parts of periphery; spasmodic palpitation of heart; sleeplessness; emaciation with ravenous appetite.

Remarkable and unaccountable sense of weakness and loss of breath in going up-stairs; leucorrhoea corroding the linen; food does not nourish or strengthen her; patient irritable, cross and sulky, hates to be touched anywhere.

Iris vers.—Biliousness, despondency, low-spirited, easily vexed; confusion of mind with mental depression; habitual headaches from gastric or abdominal causes.

Kali ars.—Scolding, morose, retired, quarrelsome and discontented; jealous, indifferent to everything, scarcely answers questions, or replies in a peevish tone; eyes have a fixed look;

Melancholia; discontented; face looks frightened and anxious, a loud noise or unexpected motion throws here whole body in a tremor.

Kali-bich.—Anthrophobia; weakness, aversion to business, indifference, irritability, anxiety arising from chest; averse to motion, inclination to lie down.

Anthropophobia anxiety arising from chest; ill-humor even to disgust of life, indifference with distress in stomach; fretfulness, weakness, aversion to business; frequent vanishing of thoughts with senseless staring at an object; great weakness of memory.

Kali brom.—Imagines he is especially singled out as an object of Divine vengeance, thinks all her friends have deserted her, is full of religious delusions and **a feeling of moral deficiency;** nervous restlessness, cannot sit still, must move about or otherwise occupy himself; insomnia; frequent shedding of tears; low-spirited, childish, giving way to her feelings; indifference and almost tired of life; profound anaemia.

Profound melancholia, often from anaemia, depressed, low-spirited, with weeping; extreme despondency; that his honor is at stake, that he is to be murdered; constant worry, fears to see people or to be spoken to, always < when trying to sit quietly; inability to concentrate the mind on any subject; failure of mental and bodily strength with consequent despondency; pricking sensation all over body; constantly busy tying his shoes, fumbling in his pockets, picking threads, etc.

Kali-carb.—Alternating mood, at one time good and quiet, at another excited and angry at trifles; constantly in antagonism with herself, frequently despondent; frets about everything, peevish, impatient, contented with nothing; great aversion to being alone.

Tearful humor, with feeling of loneliness and desire for company; timid and apprehensive of the future, easily frightened, with shrieks about imaginary hallucinations; peevishness, with intolerance of the human voice; obstinacy; changeable humor; deficiency of expression; is at a loss to say what she wishes; dread of labor; paresis, trembling; horrid dreams, with frequent awaking and urinating.

Fear of being alone and that she will die; she starts with a loud cry at any imaginary object, as if a bird flew towards the window.

Kali iod.—Very great irritability and unwanted harshness of demeanor; his children, to whom he is devotedly attached, become burdensome to him; very passionate and spiteful temper.

Melancholia; irritable and harsh; torturing feeling of anguish preventing sleep; inclined to sadness and weeping, with constant apprehension of impending evil.

Great anxiety about their present state of health, a kind of sinking and faintness with mental depression.

Kali mur.—Sad, apathetic, with chilliness in evening; habitual loss of appetite; he aboslutely refuses to take food or imagines he must starve; intoxication from the smallest quantity of wine or beer, causing congestion, > from nosebleed.

Kali phos.—Religious melancholia with fear of hell; refuses food and drink and tears everything; hypersesthesia of senses with anaemic weakness and failure of strength as after mental overstrain, depressing emotions, or from exhausting drainings affecting nerve-centres of spinal cord; hysteria with globus.

Suspiciousness; mental depression, showing itself by vexation, irritability; fearfulness, weeping mood, timidity; religious mania; weariness of life and fear of death; Homesickness and morbid sensitiveness.

Nervous attacks from sudden or intense emotions or from smothering passion in a highly nervous and excitable person. Globus hystericus. Hysterical fits of yawning, of laughing or crying.

Kreosotum—Stupid feeling in head, with vacant gaze, neither seeing nor hearing; sorrowful mood, inclined to weep, and longing for death; music and other emotional causes impel him to weep.

Lac caninum—Thinks she is looked down upon by everybody, that she is of no importance (*Pallad.*); doubts her own ability and success; weeps easily, exceedingly nervous and irritable.

Lac defloratum—Depression of spirits, does not want to live and does not want to see or to talk to any one; no fear of death, but is sure to die.

Lachesis—Quiet sorrowful lowness of spirits relieved by sighing; repugnance to society and dislike to talk; solicitude about the future, with disgust of life; inclination to doubt everything; mistrusts and misconstrues everything in the worst way; indolence, with aversion to every kind of labor and motion; insane jealousy.

Hyperthymia; thinks herself under superhuman control; great weakness of memory and forgetfulness; incapability of thinking; mental laziness; amentia; delirium from watching, fatigue after fevers of a low type, from loss of fluid, excessive study; loquacious, with mocking jealousy; frightful images, satirical; talks, sings, whistles, makes odd motions, jumps rapidly from one object to another; ecstasy unto crying; peevish, morose and quarrelsome; great inclination to grief, looks at everything in the blackest color; anxious timidity, as if some great evil were impending; doubts all truth and experience; dread of recovery and of death, fears to go to bed; suicidal mood, tired of life, with fear of death; thinks she is dead and that preparations are made for her funeral; great malice and spiteful tricks, all his thoughts tending to the injury of others, even murder, accompanied by cardiac affections, lassitude, chilliness, emaciation, sickly pale complexion; lasciviousness and sexual desire, with weakness of the parts; restless and uneasy, wants to be off somewhere all the time; climaxis.

Chronic complaints from long-lasting grief and sorrow (*Ph-ac.*); great sadness and anxiety; throbbing headache.

Dread of death, fears to go to bed; fears she will be damned; thinks herself pursued by enemies or robbers; fears the medicine as poison; fears insanity.

Malice; thinks only of mischief; undertakes many things, perseveres in nothing; complaints of trifles; exalted mood, with increase of well feeling; morbid talkativeness in chosen language, but jumping from one subject to another; haughtiness, mistrusts those around him.

Sensation as if a lump were rising in throat; cannot bear the least pressure externally anywhere; she wakes from sleep distressed and unhappy, as if from loss of breath.

Uneasy about state of his health; idea that he is disliked by his family; inability to perform any mental or physical labor; suicidal mood, tired of life; foul breath; dyspepsia, < as soon as he eats; liver complaints, constipation.

Unhappy love, with jealous, suspicious despair; weary of life; pain in heart; fainting, apparent death; mistrust, suspicion; worse towards evening.

Lactic acid.—Intermittent hysteria; nauseated in the morning when swallowing and gets worse until 9 a.m. when she vomits large amount of tough phlegm, sometimes had to remove it with finger, lasting till 9 p.m.

Laurocerasus—Extreme despondency or lively, joyous mood; forgets very easily from the constant confusion in his head; nervous agitation; rotary vertigo; sensation of coldness in forehead and vertex;

Indolence and indisposition to either physical or intellectual labor, so that patient becomes disgusted and tired of his life; fear and anxiety about imaginary evils; disposition to sleep; titillation in face, as if flies and spiders were crawling over face; want of energy of vital powers, no reaction, a paralytic weakness.

Ledum—Fears death and fears to go to sleep lest she will die.

Leptandra—Hepatic derangement. Languid, tired feeling, with great prostration; gloomy, desponding, drowsy; physically and mentally depressed.

Lilium tig.—Indecision of character, and depends entirely upon others; dislikes being alone, but has no dread of being so; opposite mental states, feels nervous, irritable, scolding, and still in a pleasant humor; constant inclination to weep; has to keep very busy to repress sexual desires; great bearing down in pelvic regions, as if everything from the chest down would fall out; the heart feels as if it were full of blood, with depression of spirits and apprehension of impending evil; blurred vision.

Uterine dementia; doubts her salvation, walks for day and night, < by consolation, weeps much and is very timid; curses and uses obscene language; head confused and heavy; vertigo < walking.

Fear and apprehension of having some incurable disease (*Cact.*), of becoming insane; low-spirited, can hardly keep from crying.

Nervous depression; indisposition to any exertion of mind and body; aversion to food or capricious appetite; bearing down and pain in lower abdomen; fluttering of heart, with irregular pulse.

Lithium carb.—Disposition to weep about his lonesome condition; difficulty in remembering names; sensation of entire helplessness, especially at night.

Lobelia infl.—Fear of death from difficulty of respiration; restless sleep, with anxious and sad dreams; excessive weakness of the stomach, extending into the chest, with oppression of chest; sudden shocks through the head.

Apprehension of death and difficult breathing; desponding and sobbing like a child; vertigo, with deathly nausea; scratching and burning, with dryness in throat; muscular relaxation with great prostration ; sensation as if heart would stop beating, etc.

Lycopodium—Melancholy and hypochondriasis in mild characters; loss of confidence in himself and in others; miserly disposition; oversensitive and irritable, even to the most violent rage; obstinate, defiant, arbitrary; extreme indifference and insensibility to external impressions; torpor of mind; laughing and weeping in alternation; difficult digestion, intestinal and hepatic torpor; absent-minded;

uses wrong words; great weakness; early and profuse menses; baldness; mental disturbances in the latter stages of phthisis pulmonalis, with emaciation from malassimilation and night-sweats. *Talks imperiously. Manner stiff and pretentious.*

Want of self-confidence; fear of phantoms in the evening, with anguish; parsimonious, greedy, avaricious, malicious and pusillanimous; nervous, irritable and peevish; seeks disputes, which is followed by supreme indifference; hypochondriasis; confusion of thoughts and forgetfulness, using wrong words, supposing himself to be at two places at once; fear of going to bed in the evening, is sure to hear somebody in the room; satiety of life, particularly mornings in bed, dread of men, wants to be alone or dread of solitude with irritability; abdominal and mental torpor.

Fear of imaginary phantoms, of terrifying images; dread of solitude with irritability and melancholy; fear about one's salvation; forgetfulness, anguish and excitement when alone, with restless moving about.

Hepatic troubles after mortification, with relief from weeping; dread of people, wants to be alone and still is irritable and melancholy when alone; vehement, angry, headstrong; constipated. Oversensitiveness of senses.

Low-spirited, taciturn, irritable and nervous; hates company and still dreads to be alone.

Sensation of satiety and of fulness up to the throat; flatulency, particularly in left hypochondrium; cutting pains across adbomen, from right to left; frequent and copious micturition; urine pale, especially at night; violent burning in vagina during and after coitus; tickling through the genitals; itching of the pudenda; much milky leucorrhoea.

Lyssin (Hydrophobinum)—Cannot rid himself of the tormenting idea that something terrible was going to happen to him; fits of abstraction, he takes hold of wrong things, does not know what he wanted; uses words which have but a remote similarity of sound; two distinct trains of thoughts seem to be operating at the same time; imagines to be abused by others and tries to defend himself.

Magnesia mur.—After dinner she is seized with nausea, trembling and fainting spells; anxious and restless, < from mental exertion; congestive headaches with sensation as of boiling water in cranium, especially about temples, > by pressure and by wrapping up the head warmly (*Sil.*); globus hystericus, > by eructations; bearing down in uterine region and uterine spasms, menses black and pitchlike, with pain in back when walking and in thighs when sitting; leucorrhoea after every stool and after uterine spasms; constipation, stools passed with difficulty, being so dry and hard that the lumps crumble as they pass the anus; inability to urinate without pressing on abdominal walls; palpitation of heart while sitting, going off on motion and exercise; unrefreshing sleep or sleeplessness.

Apprehension, sad, homesick, weeps, loneliness, with frequent weeping; hysterical and spasmodic complaints; sleep unrefreshing.

Mancinella—Melancholy homesickness; about midnight, attacks of fear and trembling; afraid of evil spirits, of being taken hold of by the devil; sleeplessness; pressing in cardiac region, hard beats of heart, followed by faintishness, with darkening before the eyes; pulse slow and soft; tetters; Bashful; pemphigus, skin peels off in large plates.

Melilotus—Hypochondriasis; full of hallucinations; is possessed by the evil spirit; bloatedness of abdomen, with a crawling sensation as of worms; horrible, oppressive headache; nausea and faintishness; muscular jactitation; redness of face, with active melancholia, even to fury.

Religious melancholia with weeping and indolence; reluctant to rise in morning, sits and does nothing; face always hot and flushed, throbbing of carotids; constipation; > by nosebleed or any other haemorrhage.

Mercurius auratus.—Syphilitic melancholia; apprehensive of some fearful accident; filthy habits, eats manure; imagines he is enduring the tortures of hell.

Mercurius sol.—Inexpressible pain of soul and body, anxious restlessness, as if some evil impended, worse at night, with praecordial anguish; sweat of the hands and heat of the face; disgusted with himself, has not enough courage to live; constant suspicion, considering everybody his enemy.

Desire to run away to foreign countries; complains of everything; anxiousness; hunger, with weak digestion; diarrhoea, with tenesmus; pains in limbs at night; weak and trembling after slight exertion; fear in the night; nightsweats.

Excessive restlessness and anguish, particularly at night, of impending misfortune; indifference to everything, even to taking his food; homesickness, with irresistible desire to travel; homesickness, with desire to escape and to run home; mania, with tearing everything to pieces, and aversion to fluid; amentia, with absurd talk and actions; tricks, foolishness and mischievous jokes of all kinds, with senseless, disgusting actions; buffoonish insanity; suspicious, disturbed mood; *lassitude and prostration,* great heaviness of head, cutting pains in abdomen, *restless sleep, full of heavy dreams.*

Fear and weakness, timidity and nightly complaints, wants to go outdoors, far away, discontented, complaining of weak digestion and continual hunger; heaviness in abdomen with long-lasting anxiety; trembling after slight exertion; sleep prevented by fearful visions; fear of losing his mind; complains of everything and everybody.

Grief with fear at night, disposition to quarrel, complaining of his relations and surroundings; sleep prevented by seeing frightful faces.

Mezereum—Hypochondriacal sadness; great disgust for life and longing for death; sensitive peevishness, with pale, miserable, sunken look; indetermination; attacks of thoughtless staring, fixed look for hours together; apprehensiveness felt at the pit of the stomach, indifference to everybody and everything.

Morphium—Fear and trembling before and during a thunderstorm.

Moschus—Suitable to spoiled, sensitive natures and hysteric women; tearful vexation and peevishness, with violent quarreling, even to the most extreme malice and rage; great bustling, during which everything falls out of his hand from weakness; thoughtlessness, with foolish gestures and complaints of pain; sudden loss of memory, with complete inability to collect his senses; great tendency to get frightened, trembling, palpitation of heart and dread of death.

Great and constant anxiety, with thoughts of death; headache as if a weight were lying upon it; everything tastes bad, aversion to all food; tension in abdomen; profuse diarrhoea with retraction of abdomen; fainting.

Hysteria, especially for the paroxysm, even if insensible, cries one moment and bursts into uncontrollable laughter the next; palpitation of heart, as from anxious expectation;

nervous, busy, but weak, soon drops things; tremoulous nervousness; fainting spells, with pale face and coldness; sleepy during day; rush of blood to head, with staring eyes; dizzy, unsteadiness as of something rapidly moving up and down; tension, stiffness, pressure in back and limbs; tonic spasms; uneasiness in legs, < while sitting; tympanitis, with fainting; spasmus glottidis, as if it closed upon the breath; cramp in lung, beginning with inclination to cough, gradually increasing and making him desperate; suffocative constriction in chest; copious pale urine; fear of death, with pale face and fainting; scolding disposition, until her lips turn blue, her eyes stare and she faints away; menses too early and too profuse, preceded by drawing, dragging sensation towards genitals; sexual desire increased by local titillation; great desire for beer or brandy; rotary vertigo with dim vision.

Murex—Great depression of spirit, she considers herself hopelessly ill, goes to bed and remains there; great debility of the muscles; sinking of stomach; sensation of dryness or constriction of uterus.

Mygale.—Constant talk about business, restless at night; despondent with anxious features; tremulousness of whole body in the evening; nausea, with strong palpitation of heart; dimness of sight; general weakness and fear of death.

Naja tripudians—Depression and forgetfulness; consciousness of some duty to be performed, but attended with an unaccountable inclination not to do it; sadness with intense frontal headache, fluttering of heart and spinal pains.

Suicidal insanity, broods constantly over imaginary troubles; sleep full of frightful dreams, and wakes with dull pain in the head, and fluttering of the heart; uneasy dryness of the fauces; grasping of throat, with sensation of choking, and lividity of the face.

Anxiety with dragging at praecordia, occurring in cases of great grief; excessive nervous palpitations; headache with coldness of feet, affecting especially right side.

Natrum carb.—Aversion to mankind and society; sadness, depression of spirits, head feels stupefied if he tries to exert himself; avarice (Lyc., Calc. fluor.); restless, with attacks of anxiety, especially during a thunder-storm, playing piano for a short time causes painful anxiety in chest, trembling of body and weariness; must lie down; phlegmatic indolent disposition, with repugnance to speaking, to work, or any occupation.

Hypochondriasis, great weakness of the digestive organs, with very bad humor after a meal; troubles after drinking; phlegmatic flaccidity; dislike to talk and work, want of sympathy and disgust of life; trembling and feeling of faintness; great sadness, constant sighing; clumsy manner and awkwardness; < from music and during a thunderstorm; great timidity; avarice.

Depressed and exceedingly irritable, especially after a meal; < after a vegetable diet, especially starchy food; the degree of hypochondriasis can be measured by the stage of digestion; averse to society, even to that of his own family; dyspepsia, with sour belching, waterbrash, retching in the morning; griping colic just after a meal.

Natrum mur.—Crowding of gloomy thoughts which recall insults long since suffered, with want of self-reliance and palpitation of heart; great inclination to weep, and condoling only makes things worse; timid inquietude about the future, with inclination to remain for hours buried in thought; indifference from hopelessness and mental languor, wishes only to remain quiet and to sleep; sallow complexion; excessive sadness during menses, with palpitation and morning headache; he loses flesh though living well.

Melancholy; likes to dwell on past unpleasant occurrences; weeps on being merely looked at, and rejects consolation (puls., patient seeks consolation), joyless indifference and indolent indisposition to talk; quarrelsome fretfulness, gets into a passion about trifles; attacks of great cheerfulness and merry disposition, with inclination to laugh, dance and sing; great distraction in all his actions and constant wandering in his thoughts; weakness of memory and forgetfulness; awkwardness; sexual desire, with frequent erections and pollutions; palpitation of heart, predominant chilliness, inclined to sweat; suits anaemic women with thin, worn face and general emaciation.

Chronic effects of fright; horror, full of apprehensions and hurriedness, with anxiety; dreams of robbers in the house, starts and talks in sleep.

Chronic effects of grief, with vertex headache (*Phos.ac.*); sadness, weeping, emaciation.

Delaying and decreasing menses; somnambulism; debility; excessive thirst; great inclination to weep; much mucus in the urine; aversion to bread; all symptoms relieved as soon as she gets into a perspiration; haunted with thoughts that something unpleasant will happen.

Despairing, hopeless feeling about the future, with dryness of mouth, irritable mucous membranes, sore and slightly ulcerated tongue, chronic constipation with hard stools; foul breath; hypochondriasis < by dyspepsia and constipation, > when bowels move freely.

Sad, weeping, consolation aggravates, with palpitation and intermittent pulse; gets angry at trifles; hateful and vindictive; weariness in head, dull, heavy aching and distention of abdomen.

Natrum sulph.—Great restraint necessary not to do himself bodily harm; aversion to life; great sadness and despondency, with irritability and dread of music, which makes her weep and melancholic; mental troubles coming on from a jar or knock on the head or a fall or injuries about the head, causing concussion or other affections of the brain; Music unbearable, makes him melancholic even of a lively kind makes him weep.

Suicidal tendency, must exercise restraint, attended with wildness and irritability, due to gastric, bilious conditions, < in wet weather and damp dwellings, and > in warm, dry weather.

Nitric acid.—Dread of contentions, quarrels and lawsuits; frequent sorrowful thoughts of past events; fearful and easily frightened; disgust of life, with longing for death, which, however, is dreaded; reserved and does not wish to talk.

Nux moschata.—Dementia, irresistible inclination to laugh; insane intoxication; wandering talk, with extraordinary gestures and loud voice; foolish gestures, with absence of mind; indolent march of ideas and slow recollection, fatuity; sleepiness and fainty, weak digestion; cool, dry skin.

Hysteria with frequent emotional changes and enormous bloating of abdomen after a slight meal; excessive dryness of mouth and throat even when they show their normal degree of moisture; mind bewildered, dreamy, finally deep stupor with loss of motion and sensation; errors of perception, a momentary unconsciousness she thinks as having been of long duration; laughing and jesting alternate with sadness and weeping, both without cause; prostration and tendency to faint; pulse and breath hardly perceptible; mental and bodily agony; head jerked forward, Jaws clinched, heart as if rasped, oppression of heart with choking sensation, tonic and clonic spasms, unconscious.

Palpitations from sadness; weeping mood, gloomy, fears to go to sleep; sleepy from mental overexertion; gastric ailments; hysteria; staggers in walking; falls often.

Nux vomica—Insanity, with perverted talk and actions, frightful visions at night, murmuring delirium; disgust of life, with palpitation of heart; peevish and solicitous about his health; stubborness and obstinate resistance; irascible and violent, with malice and spiteful tricks; dislike to mental work after mental overexertion; oversensitivenss to external impressions. Depression following overstimulation. (irascible = hot tempered and irritable)

Mental recklessness, desperation and hot, irritable temper; wants to kill those she loves best; nervous excitement and mental worry, inability for mental work; taciturn, desire for solitude; **afraid he might not have enough to live on** and great propensity to end his existence; abdominal plethora and constipation.

Ill-humor, despondency, aversion to life, disposition to vehemence; indisposition to work or to perform any mental labor; fatigue of the mind after the least mental exertion; unrefreshing sleep, aggravation of the distress in the morning; dullness of the head, with aching pains, or sensation as if a pin were sticking in the brain; aversion to the open air, constant desire to lie down, with great exhaustion after walking; painfulness and distention in the region of the hypochondria, epigastrium and the pit of the stomach; constipation, slow action of the bowels, haemorrhoidal disposition, feels better when bowels move, etc. (*Sulph.* is frequently used after *Nux.*)

Oversensitivenss to emotional and external impressions; sedentary habits; hypochondriac mood of those who dissipate and keep late hours, with abdominal troubles and constipation; very easily bewildered; everything he attempts goes wrong; pain in small of back, cannot sit up.

She seldom sleeps after 3 a.m., but dozes after 5 and late in the morning, the latter sleep unrefreshing; constipation or large difficult stools; dyspepsia well developed, cannot bear any kind of stimulants or high-seasoned food; feels best on plain, simple food; menses irregular, never at the right time; sensation of constriction about hypogastrium.

Oenanthe crocata—Profound disturbance of intellectual faculties, mania, delirium tremens, most painful spasms; excessive excitement, she talked to herself, swore and blasphemed, while at the same time she was seized with convulsive laughter; extreme restlessness; confusion of intellect, even stupor and coma; convulsions of the mouth, face and extremities with unconsciousness, restlessness, exhaustion and debility after the fit; cold sweats.

Oleander—Absentmindedness and slowness of perception; utter indolence and aversion to do anything, will not dress or eat; cannot bear the slightest handling and becomes greatly enraged if touched by any one; breathing oppressed and heavy; head hanging down constantly; itching of scalp with constant tendency to scratch the head; rumbling and flatulence of bowels, with hard difficult stool; urine brown, normal in quantity.

Opium—Fantastical insanity, with frightful visions congregating around his bed and tormenting him; talks in a confused manner; commits indecent actions; cheerfulness and feeling of great strength; vivid hallucinations of sight; contempt of death; rioting hilarity, with buffoonery and subsequent angry savageness or tearful sorrowfulness; instability and imbecility of will; indifference to joy and suffering; complete dementia, does not recognize his own relatives; excessive debility, stupor, frequent sweats and eruptions on skin; diminished secretion of urine. Suitable to old bummers, to old people inclined to applexy and paralysis; heavy, unrefreshing sleep or sleepless but stupid (*Gels.*).

Hallucinations of spectres and animals with great fear; imagines parts of body very large; imbecility of will, as if annihilated.

Immediate effect of fright, stupefied, with internal heat, rush of blood to head, dim sight with twitches and starting; diarrhoea with involuntary discharge of faeces; suffocation with anxiety; limbs become numb and torpid; convulsions of children; tonic spasms, the whole body stiff; debility with cold sweat, fainting.

Palladium—Mental exhaustion, everything is too much exertion; time seems long to him; wounded pride, easily out of humor and uses then strong expressions; fond of good opinion of others; < from any mental exertion or excitement, as on the day following an evening entertainment.

Mortification after wounded pride, not getting the praise of others which she expected; great inclination to weep and to be sulky.

After wounded pride, not getting the praise of others she expected, is greatly inclined to use strong language and violent expressions, and feels, next day, headache and worse from the excitement.

She imagines herself neglected; greatly inclined to use strong language and violent expressions (*Mosch.*); excited and impatient; distended abdomen, from flatulency; stools hard, like chalk; pain and weakness, as if the uterus were sinking down; every motion painful; great sleepiness, and feels better after sleep.

Paris quad.—Loquacious vivacity; jumping, with a good deal of self-complacency, from one subject to another, merely for the sake of talking; indisposition to any mental labor.

Petroleum.—Fear of death; great irresoluteness, no desire for work and dissatisfied with everything; sensation as if there were a cold stone in the heart; emaciation; profuse night-sweats; mucous diarrhoea.

Thinks that another person lies beside him or that one limb is double; sadness and despondency; weakness of memory; violent starting from trivial causes; head feels numb, as if made from wood and bruised; vertigo and nausea when stooping or when rising from a recumbent position; twitching of limbs; weak unto faintness.

Phosphoric acid.—Long-lasting cases: Chronic effects of grief, with night-sweats from sheer exhaustion, heavy pressure on top of head, as if a great load lay there; indifference and unwillingness to speak; homesickness, with inclination to weep; hysteria during climaxis.

Chronic effects from disappointed love; hectic fever flushing of the face, especially afternoon and night with sweating; crushing weight on vertex; uterine and ovarian complaints in consequence of the depressing emotion.

Dread of the future, brooding over one's condition, taciturn, talking is irksome; confusion of head, weakness of mind, distention of abdomen, < by emission of flatus; pressure in several places of lower abdomen; painless diarrhoea or constipation.

Homesickness, with inclination to weep; nightsweats towards morning; drowsiness; emaciation; chronic congestions to the head; hair turns gray early; intolerance of music; great thirst, but no appetite; weak chest; unable to talk; diarrhoea; crawls over the back; constant inclination to sleep.

Sweat towards evening; mental and bodily depression; frequent sighing; weakening pollutions, diarrhoea; weakness of chest with inability to speak long; sleepy in daytime; epilepsy.

Phosphorus—Sadness recurring regularly at twilight, anxiety and irritability; melancholy, only > by vehement weeping; depression with foreboding of calamity; tearfulness and restlessness, which seem to arise from left chest and attended by palpitations; prostration from least unpleasant impression; indifference, even towards his own children.

Softening of brain, with persistent headache; slow in replies; irritable weakness and somnambulism; great fear and anxiety, especially towards evening, with frightful delusions and hallucinations, < especially hearing and smell, followed by prostration; disgust of life and repugnance to the world; great irritability of mind and tendency to be easily startled; changeable humor, spasmodic laughter and weeping; satyriasis and nymphomania in old people, with insane shamelessness, expose themselves and want to go naked; delirious fancies about his own person (second and third stages of dementia paralytica) with mania de grandeur; tuberculosis.

Apathy and sluggishness, alternating with mirth and laughter; uneasy about his health; anguish when alone, especially at twilight, or in stormy weather, with timorous disposition. Hepatic or renal affections.

Fear of terrifying images.

Increase of sexual desire; great sense of weakness in abdomen, aggravating all other symptoms; eructations of wind after eating; sleepy after dinner; erotic melancholia, hysterical laughter.

Irritable weakness, with ecstasy; thinks his body is all in fragments and wonders how he is going to get the pieces together; imagines himself a great person; shameless sexual excitement; erotic mania, followed by apathy and coma.

Picric acid.—Neurasthenia with anaemia; dementia; imbecility with total abolition of memory and reason; great indifference; lack of will-power to undertake anything; desire to sit still without taking any interest in anything; mental prostraion after the least intellectual work; anaesthesia and weakness of lower extremities; > in recumbent position (*Picrate of Ammonia*).

Piper meth. (Kava Kava).—Nervous prostration, constant fear of something happening; hallucinations and dullness after headache; dizziness and black spots before eyes, ringing in ears; fantastic ideas and a strong desire to skip about.

Platina—Melancholia activa, the mind rises in defiant and distorted superiority over vexation and sorrow; personal demonstrative apprehension, alternation of weeping and boisterous mirth; indifference to others, but anxious about herself, ill-humor, dizziness, she dare not move her eyes; < in daytime, with palpitation of heart and internal and external coldness, except the face, > in open air; mental symptoms associated with hysteria and disorders of sexual organs.

Nymphomania; puerperal melancholia and mania; indifference, does not care for anybody; low-spirited, reserved, fearful; inconsolable violent weeping; praecordial anguish, with palpitation and fear of death and of imaginary forms, ghosts; nervous excitement, pride, arrogance, considers everybody below her; vacillation; attacks of cheerfulness, increased feeling of strength; inclination to embrace everybody; slight vexation affects the patient for a long time; anxious when in company; dullness or absence of mind; ill-humor in the morning (*Pallad.*, evening); everything seems too narrow and strange; the thought of death horrifies the patient, any serious thought is displeasing; mental symptoms associated with gastric symptoms, both originating in sexual sphere, worse afternoon and evening; alternate appearance of the symptoms of body and mind, as soon as one group predominates, the other ceases.

After trying to speak in company, anxious heart-beating; pride and overestimation of one's self; fault-finding.

Demonstrative self-exultation and contempt for others (*Pallad.*, self-love and feels therefore easily slighted); cramp pain in forehead, as if between screws; violent boring in centre of forehead, gradually decreasing and finally disappearing; impeded respiration from weakness of chest; hysterical asthma, with heavy, slow breathing; clavus hystericus, spasms preceded or followed by constriction of oesophagus; sudden arrest of breathing when walking against the wind; strange titillating sensation from genital organs upward into the abdomen; great alternation of sadness and cheerfulness; spasms with wild shrieks; apprehension of death with disposition to weep; very fretful and irritable; chilliness and shuddering mingled with fugitive heat; menses in excess, dark and thick; mental and physical sexual excitement. Hysteria in males from prepubic masturbation with melancholy, sleepish look, hollow eyes, pale and sunken face; limbs are usually drawn down and spread apart.

Fear of the near approach of death, very sad, < evenings; indifference or contempt of others; fear of losing his mind; very much dejected and lachrymose; aversion to food, face red; pride and contempt for others.

Nymphomania; hysteria, with great lowness of spirits; nervous weakness and vascular excitement; imagines that everything around her is small, and everybody around her inferior in body and mind; involuntary disposition to whistle and sing; canine hunger, and eats greedily.

Plumbum—Deep melancholy, with timidity, restlessness, anxiety at the heart, with sighing and trembling; imagines he hears voices and thinks he is to be shot or poisoned (*Lach., Rhus., Ver-vir.,* fear of being poisioned), sees frightful things which chase him out of bed; dislike to talk or to work; maniacal rage with cries, brawling and convulsions; absence of mind, stupidity; pale, miserable, cachectic appearance, colic, dry skin, dry short cough, sleeplessness or somnolency. Cirrhosis renalis.

Podophyllum—Depression of spirits and disgust of life from abdominal affections.

Polygonum punct.—Slight vertigo, with sensation in extremities as of a galvanic shock passing through them; constant desire to urinate; amenorrhoea; warmth and a peculiar sensation of tingling through the whole body.

Pothos foetida.—Hystero-epilepsy; inflation and tension in abdomen; temporary blindness; sudden feeling of anguish, with oppression of breathing and sweat, > after stool.

Spasmodic and erratic pains in head and abdomen, now here, now there; tension and inflation of abdomen; spells of bloating, with oppression rising from abdomen to chest, precede the fit.

Psorinum—Religious melancholia, full of fears and evil forebodings; every moral emotion causes trembling; walks up and down the room wringing his hands and moaning continually, except at his meals which he relishes; irritable; peevish, noisy, passionate, easily startled, restless and then again cheerful, takes pleasure at his work; frightful dreams which follow him up after awaking.

Pulsatilla—Religious melancholia which finds consolation in prayers; grief and sorrowful timidity on account of his worldly and eternal affairs; anxious and weary of life, sad and gloomy, easily bursting into tears; dissatisfied; very easily frightened; anxious dreams with praecordial anguish and ideas of suicide; mild, yielding disposition, clinging to others and seeking consolation; earthy, dark ring about eyes; dislike to bread and meat; nausea and bitter, slimy vomiting, flushes of heat, pale face and cold hands.

She prays constantly for the salvation of herself and of others; great solicitude about her affairs, is full of sorrows, folds her hands and sits like a statue; dread of darkness; irresolution, desires for different things, without knowing what; hastiness and inability to collect her senses; chilliness, flushes of heat, with inclination to vomit, cold hands and pale face; sleep full of fantastic dreams; palpitations; great excitement in sexual organs.

Diarrhoea after fright, stools greenish, yellow, mucous; fear of ghosts in the evening; dread of men; tremulous anguish, as if death were near; bad effects from suppressed menses.

Sad, bursting into tears, anxious, weary of life, thinks with pleasure of drowning; dissatisfied with everything; easily enraged and easily pacified again; frequent profuse nosebleed; earthy color of face, with dark rings around eyes; flat taste, nausea and bitter slimy vomiting; labored breathing; heavy legs; anxious dreams; hard, scanty stool.

Tensive, cutting pain in uterus, which is very sensitive to touch and during coitus; crampy condition of vagina; constriction in throat, felt something there impeding speech, especially at night in bed; tired, worn-out feeling; constant change in her feelings and in her symptoms; flat, slimy taste, especially in the morning; vomiting of mucus; gastric disturbance from rich, fat food; violent cardialgia in mild, tearful women inclined to be fleshy, with scanty menses; mucous diarrhoea; profuse, watery urine; thirstlessness; a languid, pituitous state all through her system.

Ranunculus bulb.—Dread of labor; ill-humor and disposition to quarrel and scold; fear of being alone, afraid she will be haunted by ghosts.

Fear of electricity; fear of being alone, of spirits in the evening; twitching of muscles, with oppression of breathing, after fright, < evenings or after eating, from change of temperature, especially from heat to cold.

Rhododendron—Great indifference, aversion to all kinds of exertion, while talking he easily forgets what he is talking about; in writing omits words and sentences.

Rhus tox.—Anxiety and timidity, < at twilight, restless, change of place, wants to go from bed to bed; fear of being poisoned; suicidal mood, wants to drown himself; stupefaction, cannot recollect the most recent events.

Often cries without cause; imagines people find fault with her, feels heavy; eyes dim, shuns light; chilly hands and feet; diarrhoea.

Ruta—Fear of being captured and imprisoned; anxious and lowspirited; tottering as if thighs were weak.

Sabadilla—Melancholy from deep-seated abdominal irritation, suffers from imaginary diseases, considers herself pregnant when she is merely bloated up by flatus; he fears the shrinking of all his sexual parts, is easily frightened; hysteria following maniacal rage, only quieted down by washing head in cold water.

Cheerful disposition, which is not natural to him; imagines all sorts of strange things about his body; is absorbed in revery the whole day; mind excited, almost strained, with fanciful notions and the body cold.

Illusions about state of internal organs, that stomach is disorganized, ulcerated, etc., with features expressive of great anxiety; not disposed to work; heaviness and dullness of head; great anguish about heart.

Sabina—Very nervous and hysterical; habitual threatening abortion in third month; music is intolerable to her; very tired and lazy; flushes of heat in face, with chilliness all over and coldness of hands and feet; lustreless eyes.

Sambucus—Children have frightful hallucinations, weep, move arms and hands about, turn blue in the face with wheezing; frequent copious urination; heat without thirst.

Sanguinaria—Migraine; excessive irritability to odors, which make her faint; cannot bear sounds, the slightest jar annoys her; seeks a dark room for relief; > from sleep.

Secale—Paralytic mental state; insanity with inclination to bite, with inclination to drown himself; impaired power of thinking; apathy and indifference; treats his family with contempt and sarcasm; wandering talk and hallucinations; great anguish, wild with anxiety; senile dementia, senile gangrene.

Excessive sadness, which gradually changes to imbecile cheerfulness; talks and acts foolishly; rage, followed by continuous deep sleep.

Selenium—Abject despair, uncompromising melancholy; Bone and teeth are affected; Compalints incident to old age, particularly at the critical age; full of melancholy, with profuse micturition; dread of society; exhaustion even from light labor; rage and cruelty in his dreams, as if he were a hyena or a wild beast. Lascivious thoughts, with impotency. Mental labor fatigues. *Extreme sadness.* **Even for crossing the street to go to the opposite house in the hot sun he has to cover his head.**

Senecio—Inability to fix the mind on any one object for any length of time; depression of spirits, alternating with very cheerful mood; meditative, but don't know of what he thinks, especially in the evening; hysteria; great sleeplessness, or sleep with vivid unpleasant dreams.

Lowness of spirits, sleeplessness; globus hystericus; amenorrhoea, dysmenorrhoea.

Sepia—Loathing of life from prostration of mind and body; fears to starve, is peevish and feels mortified, easily frightened and full of evil forebodings; inability for mental labor and aversion to the usual duties; indifference to persons formerly loved, and especially to household matters (*Citric. ac.,* indifference to household affairs from weakness); restless and fidgety in company and still afraid of being alone; greedy and miserly (*Lyc.*); violent bursts of anger, with furious gestures; constant contradiction of himself; frequent alternation of gaiety and sorrowfulness; portal stagnation, humid tetters; arthritic affections of joints.

Organic diseases of female genital organs (*Lilium tig.* functional); full of despair, down-hearted, with suicidal ideas; great disinclination to work and motion; sadness, worrying about her health and the future, with frequent attacks of weeping, and indifferent about the health or affairs of her own family; < evenings and in open air; fits of involuntary laughter and weeping; dread of being alone; very irritable, inclined to be vehement; weak memory, difficulty in expressing her thoughts and dislike to mental labor; relief by violent exercise, as walking; indifference to her household affairs, to which she was formerly attentive.

Aversion to society and indifference to business and to one's own family; desponding, weary of life, often ushered in by an attack of indigestion; extremely irritable and peevish; sour eructations and formation of gas in abdomen; gone, sinking feeling in epigastrium, which food does not fill up, except, perhaps, at supper.

Paroxysms of something twisting about in her stomach and rising to throat; tongue stiff, she is sleepless and rigid; like a statue; painful sensation of emptiness in the pit of stomach; putrid urine; icy-cold hands and feet; sudden fainting with profuse sweats and undisturbed consciousness, without being able to stir or to speak; involuntary fits of weeping and laughter; sensation of coldness between shoulders, followed by general coldness; convulsive twitchings of right side and difficult breathing; piercing, boring, throbbing headache.

Silicea.—Want of vital warmth, even when taking exercise; secret disgust for life; faint-hearted, anxious mood; stings of conscience, as if he had committed a crime, worse during growing moon.

Longing for his relations and home; pensiveness; confused restlessness in doing anything; obstinacy, disposition to take things ill; irascible; imagines to be in two places at the same time; monomania about pins, which she sees everywhere and dreads; great prostration and nervous weakness; aggravation of all symptoms about full moon and in change of weather, especially during a storm; restless, with heavy dreams. Mental aberration nearer to imbecility.

Spigelia—Irritable nervousness; full of fear, anxiety, forebodings; great fear of pointed things, patient is afraid of pins.

Spongia—Irresistible desire to sing; mania with constant gaiety of spirits, especially in women and children who have a strong tendency to phthisis pulmonalis.

Stannum—Monomania, cannot get rid of an idea once fixed in her mind; visions by day of fancied things; feels like crying, which makes her only worse; silence; vexatious sensitiveness, with inclination to stormy anger, weak memory; fails to notice any desire to urinate.

Great sensation of faintness after going down-stairs, although she could go up-stairs well enough; she can hardly sit down, she must drop down suddenly; she can get up well enough; great exhaustion from talking or reading aloud; all pains gradually increase to their highest point and then gradually disappear.

Hypochondriasis abdominalis. Gastric pains which compel patient to walk for relief, though so weak that he is soon tired out; nausea and vomiting in the morning; goneness in stomach; inactivity of rectum; helminthiasis; odor of cooking causes nausea and vomiting.

Staphisagria—Inwardly gnawing grief and anger, he looks at everything from the darkest side, with desire to die; **disinclination to work and to think; dread of the future and dread of being constantly pursued by others; a sorrowfulness ending in paralysis of the intellect;** constant chilliness, even in summer, vertigo and sensation of seasickness; scurvy.

Hypochondriacal indifference, phlegmatic humor, intellectual languor; obtuseness of intellect and vanishing of thought; weakness of memory and forgetfulness, or very sensitive to least impression; is very indignant, wants to throw away everything he holds in his hands; quarrelsome, and nervetheless he is merry; great concern for the future; suffering from pride, envy or chagrin; never knows when he has eaten enough, with complete loss of taste.

Ailments from indignation over unjust charges, with vexation or reserved displeasure; fretful peevishness, with excessive illhumor; great dread of the future; sleepy in daytime and sleepless at night; feeble and faint voice; falling off of the hair.

Great sensitiveness to the least impression, feels easily offended; pushes things away indignantly; sound and decayed teeth painful to the touch of food or drink; teeth with black streaks.

Listless, sad, dreaming of the coming evils; fears about his state of health, of incurable diseases; aversion to mental and physical labor; inability to think; oversensitive to the least word.

With apprehension for the future; hypochondriacal, apathetic with weak memory, caused by unmerited insults, or by persistently dwelling on sexual subjects; great indignation about things done to others or by himself; grieves about the consequences; nervous weakness; convulsions with loss of consciousness; sleepiness in daytime.

Sticta pulm.—Hysteria after loss of blood; strange sensation about the heart, after which she felt as if floating in the air; cannot keep her legs quiet; hysterical chorea; migraine, she has to lie down, light and noise aggravate; nausea and vomiting with faintness.

Stillingia—Gloomy forebodings; depressed. **Deplorably down hearted.**

Stramonium—Melancholy, with desire for society and sunshine; welcomes the thought of death when alone; indomitable rage, with great desire to bite and tear everything to pieces.

The first sight of objects, persons, etc., alarms the patient, and he stares at it with a frightened look, till he discovers there is no need of fear; whilst sleeping quietly, the head is seen to be lifted from the pillow, or the patient will start upon his elbows and gaze about the room with a frightened look; on being asked what is wanted, an evasive answer is given and the patient lies down again; the good-natured, loquacious patient is fully occupied with his phantoms, by which he fancies himself surrounded; mania, with absolute rage, with disposition to strike and bite, alternating with convulsions; illusions as to shape, feels that he is very large in size, or that part of him is very large or double, or one-half of body cut off; converses with spirits, preaches, prays fervently; talks incessantly and absurdly, laughs, claps her hands, great sexual excitement; mania for light and company, fear when alone or in the dark; fears death and weeps all the time; alternate exaltation and depression; great bodily indolence and aversion to movement or to being touched; frequent ebullition of blood; mental and nervous troubles especially in children or in plethoric young persons.

Fear of terrifying images, of being bitten by animals, of insanity; of losing eternal salvation; nervous disorders after fright; raving madness.

Full of strange and absurd fancies; full of fear, starts back and stares wildly, even at familiar objects; does not wish to be left alone; great loquacity; puffed-up face; praying and imploring.

Loquacious delirium, with strange ideas; imbecility; talks with absent persons; behaves himself nasty and unclean; frightful fancies, all his features show fright and horror; religious mania, with pious looks; desire for light and company (reverse of *Bell.*).

Sulphur—Religious melancholy; reproaches of conscience, despair of salvation, much weeping; abdominal venous plethora, venous lethargy; inclination to consume hours in doing nothing; does not take any interest in anything;

pusillanimity and disgust for life, being too lazy to rouse himself up, and too unhappy to live, wishes to be alone, as soon as he sees anybody, he feels a weakness all over, but worse in stomach, followed by sweat on head and flushed face.

Melancholy, dwells on religious and philosophical speculations; anxiety about his soul's salvation, indifference about the lot of others; foolish happiness and pride, everything, even rags seem beautiful; fantastic mania, patient is inclined to deck himself with gaudy colors or puts on old rags of bright hues and considers them most elegant decorations; destroys her clothing, as she imagines she has everything in abundance, with emaciation even to a skeleton; wandering talk night and day; peevish, irritable, obstinate; disgust, even to nausea, of any effluvia, especially as if coming from his own body, although he has not soiled himself, the smell of the stool follows him about; < during new moon (*Sil.*, full moon).

Great fright on being called by his name; child jumps, starts and screams fearfully.

Lowness of spirits, painful anxiety of mind; solicitude on account of one's affairs, health, salvation; fixed ideas, paroxysms of anxiety, with impatience, restlessness, vehement disposition; bodily and mental indolence; absence of mind, irresoluteness; dullness of the head, with inability to perform any mental labor; exhaustion after the least mental exertion; headache, especially on the vertex; fullness and pressure in the pit of the stomach; constipation, haemorrhoidal disposition; disposition to feel very happy, etc. (*Calc.* is frequently suitable after *Sulph.*)

She comes out of her spasms feeling very happy and everything seems beautiful to her; considers herself very rich, tears up her clothes etc.; or profound melancholy and listlessness with disposition to do nothing; religious anxiety about her own salvation with perfect indifference concerning others; copious discharge of watery urine at the end of the spasm; heat of top of head, flushes of heat, coldness of feet; cannot wait at the noon hour or before for her dinner, feels faint and hungry.

Tabacum—Despondency, gloom, apprehension of sudden death; fear of death, yet attempting suicide; great timidity, fear to undertake what he has frequently done; difficulty in concentrating his mind for any length of time on one subject.

Cheerful and merry mania; sings the whole day; talks nonsense; becomes quite stupid, loses his senses; praecordial anguish, with faintness.

Tarentula hispanica—Hysteria with bitter belching and repeated yawning, > by lying down and by music; restlessness of hands and legs, constant movement, cannot remain long in one position, she pulls her hair, strikes her head with her hands, sings, dances, jokes, laughs, plays tricks or is sad and disgusted with everything; hysterical sexual excitement; sudden insane paroxysms with fox-like and destructive efforts, requiring the utmost vigilance to prevent damages, followed by laughter and apologies.

Consciousness of unnatural state of mind, hence despondency, sadness, **moral depression and relaxation** with complete loss of memory; fear of contracting disease (*Hyosc.*); mental corea; hyperaemia and hyperaesthesia of female sexual organs.

When alone she has no hysterical attack, as soon as attention is directed to her she begins to twitch; peripheral irritation, > by rubbing, motion or using the parts affected. Hystero-epileptic convulsions; anguish and oppression of chest, nearly amounting to suffocation; marked spinal irritation, the hands are kept in constant motion to work off this overexcitability; music sets her crazy; headache > from boring head into pillow; pain in sexual region with the constrictive headache; burning pain in hypogastrium and hips with sensation of great weight in pelvis; profuse menses followed by pruritus vulvae; she feels sore and bruised all over, < when moving about; great sleepiness, but her nervousness prevents her from falling asleep.

Theridion—Hysterical affections during puberty and climaxis; excessive pain in head, the least noise increases the headache; time passes too quickly, weakness, trembling, coldness and anxiety; hilarity and talkativeness, feels as if her head did not belong to her and she could lift it off; luminous vibrations before eyes; double vision; sensitive to light; faints after every exertion; anxiety about heart, with sharp pains through left chest to left shoulder; bites tip of tongue during sleep; nausea and vanishing of thoughts, greatly intensified by closing eyes.

Thuja—Fixed delusions, as if a living child were in her abdomen, as if a strange person were at his side, as if soul and body were separated, as if the whole body were very thin and delicate and could not resist the least attack, as if the continuity of the body would be dissolved, and the patient continually harping on this one fixed delusion; hurried, with ill-humor, talks hastily; angry at trifles; disgust for life; deficiency of words and slow speech; insane women will not be touched or approached; ebullition of blood, with pulsation in all the veins, palpitation, pain in head as from a nail driven in it; dreams of dead persons, perils of death, false accusation, etc.; music causes weeping and trembling of feet; she does not want anybody to come near her or to touch her, talks about being under the influence of a superior power.

Valeriana—Hysteria; exaltation and rapid change of ideas; immoderate mental excitement; thinks she is some one else, moves to the edge of bed to make room; imagines animals lying near her, which she fears she may hurt; feeling of great lassitude, with extreme sensitiveness of all the senses. Slightest exertion causes violent headache; sensation as if a string were hanging down the throat or as if something warm were rising from the stomach, arresting breathing, with tickling deep in throat and coughing; slightest pain causes fainting; fear, tremulousness and palpitation; pains simulating those of rheumatism of limbs, < while sitting > when walking; feels light, as if flying in the air (*Stict.*).

Veratrum alb.—Constant laughter, alternately with lamentations and howling, or with heat and redness of face; extreme liveliness and extravagance of ideas; singing and clapping of hands; mania, with desire to cut and tear, especially clothes, with lewdness and lascivious talk; kisses everybody, before menses; imprudent behaviour in childbed; curses all night, and complains of stupid feeling; talks much about religious things and prays; talks rapidly; sclerosis of the hemisphere, with mania de grandeur. Dislike to talk, to be left alone; anxious, restless, easily frightened, weeping; despair of her position in society, with suppressed catamenia; of his salvation; constant feeling of coldness, paralytic weakness, pain as if bruised in the brain, restless wild look, distorted face; great voracity; (voracity: wanting or devouring great quantities of food; very eager or enthusiastic in one's approach. cough, with tenacious mucus in chest, palpitations). Patient combines the wildest vagaries of the religious enthusiast, the amorous frenzies of the nyphomaniac, and the execrative passions of the infuriated demon, execrative = feel or express great loathing for; curse, swear;each of these manifestations struggling for the ascendency, and causing him to writhe and struggle with his mental and physical agonies; after short anguish the patient passes from this frenzy into one of deepest melancholy, abject despair of salvation, imbecile taciturnity and complete prostration of mind and body; utter collapse. Religious melancholy, with reproaches of conscience; suicidal melancholy; this condition frequently ends in a raving mania, with cursing and scolding, endeavors to escape, bites everybody, and tears everything that offers opposition; foolish imaginings; placid sadness, with weeping, discouragement and despair; apprehension of misfortune; conscious about his unworthiness; very taciturn; sudden paroxysms of sinking of cerebral innervation, characterized by sudden loss of power to control his movements; melancholia cum stupor, mind dull and stupid, with obstinate taciturnity.

After fright fear remaining; diarrhoea with icy coldness of the body; cold sweat on forehead; twitchings with anxiety.

Mania de grandeur; alternation of laughing and moaning; attempts a great many things, but accomplishes nothing; only conscious of himself as in a dream; rage, with great heat of the body; eats his own faeces. Suicidal tendency from religious despair.

Veratrum vir.—Great depression of spirit; mental confusion and stupefaction; will not see her physician, fears of being poisoned; sleepless, can hardly be kept in her bedroom; cerebral hyperaemia with coldness of whole body.

Mental indifference, with physical restlessness (*Acon.,* intense mental excitement); insanity from cerebral congestion; puerperal mania, silent, suspicous, careless about the future; dry, hot mouth, and still very little thirst.

Verbascum—Excessive mirthfulness; lascivious fancies; ideas crowd upon him; indisposition to mental or bodily work; liable to neuralgia.

Zincum met.—Melancholy, with thoughts of death; timidity and anxiousness, repeats all questions before answering them (*Aur.,* continually asks questions, without waiting for an answer); repugnance to the human voice and to noise; aversion to all labor; changeable humor; constant variation between angry irritability and great lively excitement; weakness of memory; difficult comprehension, with inability to all exertion; paralytic pressure on the brain, great lassitude and depression; fidgety feet.

Fear of thieves, of horrid phantoms; stares as if frightened on waking, and rolls from side to side.

Incessant and powerful fidgety feeling in the feet and lower extremities (*Stict., Tarent.*); she must move them constantly; variable mood, aversion to mental and bodily exertion; somnambulism; involuntary urination while walking, coughing or sneezing; she feels better in every respect during menstruation (*Zinc. val.*).

Sexual hypochondriasis from spermatorrhoea following long-lasting abuse of sexual organs; testes drawn firmly up against external ring; excessive irritability.

Bibliography

1. Horder Lord. The British Encyclopaedia of Medical Practice. London: Butterworth & Co; 1950
2. Kent JT. Repertory of the Homoeopathic Materia Medica. New Delhi: B Jain Publishers Pvt Ltd; 2010
3. Boericke William. Boericke New Manual of Homoeopathic Materia Medica with Repertory. New Delhi: B Jain Publishers Pvt Ltd; 2010
4. Lilienthal Samuel. Homoeopathic Therapeutics. New Delhi: B Jain Publishers Pvt Ltd; 1985
5. Yingling WA. The Accoucheur's Emergency Manual. New Delhi: Bjain Publishers Pvt Ltd; 2004
6. Wilkinson GE (Compiled by: Dr V Krishnamurthy). Wilkinsons Materia Medica. Chennai: 2012
7. Clarke JH. Dictionary of Practical Materia Medica (3 Vol). New Delhi: B Jain Publishers Pvt Ltd; 2007